THORSONS COMPLETE GUIDE TO
VITAMINS & MINERALS

An invaluable reference book giving the latest information available on the full range of vitamins and minerals and also vitamin and mineral therapy.

THORSONS COMPLETE GUIDE TO VITAMINS & MINERALS

Compiled and written by

Leonard Mervyn

B.Sc., Ph.D., C.Chem F.R.S.C
Member of the New York Academy of Sciences

THORSONS

THORSONS PUBLISHING GROUP

First published 1986
Second edition, revised
and expanded, 1989

British Library Cataloguing in Publication Data

Mervyn, Leonard, 1930-
Thorsons complete guide to vitamins and minerals. —
2nd ed., rev. and expanded.
1. Man. Nutrients: Minerals and vitamins
I. Title
613.2'8

ISBN 0-7225-2147-2

Published by Thorsons Publishers Limited,
Wellingborough, Northamptonshire NN8 2RQ, England

Printed in Great Britain by
Cox & Wyman Limited, Reading, Berkshire

3 5 7 9 10 8 6 4 2

DEDICATION

This book is lovingly dedicated to my wife Beryl in grateful recognition of her forbearance and understanding whilst I was writing it.

EDITOR'S NOTE

This book is an international guide to vitamins and minerals. While spellings and terminology are chiefly British, the content applies equally to British, American, Australian and Canadian readers.

NOTE TO READER

Before following the self-help advice given in this book readers are earnestly urged to give careful consideration to the nature of their particular health problem, and to consult a competent physician if in any doubt. This book should not be regarded as a substitute for professional medical treatment, and whilst every care is taken to ensure the accuracy of the content, the author and the publishers cannot accept legal responsibility for any problem arising out of the experimentation with the methods described.

FOREWORD

I have known and respected for more than twelve years Dr Leonard Mervyn and his scientific judgement. His basic research on vitamin B_{12} is well known to me, and I turned to the *Complete Guide to Vitamins and Minerals* hoping for a breath of fresh air in a subject area full of misleading overstatements and simplifications.

The reader will not be disappointed. We have here a clear, factually expressed encyclopaedia containing as much general information as the state of the art permits. Nutrition today has to be looked upon as a dynamic science where knowledge is changing constantly, and where even the choices we make as to what is or is not a sensible diet have to undergo modifications as science broadens its frontiers.

The book defines clearly those who may be at risk from vitamin or mineral deficiency but does not suggest rashly fortifying the diet with those megadoses which are more properly prescribed by nutritionally-qualified practitioners.

Len Mervyn's writings, like himself, are balanced and authoritative, and I feel delighted and honoured to write this short foreword. The fact that I have not so commended any other book on this subject speaks for itself. I commend it to all readers with the one proviso that, in a constantly changing science as is nutrition, you will need to update yourself every two or three years in order to make valid judgements.

It is only in this century that vitamins were identified and the importance of minerals understood. The developing story is now that of the trace elements, the micro-nutrients. Len Mervyn has told us much concerning these — truly a comprehensive source of reference.

MAURICE HANSSEN

INTRODUCTION

Whilst Nature, in her wisdom, saw fit to supply all our needs of vitamins and minerals, those micronutrients essential for health and indeed for life itself, in our daily diets, it is mankind with his arrogant attitude towards how food should be grown and treated who has in many cases demeaned what Nature has provided. Plants (and they include microorganisms) the ultimate source of all foodstuffs, are sprayed with toxic chemicals; animals destined for slaughter are injected with potent hormones and antibiotics; naturally-grown food is refined, processed and generally emasculated before being presented to the consumer as a pale shadow of its former self. Little wonder then that the more open-minded amongst our doctors and nutritionists are beginning to question what happens to the nutritive value of our food when it eventually ends up on the plate. Vitamins particularly are adversely affected by modern treatment of foodstuffs because we should never forget that these substances are delicate, discrete, unstable chemical entities that will not stand up to many processing methods. Hence whilst this book tells of the food sources of our vitamins it also warns of how these nutrients are lost or destroyed in cooking processes and refining. Minerals too are not exempt from losses in the transition of food from the field to the mouth and up-to-date information on these essential nutrients is also found here.

All that we know about vitamins and minerals is summarised here in this dictionary in a form presented for easy reference. What vitamins and minerals do, where they are found, what happens when we do not have sufficient, what are the effects of too much and what can they do to maintain or improve our general health are all explained here.

One of the more controversial subjects today is the role of supplementation with vitamins and minerals. Do we need supplements and if so, why and to what extent do we take these extra micronutrients? These questions are answered in the book under the appropriate headings but for simplicity we can divide vitamin supplementation into three categories, each of which demands a different level of potency. The reasons for taking extra minerals can be summed up in one category, that where we are deficient for one reason or another.

We know that modern processing of foods reduces their vitamin content and any losses in the factory are exacerbated in the kitchen. Certain sectors of the population have also been pin-pointed as being prone to deficiency of certain vitamins by virtue of their diets, age, sex, social and economic status and general health. Hence anyone who falls into one of these sectors or who is concerned about their diet may benefit from a general all-round supplementation of all the vitamins and minerals. This is known as the 'insurance' category and any multivitamin, multimineral supplement should ensure at least the minimum daily requirements of these micronutrients without reference to those in the diet. Fortunately, such preparations usually supply the Recommended Dietary Intakes which are quantified in the book.

The second category or level of supplementation may be needed by those whose lifestyles increase their needs for certain vitamins. Stressful situations demand increased requirements for the vitamin B complex and vitamins C and E and extra must be supplied to overcome the effects of stress. The habits of smoking tobacco and drinking alcohol denude the body of certain vitamins and some minerals by virtue of the poisons in tobacco smoke and alcoholic drinks that attack the body processes directly or produce metabolites that have similar deleterious effects.

Many medicinal drugs can reduce absorption of vitamins or cause them to be excreted in abnormal quantities so medical treatment can also contribute to decreased vitamin (and some mineral) body levels. Prime examples are antibiotics (vitamin B complex and vitamin K) corticosteroids (vitamins B_6, C and the mineral zinc), diuretics (potassium and calcium), aspirin and other non-steroidal anti-inflammatory drugs (vitamin C) and the ingredients of the contraceptive pill (vitamin B_6). In no case can diet supply all of the increased needs and supplementation at up to 5 times the Recommended Dietary Intakes is sometimes required.

The third category is that of therapeutic potencies of vitamins. Here the quantities of vitamins given are between ten and one hundred times those available even from a good diet and such amounts are needed because the vitamins appear to act as therapeutic agents. This approach represents the most controversial use of vitamins and argument still rages on the efficacy of such treatment. Amongst current uses are vitamin E in heart and blood circulatory disease; vitamin C in respiratory infections and cancer; pantothenic acid in rheumatoid arthritis and vitamin A and zinc in the treatment of various skin complaints. Whilst naturopathic practitioners continue to claim beneficial effects of use of vitamins alone, an increasing number of medical practitioners are successfully using high potency vitamin therapies to complement the medicinal drugs deemed essential in some clinical conditions.

There the matter rests at present but the fact remains that therapies suggested in this book have had a measure of success in the hands of some practitioners and the beneficial results have been reported in medical and scientific journals. They can be undertaken in the knowledge that they are safe but in cases where they best complement medical drug treatment, this is mentioned. The benefits of vitamin therapy are usually experienced by the person undergoing it. Who better to judge the efficacy of such treatment?

Mineral supplementation has no counterparts to those of vitamins. Minerals are needed only if they are deficient in the body and once that deficiency has been overcome there is little point in taking more. Poor diets and some clinical conditions are the main causes of mineral deficiencies and supplementation is often the only answer. There appears to be no justification for massive doses of minerals comparable to their equivalent in vitamin therapy and indeed such doses may even be harmful. Nevertheless, evidence is growing that despite the stability of minerals, their poor absorption and their removal and immobilization during food processing methods contribute to their chances of deficiency in many individuals.

This dictionary has been written to supply information on vitamins and minerals in a concise though comprehensive manner. This is the first time that a popular dictionary has been written supplying data on both types of essential micronutrients, vitamins and minerals. Information on each micronutrient is presented in a manner that allows the salient points about it to be easily and quickly seen. Whilst the therapeutic uses of the vitamins and minerals are summed up succinctly, more information is available under the appropriate condition heading. The contributions of various foodstuffs to our vitamin and mineral needs are presented in chart form as a percentage of what is recognized generally as the minimum requirements of adults in 100g of food. This quantity is about 3.5oz and in most cases represents an average portion. The percentage minimum daily needs or desirable daily intakes are not based on any particular government's recommendations, since these all differ, but are nearer the average of all the suggestions made by the authorities of different countries. For the purposes of the charts, 100 per cent of the minimum daily needs or desirable daily intakes are regarded as:

VITAMINS (Minimum Daily Needs)		MINERALS (Minimum Daily Needs)		SYMBOL
A		Calcium	1000mg	Ca
Carotene	750μg (2500IU)	Magnesium	400mg	Mg
D	10μg (400IU)	Phosphorus	1000mg	P
E	30mg	Iron	18mg	Fe
B_1	1.5mg	Copper	2mg	Cu
B_2	1.7mg	Zinc	15mg	Zn
Nicotinic acid	19.0mg	Manganese	5mg	Mn
Pantothenic		Molybdenum	500μg	Mo
acid	10.0mg	Chromium	200μg	Cr
B_6	2.0mg	Selenium	200μg	Se
B_{12}	3μg	Sulphur	800mg	S
Folic acid	400μg			
Biotin	300μg	MINERALS (Desirable Daily Intakes)		
C	60mg	Sodium	1200mg	Na
		Potassium	3000mg	K
		Chloride	1800mg	Cl

In all charts B_3 is used for nicotinic acid; B_5 is used for pantothenic acid.

A

A, fat-soluble vitamin. Known also as retinol, axerophthol, biosterol, anti-infective vitamin. Present in supplements and used in food fortification as retinyl palmitate and retinyl acetate. First isolated in 1913 by two groups of American workers.

One microgram retinol = 3.3 international units (I.U.)

Found only in foods of animal origin but its active precursor beta-carotene is present in fruits and vegetables.

Best Food Sources (μg per 100g)		Functions
Halibut liver oil	60,000	Sight
Liver	18,000	Skin
Margarine	800	Mucous membranes
Butter	750	Anti-infective
Cheese	385	Protein synthesis
Eggs	140	Bones
		Anti-anaemia
		Growth

Stored in liver and kidneys.

Stability in foods — see Losses in Food Processing.

Absorption — enhanced by fats and oils
— reduced by liquid paraffin

Recommended daily intakes — should be at least 750µg (2500IU) but see separate entry.
Supplementary daily intake — should not exceed 2250µg (7500IU).

Deficiency Symptoms
Spinal infections
Respiratory infections
Scaly skin and scalp
Poor hair quality
Poor sight
Burning and itching eyes
Pain in the eyeballs
Dry eyes
Eye ulceration

Deficiency Results in:
Night blindness (unable to see in the dark)
Xerophthalmia
Kidney stones
Mild skin complaints
Inflamed mucous membranes

Therapeutic Uses
Skin cancer
Gastric ulcers
Acne
Eczema
Psoriasis
Night blindness

Symptoms of Excess Intake
Loss of appetite
Dry, itchy skin
Loss of hair
Headaches
Nausea and vomiting

acetaldehyde, toxic substance found in tobacco smoke and produced by body from alcohol. Destroys vitamin B_1, vitamin C, vitamin B_6. These vitamins plus amino acid L-cysteine can overcome effects of acetaldehyde at dose levels B_1 (10mg), B_6 (10mg), vitamin C (500mg), L-cysteine (100mg) daily.

acetylcholine, derivative of choline involved in transmission of nerve impulses. Formulation depends on adequate vitamin B_1, pantothenic acid and choline. Lack of acetylcholine leads to brain damage and may be a factor in senile dementia and Alzheimer's disease.

---

achlorhydria, also known as hypochlorhydria. Lack of production of hydrochloric acid in the stomach. Believed to increase chances of developing gastric cancer. Symptom of pernicious anaemia specific to vitamin B_{12} deficiency.

Treat with betaine hydrochloride, also known as lycine hydrochloride; glutamic acid hydrochloride; dilute hydrochloric acid (2ml diluted to 200ml with water and sipped through a straw during meal).

---

acid-base balance, the balance between the amount of carbonic acid and bicarbonate base in the blood which must be maintained at a constant ratio of 1 to 20 to ensure the pH of the blood is kept between 7.35 and 7.45. In the healthy individual the blood is maintained within this narrow range of alkalinity. This pH value depends upon two mechanisms: the rate of excretion of carbonic acid (i.e. aqueous carbon dioxide) through the lungs in the expired air; and the ability of the kidneys to excrete either an acid or alkaline urine. When the lungs and kidneys are diseased these mechanisms may no longer function efficiently and an acidosis (excess acid) or alkalosis (excess alkali or base) results.

Dietary aspects of acid-base balance are less important than metabolic defects but can still influence the acidity or alkalinity of the body and hence that of the urine. For example, a rabbit has a diet consisting mainly of green and other vegetables and normally excretes an alkaline urine. A dog, which is carnivorous or omnivorous, excretes an acid urine. Vegetarian human beings usually excrete a neutral or slightly alkaline urine. Omnivorous human beings will excrete a slightly acid urine; large meat eaters will excrete a more acid urine. The reason is because meat protein is high in sulphur which the body converts to sulphuric acid before excretion in the urine. The high phosphorus content of meat ends up as phosphoric acid which also contributes to the acidity of the urine.

Dietary acids are organic acids present in fruit, vegetables and yogurt. Contrary to popular belief they do not produce acid reactions within the body (acidosis) and are in fact alkali-forming. Examples of such acids in the diet are:

1. citric acid (citrus fruits, pineapple, tomato, most summer fruits). Citric acid is oxidized by the body in its normal energy production cycle.
2. malic acid (apples, plums, tomatoes). Malic acid is oxidized by the body in its normal energy production cycle.
3. benzoic acid (cranberry, bilberry). Benzoic acid is readily excreted by the kidney (after combination with the amino acid glycine) as hippuric acid.
4. tartaric acid (grapes). This acid is hardly absorbed so does not contribute to the acid-base balance of the body.
5. oxalic acid (strawberries, green tomatoes, rhubarb, spinach). Oxalic acid can combine with calcium to form insoluble calcium oxalate so it is not absorbed. However excess oxalic acid can immobilize calcium and other minerals to an extent that may cause mild deficiency. Any oxalic acid absorbed is readily oxidized by existing metabolic processes.
6. lactic acid (yogurt). Is metabolized by the same body processes that dispose of lactic acid produced from glucose.

Foods are either acid-producing or alkali-producing, depending upon how the body metabolizes them. It is believed by some that an excess of acid-producing foods in the diet is a factor in inducing arthritis. Treatment of the condition is therefore aimed at switching to an alkali-producing diet.

Acid-forming foods are: meats of all kinds (with the exception of horse); poultry; fish and all sea foods; lentils; onions; brazil nuts; peanuts; walnuts; pearl barley; bread, all types of wheat and other cereal flours; all types of pasta; oatflakes; rice; semolina; tapioca; cocoa powder; chocolate; eggs; all cheeses.

Alkali-forming foods are: all fruits; all fruit juices; all vegetables (with the exception of lentils and onions); all vegetable juices; honey; molasses; cream; fresh milk of all types and treated milks (buttermilk, evaporated, condensed, dried); horseflesh; wine; nuts (except brazils, peanuts and walnuts).

---

acidosis, a condition in which the acidity of the body fluids and tissue is abnormally high, producing a low pH. Induced by a failure of the acid-base balance mechanism.

Lactic acidosis is due to:
1. accumulation of large amounts of lactic acid in the blood after severe

muscular exercise. Rapid breathing during the recovery phase helps to restore the acid-base balance by removing excess carbon dioxide through the lungs.

2. inadequate oxygenation of the tissues in certain diseases (e.g. heart failure);
3. loss of sodium, potassium and ketone bodies in the urine of those suffering from diabetes;
4. some liver diseases;
5. intravenous infusions of fructose.

Metabolic acidosis may be due to:
1. kidney failure;
2. lactic acidosis;
3. poisons such as ethylene glycol, salicylates;
4. acetoacetic acid that accumulates in the blood of diabetics;
5. excessive loss of alkali from the intestinal tract, as in diarrhoea;
6. ingestion of ammonium chloride.

Symptoms of acidosis include: increased depth and frequency of respiration; vague lassitude; nausea; vomiting. Apart from acidosis induced by severe muscular exertion, all other causes need medical management.

---

acne, inflammation of the hair and sweat glands. Has been treated with oral vitamin A ($2272\mu g$ or 7500IU daily) plus the mineral zinc (15mg daily as amino acid chelate). Spots may also be treated with cream containing vitamin A or retinoic acid. Also may respond to oil of evening primrose oil (500mg capsules three daily) or to other polyunsaturated oils.

Premenstrual flare-up of acne responds to 50mg vitamin B_6 daily for one week before menstruation and during it.

Zinc appears to function by restoring the hormone balance that may be upset at puberty. Evidence of low body zinc levels at puberty.

---

acrodermatitis enteropathica, a rare inherited disorder characterized by a psoriatic dermatitis, hair loss, infections of the nails, growth retardation and diarrhoea. Once fatal, it is now known to be due to malabsorption of zinc leading to low levels in the blood plasma. Complete remission is obtained with daily doses of 35-150mg zinc sulphate, providing 8-34mg zinc.

Addisonian anaemia,   pernicious anaemia. *See* B_{12} vitamin.

adrenal,   gland that produces anti-stress hormones (e.g. cortisol) from cholesterol. High concentration of pantothenic acid and vitamin C in gland needed for production.

ageing,   increases need for all vitamins, particularly vitamin B complex, vitamin C and vitamin E.

   Supplementation recommended as absorption and utilization of vitamins are impaired in old age.

alcohol,   drinking increases need for whole vitamin B complex but particularly vitamins B_1, B_6, B_{12} (10μg) and folic acid (200μg). Chronic effects of deficiency prevented by all vitamins plus oil of evening primrose oil (1500mg daily).

aldosterone,   a steroid hormone, elaborated by the adrenal cortex, that acts upon the kidney to regulate water balance by causing sodium retention and potassium loss. Used medically to treat deficient production and in the treatment of shock. Overproduction of aldosterone leads to excessive blood and tissue levels of sodium and loss of potassium, causing water retention and eventually high blood-pressure. One class of diuretic drugs act by inhibiting the action of aldosterone. *See* diuretic drugs.

alkalosis,   a condition in which the alkalinity of body fluids and tissue is abnormally high, producing a high pH. It is due to failure of the mechanisms that maintain a normal acid-base balance. It may be associated with certain diuretic therapy; loss of acid through persistent vomiting;

excessive sodium bicarbonate intake; deep breathing not associated with physical exercise. Symptoms of alkalosis are muscular weakness or cramp.

Apart from that produced by abnormally deep breathing, alkalosis usually requires medical management.

---

alopecia, baldness, loss of hair. Symptoms of pantothenic acid deficiency in animals; of biotin deficiency in mink and fox; of poly-unsaturated fatty acids deficiency.

May respond to calcium pantothenate (100mg); biotin (500µg); wheatgerm oil or safflower oil (3-5g); nicotinic acid (35mg); folic acid (200µg); vitamin B_{12} (5µg); vitamin E (10IU).

In addition, supplementary zinc (15mg daily) may help restore hair growth.

---

alpha tocopherol, *see* E vitamin.

---

alpha tocopheryl acetate, *see* E vitamin.

---

alpha tocopheryl succinate, *see* E vitamin.

---

aluminium, chemical symbol Al. Atomic weight 27.0. Third most abundant element in the earth's crust at a level of 8.8g per 100g. Occurs mainly in combination with silica (aluminium silicates) and as aluminium oxide.

Present in trace amounts in plants, animals and man but it does not appear to act as an essential element.

Storage in the body is in the lungs, liver, thyroid and brain. Later most of the dietary aluminium is excreted.

In *the diet* aluminium may be supplied from aluminium cooking pots used to cook acid-containing foods or liquids; some baking powders; food additives. Aluminium-containing preparations are widely used as antacids representing another source. Water used in dialysing solutions for those on kidney dialysis may also contribute aluminium.

Functions of aluminium in the body are not known but it is used in medicine:
1. as an antacid, to relieve the pain in gastric and duodenal ulcers and in reflux oesophagitis (heartburn) by neutralizing hydrochloric acid in the gastric secretions. Aluminium salts used for this purpose include:
(a) aluminium glycinate; (b) aluminium hydroxide; (c) aluminium phosphate; (d) aluminium sodium silicate.
2. as an astringent to form a superficial protective layer over damaged skin and mucous membrances. Preparations include: (a) aluminium potassium sulphate (alum); (b) aluminium acetotartrate; (c) aluminium chloride; (d) aluminium chlorohydrate; (e) aluminium formate; (f) aluminium subacetate; (g) aluminium sulphate; (h) ammonia alum.
3. to reduce phosphate absorption in those with chronic kidney failure;
4. to treat disorders of the mouth. Preparations include aluminium lactate.
The astringent properties of aluminium salts are also utilized in cosmetic preparations and in deodorants.

Toxic effects of aluminium on the skin include contact dermatitis and irritation in sensitive people. Internally, the mineral can cause phosphate depletion and skeletal demineralization resembling osteomalacia in those undergoing kidney dialysis; brain dysfunction in those undergoing kidney dialysis; brain degeneration characteristic of some types of senile dementia; slow learning in the young; epileptic-type fits in experimental animals; exacerbation of osteoporosis.

Levels of 12 μg aluminium per g brain tissue that give rise to brain deterioration in experimental animals are the same as those found in the brains of human beings who suffered from Alzheimer's disease or senile dementia. This suggests that aluminium may be a factor in these diseases of human beings.

Bioavailability — although aluminium is a common mineral and is present in many foods, it is very poorly absorbed from the gastrointestinal tract. Most of the aluminium in our diet passes straight through unchanged, and any that is absorbed is rapidly removed by the kidneys. In infants, however, both the gastrointestinal tract and the kidneys are still in the stages of development, and it has been suggested that (i) infants may absorb the mineral more readily than adults do and (ii) their capacity to eliminate aluminium through the kidneys is less efficient than in adults. There is a dearth of data on these two aspects of aluminium bioavailability in infants.

One survey has been carried out by the Ministry of Agriculture, Fisheries and Food. Milk-based infant formulae and soya-based formulae were purchased at retail outlets during 1987 and 1988 and the aluminium contents of the formulae (made up to manufacturer's instructions) were measured. The levels in milk-based formulae were 0.03 to 0.20mg per litre with a mean of 0.11mg per litre; those in the soya-based formulae were higher at levels between 0.64 and 1.34mg per litre with a mean of 0.98mg per litre. Plant-based foods like soya milk are usually higher in aluminium than those from animal sources. It was calculated from these figures that between the ages of 0 and 4 months, an infant fed cow's milk formulae will receive between 0.2 and 0.55mg aluminium per week, and one fed soya milk formulae will eat between 2.5 and 4.9mg of the mineral per week. Both intakes are well below the Joint FAO/WHO Expert Committee on Food Additives recommendations that the Provisional Tolerable Weekly Intake of aluminium is 7mg per kg body weight.

Studies are at present underway on the bioavailability of aluminium from common foods in adults and from various formulae foods in infants.

Alzheimer's disease,   occurs at any age and is characterized by loss of memory for recent events and an inability to store new memories. *See also* senile dementia. No medical treatment but some cases respond to 25g lecithin daily, increasing by 25g weekly until side-effects appear (nausea, abdominal bloating, diarrhoea) then stop at previous dose.

Second line of treatment consists of 20g choline chloride daily in 4 doses for 8 weeks, 6 weeks' rest, then 100g lecithin daily in 4 doses for 8 weeks. Memory, language functions and daily living improved. High potency phosphatidyl choline (6 capsules daily) in early stages.

---

amanitine,   choline.

---

amino-acid chelates,   minerals that are organically bound to amino acids. They may occur as such in foods or they can be produced from mineral salts within the small intestine from amino acids that are formed from the normal digestion of protein. It is also possible to produce amino-acid chelates by mimicking the natural process under controlled laboratory conditions. Soy or other protein that is broken down by enzymes supplies the amino acids required; coupling with the mineral is carried out by adjusting the pH of the mixture and creating the ideal conditions for specific mineral chelates. Amino-acid chelates may also be stabilized by buffering them to ensure they survive the acid/alkali changes of the digestive tract.

Many studies indicate that amino-acid chelation of minerals is a natural process that increases the rate and extent of absorption of the mineral compared with other mineral preparations; enhances the retention of the minerals; improves the extent of utilization of the minerals; protects the mineral against precipitating factors like phosphate, oxalate and phytic acid; reduces the side-effects of unabsorbed mineral on the gastrointestinal system.

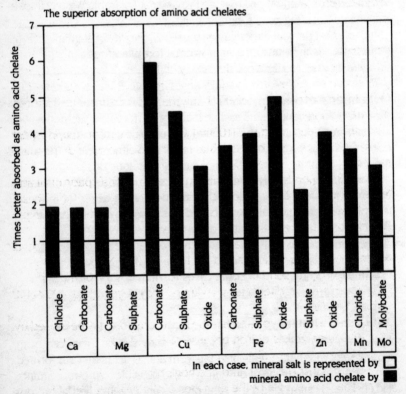

The superior absorption of amino acid chelates

aminopterin, immuno-suppressive agent. Impairs folic acid utilization.

---

ammonium chloride, a food additive that is used in yeast food and as a flavour. Provides 67.0mg chloride per 100mg. No limit on acceptable daily intake. Is a miscellaneous additive.

Used in medicine to acidify the urine when infection of the urinary tract is present; aid the excretion of certain drugs; increase the diuretic effect of mercurials; hasten lead excretion; supply chloride in chloride replacement therapy; act as an expectorant in cough mixtures.

---

amygdalin, laetrile.

---

anaemia, lack of production of normal red blood cells.

Haemolytic, due to vitamin E deficiency. In babies, treatment is 10-30IU daily in water-soluble form. In adults arises through malabsorption of fats. Need high doses orally (up to 600IU daily) or moderate doses (up to 200IU) of water-soluble form.

Iron-deficient, needs vitamin C (100mg) with each dose of iron supplement.

Megaloblastic, needs folic acid but medical diagnosis and treatment essential.

Pernicious, responds only to vitamin B_{12}. Due to malabsorption of vitamin therefore injection of B_{12} absolutely essential.

Pyridoxine-deficient, usually associated with taking contraceptive pill. Prevented by taking 25mg vitamin B_6 daily.

Riboflavin-deficient, probably caused by reduced activation of folic acid that depends on riboflavin. Prevented by 10mg vitamin B_2 daily.

Sickle cell, may respond in some cases to vitamin E (450IU) daily.

Thalassaemia or Mediterranean anaemia, may respond to 400-600IU vitamin E daily.

The iron-deficiency type which is the most common may be caused by:
1. low dietary intakes of iron because of poor diet;
2. poor absorption of dietary iron;
3. inefficient incorporation into haemoglobin;
4. pregnancy, because of the demands of the growing foetus for iron;

5. lactation, because of loss of iron through breast milk;
6. losses of iron being greater than dietary absorption, as in menstruation; in gastric and duodenal ulcers; in haemorrhoids (piles); in some drug treatments, e.g. aspirin.

A rare type of anaemia where iron is adequate may be due to a low intake of copper which is needed for incorporation of iron into haemoglobin. Most iron-deficiency anaemias respond to iron supplementation (up to 75mg elemental iron daily), but small amounts of copper (up to 2mg daily) and vitamin C (100mg with each iron dose) will help the iron to be absorbed and utilized more efficiently. If the deficiency is due to malabsorption or greatly increased losses, professional help is needed to treat the underlying cause. *See also* iron.

---

aneurin(e), B_1 vitamin.

---

angina,   full name angina pectoris, characterized by severe pain in the chest usually radiating to shoulder and arm. Treated with high doses of vitamin E (800IU and up, depending on response). Favourable response to lecithin (15g per day) also reported. Preliminary results using poly-unsaturated fatty acids from fish oils promising (eicosopentaenoic acid and docosahexaenoic acid, EPA and DHA 1500mg total daily). All vitamin therapy compatible with existing drug treatments.

---

animal galactose factor,   orotic acid.

---

anorexia nervosa,   a disorder characterized by a marked anxiety about body weight and weight gain resulting in abnormal patterns of handling food, serious weight loss and cessation of periods in women. The usual treatment is psychotherapy, but there is one case on record where zinc supplementation was successful in restoring loss of taste, increase in weight and a return to normal eating habits. Treatment consisted of 15mg zinc (as zinc sulphate) three times daily with meals. A good response was apparent after two weeks but further progress was continued only after the dose was increased to 50mg zinc (as zinc sulphate) three times daily. The main indications of zinc deficiency were loss of taste and loss of smell and these were used throughout to monitor zinc status of the female.

---

antacids, gastric acid neutralizers. Prevent absorption of vitamins A and B complex.

---

antagonists, substances that neutralize the action of vitamins or immobilize them. May be naturally occurring or produced synthetically. Used in research to induce vitamin deficiency quickly.

Examples are: *Vitamin A* — mineral oil (liquid paraffin). *Vitamin B$_1$* — alcohol; enzyme thiaminase, present in raw fish, destroys B$_1$; antibiotics; excess sugar. *Vitamin B$_2$* — alcohol; antibiotics; oral contraceptives. *Nicotinamide* — alcohol; antibiotics; leucine, amino acid in high concentrations in millet; niacytin, a bound, unabsorbable form in maize and potatoes, liberated only by alkali; excess sugar. *Vitamin B$_6$* — desoxypyridoxine; isoniazid; hydrallazine; penicillamine; levodopa. *Folic acid* — aminopterin; alcohol; oral contraceptives; phenytoin; primidone. *Vitamin B$_{12}$* — oral contraceptives; intestinal parasites; excess folic acid; vitamin B$_{12}$ acids. *Biotin* — antibiotics; sulphonamides; avidin in raw egg-white. *Choline* — alcohol; excess sugar. *Inositol* — antibiotics. *Pantothenic acid* — methyl bromide, used as fumigant in foods; omega-methyl pantothenic acid. *Vitamin D* — mineral oil. *Vitamin E* — oral contraceptives; mineral oil; ferric iron; rancid fats and oils; excessive PUFA. *Vitamin C* — aspirin; corticosteroids; indomethacin; tobacco smoking, alcohol. *Vitamin K* — warfarin, dicoumarol.

---

antibiotics, drugs used to combat infectious diseases. Taken orally can destroy 'friendly' intestinal bacteria that are providers of some B vitamins and vitamin K. Ill-effects on digestive system relieved by high doses of vitamin B complex. Vitamin K deficiency treated with acetomenaphthone.

---

anti-grey-hair factor, para-aminobenzoic acid.

---

antihaemorrhagic vitamin,   K vitamin.

---

antimony,   also known as stibium, hence the chemical symbol Sb. Atomic weight 121.75. First isolated in 1604, it is produced in China, Mexico and Bolivia. Antimony has no known function in living organisms and is not among the more toxic elements. It is present in all human tissues with the highest levels in the lungs (0.28μg per g) and hair (0.34μg per g). High levels in lymph glands (0.34-0.43mg per g). Slightly more present in soft water (1.7μg/g ash) than in hard (1.3μg/g ash). Blood plasma levels vary from 0.52 to 5.2ng per ml. Levels in human dental enamel also show variation from 0.005 to 0.67μg/g. Higher levels tend to be in those who have been treated with antimony for bilharziasis. Environmental exposure increases body levels of antimony to 318μg/g hair compared to normal levels of 0.12μg/g hair. Illness can affect tissue antimony levels, e.g. these are elevated in the heart muscle of uraemic (kidney failure) patients and in injured heart tissue from patients with coronary thrombosis.

The significance of these findings is not known.

Dietary intakes vary widely. In 28 areas of the USA, children's diets contained between 247 and 1275μg antimony per day. English diets were found to provide mean daily intakes between 4 and 60μg/day but Italians had the lowest intake of any, 1.5μg/day. Brown sugar contains 0.08μg/g compared to refined sugar with less than 0.002μg/g.

Medical interest in antimony arose when it was found to control the disease bilharziasis, or schistosomiasis, a blood disease caused by blood flukes. In the form of potassium antimonyl tartrate (tartar emetic) it is given intravenously in treating the disease but can cause severe vomiting. Soluble antimony salts are poorly absorbed from the gastrointestinal tract. Antimony has a low inherent toxicity and up to 150μg per g food can be tolerated. Liver necrosis produced by selenium-vitamin E deficiency was not exacerbated by high intakes of antimony.

---

antineuritic vitamin,   B$_1$ vitamin.

---

antipellagra vitamin,   nicotinic acid.

---

antipernicious anaemia vitamin, B_{12} vitamin.

---

antirachitic vitamin, D vitamin.

---

antisterility vitamin, E vitamin.

---

apples, *eating* variety supplies carotene, vitamin E and B vitamins (apart from B_{12}). Vitamin C levels less than those of cooking apples. Carotene content is 30μg per 100g; vitamin E 0.2mg per 100g. Levels of B vitamins (in mg per 100g) are: thiamine 0.04; riboflavin 0.02; nicotinic acid 0.1; pyridoxine 0.03; pantothenic acid 0.10. Folic acid present at 5μg per 100g; biotin at 0.3μg per 100g. Content of vitamin C is 3mg per 100g.

Cooking variety. Minimal losses of all vitamins present in raw state when baked or stewed. Carotene present for all three states (in μg per 100g) is respectively 30, 30 and 25. Vitamin E content at 0.2mg per 100g. B vitamins present are (in mg per 100g), for raw, baked and stewed respectively: thiamine 0.04, 0.03, 0.03; riboflavin 0.02, 0.02, 0.02; nicotinic acid 0.1, 0.1, 0.1; pyridoxine 0.03, 0.02, 0.02; pantothenic acid 0.10, 0.09, 0.08. Folic acid levels are only 5, 3 and 2μg per 100g. Biotin constant at 0.2μg per 100g. Vitamin C levels are respectively 15, 14 and 12mg per 100g.

Table 1: Differing vitamin C levels in apple varieties

	mg vitamin C per 100g	
	Peeled	*Unpeeled*
Cox Orange Pippin	2	5
Granny Smith	2	8
Laxton Superb	3	10
Golden Delicious	3	10
Newton Wonder	3	10
Worcester Pearmain	10	16
Lord Lambourne	10	16
Sturmer Pippin	20	30

Concentrations are slightly reduced if sugar is used in baking and stewing due to slight diluting effect of sugar.

Varieties differ in vitamin C levels, as shown in Table 1. There is more vitamin C in the peel of the apples than in the flesh, so whole apples should be eaten.

Minerals

A low sodium food that supplies useful amounts of potassium and iron with only small quantities of the other minerals.

Eating variety supplies (in mg per 100g): sodium 2; potassium 120; calcium 4; magnesium 5; phosphorus 8; iron 0.3; copper 0.04; zinc 0.1; sulphur 6; chloride 1.

Cooking variety supplies (in mg per 100g), for raw, baked and stewed respectively: sodium 2, 2, 2; potassium 120, 130, 100; calcium 4, 4, 3; magnesium 3, 3, 3; phosphorus 16, 17, 14; iron 0.3, 0.3 0.3; copper 0.09, 0.09, 0.08; zinc 0.1, 0.1, 0.1; sulphur 3, 3, 3; chloride 5, 5, 4.

---

arsenic,   chemical symbol As. Atomic weight 74.9. Abundance in the earth's crust is 0.0005 per cent. Occurs in nature as the free metal and in combination with other metals.

Small amounts present in most body tissues as a result of dietary intakes within the range 0.4-3.9mg per day. Most dietary arsenic ends up in the liver and muscle which can have concentrations up to 49 and 195 µg per 100g respectively. Excretion is fairly rapid, so toxic levels from the diet do not build up.

The richest food sources of arsenic are shellfish. Some meats contain organic arsenic which was originally added to the animals' feeds. Poultry and pigs are given traces of arsenic to improve growth. Arsenic compounds are used as insecticides which find their way to the soil and hence to plants which, when eaten, represent another dietary source. Water, too, contributes arsenic to the diet.

Traces of arsenic appear to be necessary for the health of animals but no specific functions have been assigned to the mineral. It is likely that it is also an essential trace mineral for man but such minute amounts are needed that a deficiency is highly unlikely.

Food and drink levels of arsenic are limited by law. Beverages may not contain more than 0.5mg per litre. Dried herbs may not contain more than 5.0mg per kg. Brewer's yeast is limited to less than 5.0mg per kg. WHO (World Health Organization) recommends that drinking water should not exceed 50 µg per litre.

Excessive intakes of arsenic can be fatal. Acute intoxication is indicated by severe gastric pain; vomiting; profuse watery diarrhoea; protein excretion in the urine; numbness and tingling in the hands and feet; intense thirst; muscular cramps. Eventually nerve complaints, kidney disease and brain damage result.

Chronic poisoning is characterized by oedema of the face and eyelids; generalized itching; sore mouth; inflammation of the eyes and nasal membranes; loss of appetite; nausea; vomiting; diarrhoea. Continued administration for long periods leads to dryness of the skin, dermatitis, pigmentation and hardness. Loss of hair and nails usually follows. Late symptoms include anaemia, cirrhosis of the liver; jaundice, neuritis.

Prolonged administration of sublethal amounts of arsenic may lead to cancer of the skin and lungs. Lethal intake can be as low as 100mg arsenic trioxide if taken in one dose.

Therapy with arsenic at oral doses of 1-5mg arsenic trioxide was originally used for syphilis. Externally it has been used in treating dermatitis, eczema and syphilitic skin diseases. The therapeutic use of inorganic arsenic compounds is no longer recommended.

---

arteriosclerosis,   hardening of the arteries. Treated with lecithin (15-20 grams daily), vitamin E (400IU twice daily), vitamin C (up to 3 grams daily) and vitamin A (7500IU daily). As preventative treatment, particularly in diabetes, supplement diet with lecithin (5 grams), vitamin E (400IU), vitamin C (500mg) and vitamin A (7500IU) daily.

---

arthritis,   Rheumatoid arthritis may respond to calcium pantothenate with regime of 500mg daily for 2 days; 100mg for 3 days; 1500mg for 4 days and 2000mg per day thereafter for a period of 2 months or until relief is obtained. Daily intake is then the minimum needed to maintain relief.

Rheumatoid and osteo arthritis may respond to vitamin C, 4000mg daily in divided doses. Both types of arthritis may respond to high doses (3-6g daily) of nicotinamide (preferred) or nicotinic acid. Supplementary preventative intakes are 100mg calcium pantothenate, 500mg vitamin C and 100mg nicotinamide daily.

Rheumatoid, inflammation of the joints. *Osteo*, degenerative joint disease characterized by calcified out-growths from cartilage. Both types have been reported as responding favourably to calcium supplementation at intakes between 500 and 1500mg daily. Reasons are not known, but even the calcified out-growths of osteo-arthritis, due to a high local concentration of the mineral, may disappear when low calcium levels elsewhere are remedied. Such low levels may originate in the bone reserves, as in osteoporosis, which is associated with some cases of arthritis.

Localized copper deficiencies may also be a factor in arthritic conditions, particularly the rheumatoid type. Copper bangles may contribute copper through the skin (*see* copper bangles). Some oral copper complexes, e.g those with aspirin, also appear to have an anti-inflammatory action greater than the aspirin itself. Organic forms of copper were more efficient than copper salts in relieving arthritic symptoms in experimental studies on animals.

---

ascorbic acid,   C vitamin.

---

aspirin,   analgesic and temperature-reducing drug. Reduces vitamin C body levels by destruction and excessive excretion. Causes gastric bleeding. All side-effects of aspirin can be reduced by taking 100mg vitamin C with each tablet. Also improves absorption of aspirin. Impairs thiamine and folic acid utilization.

---

asthma,   respiratory disease characterized by attacks of difficult breathing with a feeling of constriction and suffocation. Treatment with vitamin B_6 effective in some children and adults. Usual dose is 100mg twice daily. Once relief is obtained (usually after one month) maintenance dose can be lower depending on individual. More likely to help B_6-dependent children. Can be taken with all anti-asthmatic drugs. Vitamin C can also help some asthmatics by reducing symptoms of attack. Usual dose 1 gram orally every six hours.

---

atherosclerosis, fat deposition within the walls of the arteries causing constriction of the blood vessel.

Treatment with vegetable oils, margarine (PUFA) and soya lecithin. Avoid saturated animal fats. Also vitamin B_6 (25mg) daily to ensure body synthesis of lecithin plus vitamin C (100mg) and vitamin E (800IU) daily.

Prevention by replacing animal fats with vegetable oils and margarines and daily intakes of soya lecithin (5g); vitamin B_6 (10mg); vitamin C (500mg); and vitamin E (400IU). Recent studies implicate fish oils containing polyunsaturated fatty acids in the form of fatty acids EPA and DHA in preventing and treating atherosclerosis (900-1800mg daily).

---

athletes, combination of mental and physical stress associated with competition and training increases requirement of vitamins and minerals, as does high calorie intake. Particular requirements for extra vitamin B complex to ensure full use of extra calories; to ensure adequate supply of anti-stress hormones from adrenals; to supply extra pyridoxine required by most female athletes. Vitamin C also essential for production of anti-stress hormones and in ensuring full potential of muscle energy. Vitamin E essential to ensure adequate supply of oxygen to muscles. Similar function also attributed to pangamic acid.

Minimum needs probably met by up to 1500mg vitamin C, 1000IU vitamin E, 150mg pangamic acid and high potency vitamin B complex.

Female athletes should take extra iron (10mg daily) to insure against anaemia and extra calcium (up to 1000mg daily) to prevent osteoporosis.

---

autism, personality disease in children who become withdrawn and cease to communicate with outside world.

Has been treated with megavitamin therapy including vitamin C (1, 2 or 3g); nicotinamide (1, 2 or 3g); B_6 (150-450mg); calcium pantothenate (200mg) plus high-potency B complex preparation daily depending on age of child. Sometimes vitamin B_6 alone is sufficient. Medical monitoring essential.

---

avidin, unique protein in raw egg-white that binds biotin rendering it unavailable for absorption. Cooking eggs destroys avidin and liberates biotin.

---

axerophthol,   vitamin A.

B

B₁, water-soluble vitamin. Member of the vitamin B complex. Known also as thiamin(e) and aneurin(e). Supplied in supplements and in food fortification as hydrochloride or nitrate. First isolated from rice polishings by Drs B. C. P. Jansen and W. F. Donath in 1926.

Best Food Sources in mg per 100g	
Dried brewer's yeast	15.6
Yeast extract	3.1
Brown rice	2.9
Wheatgerm	2.0
Nuts	0.9
Pork	0.9
Wheat bran	0.9
Soya flour	0.8
Oatflakes	0.6
Wholegrains	0.5
Liver	0.3
Wholemeal bread	0.3

Functions

Acts as coenzyme in converting glucose into energy in muscles and nerves.

Stability in Foods

Very unstable — see Losses in Food Processing

Symptoms of Excess Intake

Oral: none reported
Injection: may cause hypersensitivity reactions very rarely

Recommended daily intakes — relates to calories in diet (0.096µg per 240 calories) so is about 1.5mg but see separate entry.

Deficiency Symptoms

Easy fatigue
Muscle weakness

Loss of appetite
Nausea
Digestive upsets
Constipation

Irritability
Depression
Impaired memory
Lack of concentration

Tender calves
Tingling and burning in
   toes and soles

Deficiency Caused by

High empty-calorie diets
Pregnancy
Breast feeding
Fever
Surgery
Physical and mental stress
Alcohol
Habitual antacid drugs

Therapeutic Uses

Beri-beri
Improvement of mental ability
Insect repellant
Indigestion
Improving heart-functions
Alcoholism
Lumbago, sciatica, trigeminal
   neuralgia, facial paralysis
Optic neuritis (50-600mg daily)

Deficiency Results in

Beri-beri (rare in Europe and
   the West)

B$_2$, water-soluble vitamin, member of the vitamin B complex. Has strong yellow colour, enough to cause high-coloured urine but is harmless.
   Known as riboflavin(e), lactoflavin(e), vitamin G.
   Isolated from whey by Dr R. Kuhn in 1933 after recognition in yeast by Dr O. Warburg in 1932.

Symptoms of Excess Intake

None have been reported except strong yellow colour in urine which is harmless.
So safe it is used as a food colourant.

Recommended daily intakes — should be at least 1.7mg but see separate entry.

Best Food Sources
in mg per 100g

Yeast extract	11.00
Dried brewer's yeast	4.30
Liver	2.50
Wheatgerm	0.68
Cheese	0.35
Eggs	0.47
Wheat bran	0.36
Meats	0.22
Soya flour	0.31
Yogurt	0.26
Milk	0.19
Vegetables (green)	0.15
Pulses (beans)	0.15

Functions

Acts as coenzymes flavin mononucleotide (FMN) and flavin dinucleotide (FDN) in converting protein, fats and sugars into energy. Needed to repair and maintain body tissues and mucous membranes. Acts in conversion of tryptyphane to nicotinic acid along with vitamin B_6.

Stability in Foods

Destroyed readily by light and in alkaline solution — see Losses in Food Processing

Deficiency Symptoms

Bloodshot eyes
Feeling of grit under eyelids
Tired eyes, sensitive to light

Cracks and sores in corners of mouth
Inflamed tongue and lips

Scaling of skin around face
Hair loss

Trembling
Dizziness
Insomnia
Slow learning

Deficiency Caused by

Alcohol
Tobacco
Contraceptive pill

Therapeutic Uses

Mouth ulcers
Gastric and duodenal ulcers
Eye ulceration

B₆, water-soluble vitamin, member of the vitamin B complex. Known as pyridoxine but also exists as pyridoxal and pyridoxamine — all equally active. Present in supplements as hydrochloride and phosphate.

Anti-depression vitamin.

Isolated from liver by Professor Paul Gyorgy at the University of Pennsylvania, USA, in 1934.

Best Food Sources in mg per 100g	
Dried brewer's yeast	4.20
Wheat bran	1.38
Yeast extract	1.30
Wheatgerm	0.92
Oatflakes	0.75
Pig's liver	0.68
Soya flour	0.57
Bananas	0.51
Wholewheat	0.50
Nuts	0.50
Meats	0.45
Fatty fish	0.45
Brown rice	0.42
Potatoes	0.25
Vegetables	0.16
Eggs	0.11

Functions

Acts as the coenzyme form Pyridoxal-5-phosphate in amino acid metabolism and in all other functions. Needed for formation of brain substances. Needed for formation of nerve impulse transmitters.
Blood formation.
Energy production.
Anti-depressant.
Anti-allergy.

Stability in Foods

Generally stable except in heated milk. See Losses in Food Processing.

Recommended daily intakes — should be at least 2mg but see separate entry.

Symptoms of Excess Intake

Noted only with minimum daily intakes of more than 200mg taken for at least one year. Unstable gait with numbness in the feet and hands. Changes in the feeling in the lips and tongue.

Deficiency Symptoms

Splitting of lips
Inflamed tongue
Scaly skin on face

Inflamed nerve endings
Migraine
Mild depression
Irritability

Breast discomfort
Swollen abdomen
Puffy fingers
Puffy ankles

Deficiency Results in

Convulsions in infants
Depression
Skin disease   } in adults
Anaemia

Premenstrual tension
Kidney stones
Atherosclerosis

Dependency States
(requiring high intakes)

May Include

Asthma
Urticaria
Mental retardation
Premenstrual tension
Convulsions

Deficiency Causes

Contraceptive pill
Many drugs (e.g. isoniazid,
hydrazine, penicillamine)
Alcohol
Smoking

Therapeutic Uses

Premenstrual tension
Depression induced by the
   contraceptive pill
Morning sickness
Travel sickness
Radiation sickness
Antidote to hydrazine
Infantile convulsions
Skin lesions of face
Anaemia
Bronchial asthma
Skin allergies

Therapeutic Dosages

Should NOT exceed 25mg
daily in treating nausea
(morning sickness) of
pregnancy.

Should NOT exceed 200mg
daily in all other uses.

Incompatible with drug levodopa

B$_{12}$, contains cobalt, hence known as cobalamin. Water-soluble vitamin. Member of vitamin B complex. Known as anti-pernicious anaemia vitamin; cyano-cobalamin; hydroxocobalamin; aquacobalamin; LLD factor; extrinsic factor; animal protein factor. Deep red crystalline substance. Last true vitamin discovered. Isolated from liver in 1948 by Dr E. Lester Smith in the UK almost simultaneously with Dr K. Folkers in the USA. Now obtained by deep fermentation.

Best Food Sources in μg per 100g	
Pig's liver	25.0
Pig's kidney	14.0
Fatty fish	5.0
Pork	3.0
Beef	2.0
Lamb	2.0
White fish	2.0
Eggs	2.0
Cheese	1.5

Confined to foods of animal origin with possible exception of spirulina algae.

Absorption from Food and Oral Supplementation

Needs unique mechanism involving specific protein in stomach called Intrinsic Factor and Calcium.
Maximum of 8μg absorbed by this mechanism. Only 1 per cent of oral dose absorbed by simple diffusion.

Symptoms of Excess Intake

None reported from oral use. Very rarely an allergic reaction from injections.

Recommended daily intake — should be at least 3μg but see separate entry.

Functions

Acts as two coenzymes methylcobalamin and 5-deoxyadenosylcobalamin. Needed for synthesis of DNA (deoxyribonucleic acid) the basis of all body cells. Maintains healthy myelin sheath (nerve insulator). Detoxifies cyanide in food and tobacco smoke.

Deficiency Symptoms

Smooth, sore tongue

Nerve degeneration causing tremors, psychosis, mental deterioration

Menstrual disorders

Hand pigmentation (coloured people only)

Typical symptoms of anaemia

Deficiency Results in

Pernicious anaemia

Deficiency Causes

Non-absorption due to lack of intrinsic factor
Sprue
Intestinal parasites
Veganism
Pregnancy
Old age
Alcohol
Heavy smoking

Therapeutic Uses

Pernicious anaemia (must be given by intramuscular injection)
Moodiness
Poor memory
Paranoia
Mental confusion
Tiredness
Appetite stimulant

Storage

In liver and kidneys

B$_{12}$b, hydroxocobalamin.

B$_{12}$c, nitritocobalamin.

B complex,   mixture of the B vitamins that tend to occur together in foods of animal, plant and micro-organism origin. Strictly speaking complex consists of eight members: thiamine (B_1), riboflavin (B_2), nicotinic acid (B_3), pantothenic acid (B_5), pyridoxine (B_6), biotin, folic acid and B_{12}, all of which are true vitamins. Some authorities include choline and inositol which can however be synthesized by the body.

PABA, pangamic acid, orotic acid and laetrile are part of the B complex in foods but are regarded as factors not vitamins.

---

backache,   when due to spinal disc injuries can be relieved or prevented by vitamin C (100mg, three times daily) or possibly more, up to 2000mg daily.

---

bacterial vitamin H,   para-aminobenzoic acid.

---

baker's yeast,   Saccharomyces cerevisiae. *Fresh, compressed variety* contains following vitamins (in mg per 100g); carotene (trace); thiamine (0.71); riboflavin (1.7); nicotinic acid (13.0); pyridoxine (0.6); folic acid (1.25); pantothenic acid (3.5); biotin (0.06); vitamin C (trace); vitamin E (trace).

Dried variety contains following vitamins (in mg per 100g): carotene (trace); thiamine (2.33); riboflavin (4.0); nicotinic acid (43.0); pyridoxine (2.0); folic acid (4.0); pantothenic acid (11.0); biotin (0.2); vitamin C (trace); vitamin E (trace).

Rich source of RNA and DNA which together account for 12 per cent of dried yeast.

Mineral
Rich source of potassium, phosphorus, iron, copper and zinc, plus chromium and selenium. All contents are increased over threefold in the dried variety.

Fresh, compressed variety contains the following minerals (in mg per 100g): sodium 16; potassium 610; calcium 25; magnesium 59; phosphorus 390; iron 5.0; copper 1.6; zinc 2.6.

Dried variety (in mg per 100g) contains: sodium 50; potassium 2000;

calcium 80; magnesium 230; phosphorus 1290; iron 20.0; copper 5.0; zinc 8.0.

---

bananas, edible part only. In the raw state carotene level is 200μg per 100g; vitamin E is 0.2mg per 100g. B vitamins present are (in mg per 100g): thiamine 0.04; riboflavin 0.07; nicotinic acid 0.8; pyridoxine 0.51; pantothenic acid 0.26. Folic acid level is 22μg per 100g but biotin is absent. Useful source of vitamin C at 10mg per 100g.

Mineral

Virtually sodium free with a very good level of potassium. Other minerals are present but in low concentration. Edible part only (in mg per 100g) contains: sodium 1; potassium 350; calcium 7; magnesium 42; phosphorus 28; iron 0.4; copper 0.16; zinc 0.2; sulphur 13; chloride 79.

---

barbiturates, sedatives and tranquillizers. Enhance excretion and metabolism of vitamin C levels and reduce conversion of vitamin D to 25-hydroxy vitamin D.

---

barium, chemical symbol Ba. Atomic weight 137.3. Has no use in the metabolism of animals or man, but in the form of its soluble salts is highly toxic. A fatal dose of barium chloride may be as low as 1g. Symptoms of poisoning include vomiting; colic; diarrhoea; slow irregular pulse; high blood-pressure; convulsive tremors; muscular paralysis.

Has been used in female contraceptive devices but these were regarded as presenting a potential cervical cancer risk in susceptible individuals. Still used in the form of insoluble barium sulphate in 'barium meals', where it shows up the gastrointestinal tract on X-rays for investigational purposes.

Despite the fact that barium performs no known essential function in man, the average individual contains 22mg of the mineral, most of which is in the bones. In heart disease there is a decrease in barium levels in blood and serum with an increase in the injured heart muscle. Other disorders that decrease blood barium levels are duodenal ulcer, chronic cholecystitis, cancer of the liver and liver cirrhosis.

Barium is poorly absorbed from conventional diets and little is retained in the body. A study of English diets found a daily intake between 400 and 900μg per day; in the USA intakes are similar at 750μg per day. Various other studies put the mean intake in general at 510μg per day. Barium levels in foodstuffs are associated usually with those of calcium and strontium. Vegetables and fruits can provide between 3 and 80μg per g dry weight but the richest sources by far are nuts. Brazil nuts contain between 700 and 3200μg per g but this was not accompanied by unusual levels of strontium.

Barium has a low order of toxicity when taken orally, probably because its salts are insoluble although barium chloride is soluble and poisonous. Toxicologists, on the basis of animal studies, suggest that the level of soluble barium in a diet should not exceed 20μg per g food. When the drinking water contains barium at levels of 1.1 to 10ppm (mg per litre) there appeared to be increased risk of cardiovascular disease in humans. When rats were exposed for life to 10 to 100ppm barium in their drinking water, blood pressure was significantly increased.

Basedow's disease, *see* hyperthyroidism.

---

beans, *see* pulses.

---

beansprouts, canned variety are devoid of vitamins A, D, E and carotene. Poor source of B vitamins with levels (in mg per 100g) of: thiamine 0.02; riboflavin 0.03; nicotinic acid 0.5; pyridoxine 0.03; pantothenic acid not detected. Traces only of folic acid (12μg per 100g) and biotin. When canned, provide only 1mg vitamin C per 100g; when fresh, vitamin C level is 30mg.

Mineral
Useful source of iron and potassium but sodium content is introduced during canning. Minerals present in canned variety (in mg per 100g) are: sodium 80; potassium 36; calcium 13; magnesium 10; phosphorus 20; iron 1.0; copper 0.09; zinc 0.8; chloride 120.

---

bed sores, decubitus ulcers or pressure sores. Healing rate increased with vitamin C (500mg daily).

---

beef extract, richest source of the B vitamins but devoid of carotene, vitamin E and vitamin C. B vitamins present are (in mg per 100g): thiamine 9.1; riboflavin 7.4; nicotinic acid 85; pyridoxine 0.53. Folic acid level is 1040μg per 100g; vitamin B_{12} content is 8.3μg per 100g.

Mineral
Very high sodium content because of salt addition but potassium also very high because of concentration of extract from original beef. Rich in iron, zinc, copper and phosphorus with useful quantities of calcium and magnesium. Mineral contents (in mg per 100g) are: sodium 4800; potassium 1200; calcium 40; magnesium 61; phosphorus 590; iron 14.0; copper 0.45; zinc 1.8; chloride 6800.

---

beer, beers and lagers of all kinds, whether bottled or draught, provide useful quantities of the B vitamins (apart from thiamine), including vitamin B_{12} which has been produced by the fermenting micro-organism. Fat-soluble vitamins are absent although there is a trace of carotene in all types. B vitamins present are (in mg per 100ml): thiamine, traces only; riboflavin (range 0.02-0.06); nicotinic acid (range 0.39-1.20); pyridoxine (range 0.012-0.042); pantothenic acid 0.10. Folic acid level is in the range 4-9μg per 100ml; biotin level is constant at 1μg per 100ml. Vitamin B_{12} is present in the range 0.11-0.37μg per 100ml. All beers and lagers are devoid of vitamin C.

Mineral
Can supply useful potassium and iron intakes depending upon type, but is generally low in sodium and other minerals. In beers and lagers of all kinds, bottled or draught, quantities of minerals (in mg per 100g) are in the ranges of: sodium 2-23; potassium 33-130; calcium 3-14; magnesium 3-20; phosphorus 3-40; iron 0.01-1.21; copper 0.01-0.08; zinc 0.01-0.04; chloride 4-57.

---

beriberi, disease due specifically to lack of vitamin B_1. Characterized by loss of mental alertness, respiratory problems and heart damage. Early symptoms are fatigue, loss of appetite, nausea, muscle weakness, digestive upsets. Mental symptoms include depression, irritability, impairment of memory, loss of powers of concentration. Water retention leading to heart and circulation problems. Therapy with 25mg vitamin B_1 daily.

---

beryllium, chemical symbol Be with an atomic weight of 9.01. Occurs as the semi-precious stone beryl and in emeralds and aquamarine.

When taken orally, beryllium is so poorly absorbed that it has a very low level of toxicity. When mice were give the mineral at a level of 5µg per ml drinking water for life, there were no adverse effects on lifespan, longevity, incidence of tumours, serum cholesterol or serum uric acid. In massive doses, like many trace elements, beryllium can be toxic when given orally, causing severe rickets that does not respond to vitamin D. The enzyme alkaline phosphatase is also inhibited in several tissues.

When inhaled, some beryllium compounds are very toxic, causing cancer, particularly tumours of the bone. Similar effects are seen after large amounts have been injected. The disease berylliosis, caused by inhaling beryllium, was diagnosed in workers concerned in the manufacture of fluorescent tubes. The result was fibrosis of the lungs and because of this the mineral's use was banned in 1948. Very low levels of beryllium are present in all human tissues and in the blood but these apparently cause no problems.

---

beta tocopherol, *see* E vitamin.

---

bile acids, constituents of bile needed to emulsify fats in digestive process. Produced from cholesterol by the action of enzyme dependent vitamin C so the conversion represents an important mechanism for reducing blood cholesterol levels.

---

bioavailability, commonly refers to the degree to which the vitamin or mineral becomes available to the target tissue after administration. As the number and complexity of fabricated foods in our food supply increase, information on bioavailability of the micronutrients becomes more significant. Processing and refining can alter digestibility and absorption, thus affecting nutrient bioavailability. Individual variability, malabsorption conditions, ageing effects, nutrient interactions and the form in which the nutrients occur complicate the problem. In addition, certain substances in foods may inhibit or enhance the absorption of other nutrients.

Vitamin A — ingested vitamin A requires release from the food by the action of pepsin in the stomach and digestive lipases (fat-splitting enzymes) in the small intestine. Absorption takes place in the small intestine. The presence of fat in the food stimulates bile flow which in turn facilitates transport of the vitamin into the intestinal mucosal cells. The presence of vitamin E and vitamin C in the diet serves to protect vitamin A and improves its bioavailability. Dietary proteins also improve absorption of vitamin A — in protein malnutrition, vitamin A bioavailability is impaired. There is interaction between vitamin A and zinc whereby a zinc deficiency in the diet impairs the absorption, transport and metabolism of vitamin A. Dietary vitamin A is absorbed with an efficiency of 80 to 90 per cent but may be lower with higher doses. This is decreased with diseases such as sprue, coeliac disease, hepatitis, cirrhosis and gastrointestinal infections. The cholesterol-lowering drug cholestyramine decreases the absorption of vitamin A by 60 per cent. Irradiation adversely affects vitamin A, reducing its availability from the food.

Beta-carotene — the factors that affect the bioavailability of vitamin A also contribute to that of beta-carotene and the carotenoids in general. However the bioavailability of beta-carotene and the carotenoids is complicated by their partial conversion into vitamin A by the intestinal cells. Hence the absorption efficiency is only 40–60 per cent at low intakes which decreases rapidly at higher levels of intake.

Vitamin D — is stable in foods whether present naturally or added by fortification. Hence cooking, storage and processing do not appear to affect markedly its bioavailability. Absorption requires lipases, bile salts and fat in the diet. It takes place in the lower ileum at a level between 65 and 75 per cent. Bioavailability is decreased in advancing age, and in gastrointestinal disease, coeliac sprue and Crohn's disease. The drug cholestyramine reduces the amount of vitamin D absorbed.

Vitamin E — although adequate dietary fat is needed to maximize vitamin

E absorption, excessive intakes of polyunsaturated fatty acids are known to decrease vitamin E absorption and utilization, perhaps because they tend to oxidize. Hence the requirement for vitamin E increases as the polyunsaturated fatty acids intake increases. Increasing the concentration of these acids in the diet without concomitant increase in vitamin E can lead to deficiency of the vitamin. Vitamin E needs pancreatic secretions and bile salts for absorption in the mid-part of the small intestine. Under normal conditions, only about 20 to 40 per cent of ingested vitamin E is absorbed, and this figure reduces as the amount in the diet increases. High levels of coarse bran or pectin can also decrease vitamin E bioavailability.

Vitamin C (*ascorbic acid*) — at intakes of 100mg or less per day, between 80 and 90 per cent of ascorbic acid is absorbed by the human. At higher intakes, bioavailability is reduced. In man, the vitamin is absorbed from the small intestine by an active transport mechanism. Some however is absorbed by simple diffusion. Diets high in pectin or zinc decrease the bioavailability of vitamin C as do high levels of iron and copper.

Vitamin B_1 (*thiamin*) — at low dietary intakes the absorption of B_1 from the intestine is an energy-requiring, sodium-dependent and saturable active transport mechanism requiring a specific carrier. At high concentrations, the vitamin is absorbed passively, mainly from the duodenum. Immediately after absorption into the intestinal cells, vitamin B_1 is phosphorylated to produce its active form. Bioavailability is high but is reduced by alcohol and when there is a deficiency of folic acid. Bioavailability may also be reduced by dietary anti-thiamin factors that include thiaminases (in raw fish, shellfish and bracken); tea (due to caffeic acid, tannic acid) and blueberries, blackcurrants, red chicory, brussel sprouts, red cabbage and red beetroot. These anti-thiamin factors appear only in the raw fruits and vegetables and appear to be destroyed when the food is cooked.

Vitamin B_2 (*riboflavin*) — usually this is well absorbed in the intestine after removal of the phosphate groups attached to the vitamin in foodstuffs. If riboflavin is complexed to certain proteins and peptides in the food, bioavailability is drastically reduced. The vitamin, once available, is absorbed in all parts of the small intestine. Factors that reduce bioavailability include alcohol, high zinc levels, copper, iron, ascorbic acid, certain antibiotics, caffeine, theophylline and high levels of tryptophane. The significance of these still requires clarification.

Niacin — normally absorbed from the stomach and small intestine by carrier-mediated, sodium-dependent, active transport mechanism at low dietary intakes, but passively absorbed at high levels. Bioavailability of niacin depends on whether the vitamin is free or bound in the food. In millet it is free and well absorbed. In wheat, cereal products and corn, it is in bound forms that are not biologically available for the human unless the vitamin is freed by processing. Bioavailability is therefore increased by treating corn with alkali or steaming or roasting it. Brewed coffee contains an appreciable amount of niacin which is of high bioavailability. The main factor reducing bioavailability of free niacin is alcohol.

Vitamin B_6 (*pyridoxine*) — all three forms of vitamin B_6 present in foods are readily absorbed by a non-saturable process. In human beings more than 95 per cent of orally-administered pyridoxine is absorbed but pyridoxal and pyridoxal phosphate have even higher bioavailability. In food, B_6 is phosphorylated and this form of the vitamin is readily absorbed intact. Pure vitamin B_6 is more readily absorbed than that in foodstuffs. Bioavailability is reduced by alcohol, particularly in those individuals with liver disease. Vitamin B_6 antagonists in foods can reduce bioavailability and such foods include linseed, mushrooms, jack beans, velvet beans and mimosa beans. The effects of these substances manifest themselves in the body rather than in the absorption process. Losses of pyridoxine (figures in brackets) leading to reduced bioavailability, occur in refining of wholemeal flour (75–90 per cent), freezing vegetables (37–56 per cent), canning of vegetables (57–77 per cent), canning of meats, fish and poultry (43–49 per cent), meat processing (50–75 per cent), cooking (55 per cent) and storage. Losses are slight in milk during processing, storage or drying but sterilization of milk leads to a marked loss in the bioavailability of the vitamin.

Heat treatment of corn and soya bean meal caused a loss in the bioavailability of vitamin B_6. The bioavailability of the vitamin from beef is superior to that from potato, cornmeal and spinach. The vitamin is 5 to 10 per cent less available from wholewheat bread than from white bread enriched with pyridoxine. High bioavailability is observed from tuna, beef, banana and filbert nuts but is low from peanut butter and soya beans. The vitamin B_6 in wholewheat bread and peanut butter was found to be only 75 and 63 per cent respectively, of that available from tuna fish. In the western diet as a whole, the bioavailability of vitamin B_6 ranged from 61 to 81 per cent with a mean value of 71 per cent.

In human studies, bran and other fibres had little, if any adverse effect upon the bioavailability of vitamin B_6. Dry-heat processing of cereals reduced bioavailabiity of all three forms of pyridoxine by 50 to 70 per cent. Only between 18 and 44 per cent of the vitamin B_6 was biologically available in a rice-based, B_6-fortified breakfast cereal. The vitamin present in non-fat dried milk was however found to be fully bioavailable.

Folic acid (folates) — there are at least 150 different forms of folic acid in the diet and not all are bioavailable to the human being. One criterion appears to be conversion of all forms to the monoglutamate before absorption can take place. The percentages of folic acid available from individual foods are as follows: Romaine lettuce (25); frozen, cooked lima beans (96); cooked beef liver (50); spinach (63); cabbage (47); wheatgerm (30); bananas (82). Even added folic acid in maize meal, rice or bread was only partially available. The absorption of added folic acid was 56 per cent for maize meal porridge, 54 per cent for rice and 29 per cent for bread. Fibre in those foods appear to impede the utilization of folate polyglutamates.

Reduced bioavailability has been observed in malabsorption syndromes such as tropical sprue, coeliac disease and Crohn's disease. Alcohol intake and ageing both lead to reduced folates' bioavailability. Many drugs have a similar effect including phenytoin, oestrogen (as in the contraceptive pill), aspirin, methotrexate, sulphasalazine, cimetidine and antacids like aluminium hydroxide and sodium bicarbonate. In addition vitamin B_{12} and zinc deficiencies can adversely affect folate bioavailability.

Vitamin B_{12} (cobalamins) — human studies with a single oral dose of vitamin B_{12} indicated that between 16 and 75 per cent of the dose was absorbed. The higher bioavailability was associated with the lower doses of 0.25 to $1.0\mu g$ of the vitamin. The intrinsic factor mechanism appears to have a saturable limit of $5\mu g$. Amounts above this are absorbed by simple diffusion and are between 1 and 3 per cent of the administered dose. Bioavailability of vitamin B_{12} approaches zero in pernicious anaemia and it can also be impaired in certain diseases, particularly tropical sprue and some parasitic infections.

Pantothenic Acid — little information is available regarding the bioavailability of pantothenic acid in food items. In human studies, those on an average Western diet demonstrated a bioavailability of the vitamin from 40-61 per cent with a mean of 50 per cent. Losses of the vitamin during food processing occur readily. Freezing of vegetables gave rise to losses between

37 and 57 per cent whilst canning losses ranged from 46 to 78 per cent of the original fresh foods. Losses in canned meat, fish and poultry were less. Processed meats lost between 50 and 75 per cent of the vitamin originally present. Processed and refined grains lost between 37 and 74 per cent of their original content in the wholegrain product. Refining of flour caused 55–58 per cent losses.

Storage can lead to losses of pantothenic acid and hence reduce its bioavailability. Frozen green beans lost 53 per cent of their pantothenic acid content after 12 months storage whilst frozen green peas lost 29 per cent during the same period. Canned vegetables continue to lose their pantothenic acid to the extent of between 30 and 85 per cent depending on the time of storage.

Biotin — little is known about the bioavailability of biotin. Studies are complicated by the natural synthesis of the vitamin by the intestinal bacteria. More biotin is often excreted than is eaten suggesting that intestinal synthesis is highly efficient in the healthy individual. This source alone is probably sufficient for most people's needs and the bioavailability of the bacterial vitamin appears to be high.

Most of the above studies on vitamins have been carried out on those present naturally in foods. However, recent studies indicate that the bioavailability of vitamins added to foods is equivalent to that of vitamins indigenous to foods. Several processes have been developed which have extended the shelf life of vitamins added to foods or present in supplements. When this happens, the bioavailability of such vitamins is increased.

Minerals

Most studies on bioavailability have been carried out on the minerals iron, calcium and zinc.

Iron — bioavailability of iron depends upon the type it is. There are two types, called haem iron, which is found only in foods of animal, fish or fowl origin and non-haem iron, which is present in foods of plant origin but also occurs in meats, fish and poultry.

Haem iron is better absorbed by the human body because it can be taken up by the absorbing (mucosal) cells of the intestine intact, and after combining with various specific proteins is transferred to the blood from where it is carried to all parts of the body. Non-haem iron cannot be absorbed from the diet intact because it must first be separated from the substance with which it is combined leaving the iron in an ionic or positively-charged form. Specific receptors in the intestinal cells are needed to remove the ionic iron from the intestine and carry it into the cell itself where it attaches to specific protein carriers similar to those used for haem iron. From then on it is treated like haem iron. Hence non-haem iron is less bioavailable than haem iron because it is taken up less efficiently from the diet into the intestinal cell.

Haem iron absorption is not affected by other factors in the food and does not require any other factor to ensure its absorption. Non-haem iron absorption is adversely affected by high fibre levels, phytic acid, coffee, tea and lack of animal protein in the diet.

Non-haem iron absorption is enhanced by vitamin C and by haem iron. Hence the presence of animal protein (which provides haem iron) in the diet increases the bioavailability of non-haem iron. The inhibitary effect of high fibre levels and beverages on the bioavailability of non-haem iron can be overcome by the simultaneous presence in the food of vitamin C. At least 50ng vitamin C each meal is the amount required to ensure adequate intakes of iron from plant foods containing it. Vegetarian diets usually provide high levels of vitamin C so there is adequate vitamin present to ensure good bioavailability of the mineral. Supplementary iron is usually absorbed to a similar extent to that of non-haem iron so vitamin C helps here also. Supplementary iron is usually presented in the ferrous form because its bioavailability is superior to that of iron in the ferric form.

Calcium — the main factor in increasing bioavailability of calcium is vitamin D. Without this vitamin, calcium in any form cannot be absorbed from the intestine. However, even in the presence of adequate vitamin D, other factors in the food and the form in which the mineral is presented can contribute to its bioavailability. Also important is the presence of gastric acid, including hydrochloric acid, in the stomach.

Lack of gastric hydrochloric acid, which can occur in certain diseases and is associated with ageing, can reduce the bioavailability of calcium from the food since solubilization of the mineral by the acid is often a prerequisite for absorption. In achlorhydric individuals (i.e. lacking gastric hydrochloric acid) calcium citrate was found to be ten times more bioavailable than calcium carbonate but in those with normal levels of gastric hydrochloric acid, both types of calcium supplements were absorbed equally well. These results were found when the supplements were fed on an empty stomach. When taken along with a meal, there was little difference in the bioavailability of calcium as citrate or as carbonate whether the individual was achlorhydric or not. In both cases the amount absorbed was almost normal.

Milk is an important source of dietary calcium but the mineral is absorbed no better from milk than from certain calcium supplements. Percentage calcium absorbed is as follows: calcium acetate (32); calcium lactate (32); calcium gluconate (27); calcium citrate (30); calcium carbonate (39) and whole milk (31). These figures apply to those with normal contents of gastric hydrochloric acid.

High protein intakes can affect adversely the bioavailability of calcium. More calcium was assimilated where 800ng and 1400ng of the mineral were eaten with 95ng protein but not with 142g protein. At daily intakes of 500ng calcium, the bioavailability of the mineral was not affected by any level of protein eaten. High protein intakes appear to cause excessive loss of calcium in the urine so increased bioavailability due to protein is offset by later larger losses in the urine. Highly purified protein intakes lead to greater losses of calcium than does protein eaten as foodstuffs such as meat, fish, fowl or high protein plant foods. This may be because the latter contains large amounts of phosphorus not present in the purified protein. Excessive intakes of purified protein should thus be accompanied by extra calcium.

Factors that inhibit the bioavailability of calcium include high phosphorus intakes but this applies only to babies whose ideal calcium:phosphorus ratio is 1.5:1. In older children and adults, early fears that the present calcium:phosphorus ratio of 1:1.5 in modern diets may reduce calcium bioavailability have not been realized. Other food constituents that may reduce the bioavailability of calcium are high dietary fibre levels, high phytic acid or oxalic acid levels and high intakes of saturated fat. Certain drugs may also reduce calcium bioavailability and these include corticosteroids, diphosphonates, glutethimide, phenytoin and other anti-convulsant drugs, antacids, diuretics, phenolphthaleine and colchicine.

Zinc — absorption of zinc occurs through the small intestine but some is taken up through the duodenum and the jejunum and in animals even from the colon. In the human between 7.5 and 14.4ng of zinc is estimated to enter the bowel daily and to be reabsorbed. Mechanisms of absorption are not understood but there are likely to be two pathways, one for small dietary amounts and the other for larger therapeutic quantities. Absorption is increased by stress, endotoxaemia, steroids and in pregnancy and lactation.

The bioavailability of zinc from human milk is better than that from cow's milk formula shown by the superior response of the zinc deficiency disease acrodermatitis enteropathica to human milk. The high citric acid and picolinic acid contents of human milk are believed to contribute to improved bioavailability. Zinc has low bioavailability from synthetic diets based on soya, crystalline amino acids, hydrolysed casein and comminuted chicken. In humans, zinc is better bioavailable when presented in animal-based foods than in those derived solely from plants. Low bioavailability from plants and cereals reflects the high fibre and phytic acid contents of these foodstuffs. Recent studies suggest that dietary fibre is less important in this respect than phytic acid content. Bioavailability of zinc improves with the protein content of the diet. Adverse effects of some vegetable components can be offset by consumption of a mixed diet containing animal protein.

Interactions with other nutrients are extensive but little understood. Iron and folic acid in large intakes can reduce the bioavailability of zinc in the diet. Antenatal supplements, which often contain these two nutrients, can reduce zinc bioavailability in pregnant women. Amino acids, protein chelators, monosaccharide sugars and fatty acids in the diet can inhibit or enhance zinc intake, depending upon concentration. Some urine constituents may also enhance zinc bioavailability. Amino acids shown to increase the bioavailability of zinc include histidine, picolinic and methionine. When complexed with zinc, all are superior in their bioavailability compared to zinc sulphate.

For bioavailability of other minerals *see* individual entries.

---

bioflavonoids,   originally called vitamin P. Known also as flavones; bioflavonoid complex. Always accompany vitamin C in foods. Water-soluble factors that include rutin; hesperidin; quercetin; nobiletin; tangeritin; sinensetin; eriodictyol; heptamethoxy flavone; myricetin; kaempferol.

Richest food sources are: citrus fruits (skins and pulps); apricots; cherries;

grapes; green peppers; tomatoes; papaya; broccoli; cantaloupe; buckwheat. Entire complex present in lemons. Buckwheat richest in rutin. Central white core of citrus fruits richest source.

Stability is high, even in canned fruits and vegetables.

Functions with vitamin C in maintaining the integrity of blood vessels particularly the capillaries; as anti-inflammatory agents; as anti-infective agents.

Deficiency symptoms include small haemorrhages under the skin; easy bruising.

Toxicity symptoms have not been reported.

Therapy found to be beneficial in menstrual problems, particularly functional uterine bleeding; in varicose veins; in varicose ulcers; in haemorrhoids; in excessive bruising especially when associated with sports; in treating thrombosis; in nosebleeds; in bleeding gums. Two types of bioflavonoids with specific and distinct actions:

1. Methoxylated type, occur almost exclusively in citrus fruits. Nobiletin possesses anti-inflammatory action. Other methoxylated bioflavonoids prevent stickiness of platelets and hence thin the blood. Nobiletin and tangeretin act as detoxifying agents. Other methoxylated bioflavonoids possess anti-infective properties.

2. Hydroxylated bioflavonoids like quercetin, myricetin and kaempferol appear to prevent cataract formation. Act as anti-oxidants to preserve foods. Rutin specific in treating high blood-pressure, arteriosclerosis and haemorrhages under the skin.

---

bios I, inositol.

---

bios II, biotin.

---

biotin, water-soluble vitamin, member of the vitamin B complex. Known as vitamin H; bios II; coenzyme R. Isolated from liver by Dr Paul Gyorgy in 1941.

Natural form is D-biotin.

Best Food Sources
in µg per 100g

Dried brewer's yeast	80
Pig's kidney	32
Pig's liver	27
Yeast extract	27
Eggs	25
Wholegrains	20
Wheat bran	14
Wheatgerm	12
Wholemeal bread	6
Maize (Corn)	6
Fish	5
Meats	3
Rice	3
Vegetables	1

Functions

As coenzyme in wide variety of body actions including:
Energy production
Maintaining healthy skin
  hair
  sweat glands
  nerves
  bone marrow
  sex glands

Stability in Foods

Very stable but see Losses in Food Processing.

Deficiency Symptoms

Babies: Dry face and scalp
Persistent diarrhoea

Adults: Fatigue
Depression
Nausea
Sleepiness
Smooth, pale tongue
Loss of appetite

Muscular pains
Loss of reflexes

Hair loss

Deficiency Causes

Antibiotics
Feeding new-born child with
  unfortified dried milk
Excessive intakes of raw
  egg-whites
Stress

Therapeutic Uses

Seborrheic dermatitis
Leiner's disease
Alopecia
Scalp disease
Skin complaints
Possibly to prevent cot (crib)
  deaths

Recommended Daily Intakes	Symptoms of Excess Intake
Should be at least 300µg but see separate entry. Difficult to assess because of large-scale production by healthy intestinal bacteria.	None have been reported. 10mg given to babies with no ill-effects.

birth defects, some can be associated with vitamin deficiencies in mother. Pantothenic acid deficiency can cause still births, premature births, malformed babies and mentally retarded babies. Riboflavin deficiency can cause congenital malformations including cleft palate.

Folic acid deficiency has been implicated in neural tube defects leading to spina bifida.

bismuth, chemical symbol Bi. Atomic weight 209. Not an essential mineral for animals or man but it has found widespread use in the past in the treatment of syphilis and yaws. Its insoluble salts are still used as protective agents in the gastrointestinal tract and by application to the skin.

Acute toxic effects include gastrointestinal disturbance; loss of appetite; headache; malaise; skin reactions; discoloration of mucous membranes; mild jaundice; blue line on the gums. Kidney changes may occur.

Chronic toxic effects include a nerve syndrome characterized by deterioration of mental ability, confusion, tremor, impaired co-ordination. Noticed mainly in colostomy and ileostomy patients taking insoluble bismuth subgallate over prolonged periods.

Medical uses of bismuth include:

1. treatment of syphilis by injection of the element or its salts;
2. antacid action in treating indigestion;
3. an astringent action in treating diarrhoea;
4. a protective action on mucous membranes and raw surfaces in those who have undergone colostomy or ileostomy.

Bismuth is widely distributed in all human tissues but at very low levels. The kidneys, lungs and lymph nodes contain respectively 0.4, 0.01 and 0.02µg per g fresh tissue. Liver contains only 0.02µg per g. Daily dietary intakes are less than 5µg. Despite these low figures, a transport mechanism for bismuth appears to exist in the body since the element is excreted into the bile from the blood.

---

bismuth carbonate,   provides 80-82.5mg bismuth in each 100mg. Dose is 0.6-2g to a maximum daily dose of 15g. Used internally as a mild antacid in treating dyspepsia and gastric and duodenal ulcers. Used externally in mild irritant skin conditions. For toxic effects *see* bismuth.

---

bismuth subgallate,   provides 46-52mg bismuth in each 100mg. Dose is 0.6-2g when used orally for its astringent properties in the treatment of diarrhoea, dysentery and ulcerative colitis. Administered by mouth to help control the odour and consistency of stools in those with colostomy or ileostomy.

Employed as a dusting powder for treating eczema and similar skin diseases. Incorporated into suppositories in the treatment of haemorrhoids. For toxic effects *see* bismuth.

---

blindness,   night, characterized by an inability to see in the dark. Specific result of vitamin A deficiency. Prevented and cured by vitamin A (2500-7500IU daily).

---

blood,   vitamins required for healthy blood production include B_{12}, folic acid, E, C and B_6.

---

blood clot,   thrombosis. In heart, coronary thrombosis. In brain, cerebral thrombosis or stroke. Supplement with vitamin E (400-800IU daily) and lecithin (15g daily). Medical treatment includes vitamin K antagonists e.g. warfarin.

---

blood-pressure,   usually measured at two levels; higher is systolic, maximum pressure of heart contraction; lower is diastolic, resting heart pressure. Hypertension regarded as diastolic pressure greater than 90mm.

High blood-pressure may respond to choline (up to 1000mg per day) itself; as lecithin (up to 15g per day). Claims also that rutin (up to 600mg daily) can help reduce high blood-pressure.

---

body content, the minerals calculated to be present in a person of 70kg (155 pounds; 11 stone) weight are shown in Table 2. These figures are only average and in no way refer to a 'normal' value. Such a term is meaningless as healthy individuals may vary in their mineral content yet show no abnormality. Mineral levels may be affected by ageing because toxic trace minerals especially accumulate in the body as it gets older; by past and current medical history; by sex; by family and religious dietary trends; by local environment which can contribute varying quantities of minerals from air, water and food; by the presence of other minerals with an antagonistic effect against the desirable ones; by the time of day the body sample is taken (e.g. before or after meals); by the analytical techniques used to measure minerals.

Table 2: Minerals present in a person weighing 70kg (155 pounds; 11 stone)

Metallic minerals	grams	Non-metallic minerals	grams
calcium	1200	oxygen	43500
potassium	250	carbon	12590
sodium	70	hydrogen	6580
magnesium	42	nitrogen	1815
iron	6	phosphorus	680
zinc	2.3	chlorine	115
copper	0.072	sulphur	100
vanadium	0.025	silicon	18
tin	0.017	fluorine	2.6
manganese	0.012	iodine	0.013
molybdenum	0.008		
chromium	0.002		
nickel	0.002		
cobalt	0.001		

body odour, due to over-activity of the sweat glands; to hormonal changes in the female; to metabolic upset, e.g. sweet smell (due to acetone) of the diabetic's skin and nitrogenous smells in the person suffering from kidney failure; to excess dietary intake of garlic. Many respond to skin application of powders containing zinc oxide or talc which absorb the substances producing the body odour; some respond to topical application of deodorants of other types. Oral treatment that is most effective includes a combination of magnesium (400mg), zinc (20mg), vitamin B_6 (25mg) and para-aminobenzoic acid (100mg) daily. These nutrients appear to act as waste scavengers, removing substances that give off acrid odours in the body.

---

boils, tender, inflamed areas of the skin containing pus at the site of infection. Pus consists of dead, white blood cells, living and dead bacteria (usually Staphylococcus aureus) and fragments of dead tissue. Standard treatment is oral antibiotics. Studies have shown that people with recurrent boils had low levels of blood zinc. When they were supplemented with 25-50mg of the element daily, blood zinc levels rose and healing of the boils was accelerated. In addition, whilst blood zinc levels were maintained, new boils did not appear.

---

bone, normal development and healthy maintenance need vitamin D and vitamin A at minimum daily intakes of 250IU and 2500IU respectively.

Bone pain of cancer has been relieved with very high doses (up to 10g daily) of vitamin C.

---

bone phosphate, edible, a food additive that consists mainly of hydroxyapatite. Used as an anti-caking agent; as a mineral supplement. Provides 39.9mg calcium; 18.5mg phosphorus per 100mg. Acceptable daily intake up to 70mg phosphorus per kg body weight. A permitted miscellaneous additive.

---

bonemeal, main constituent is calcium hydroxyapatite which provides

40mg calcium in 100mg plus 18.5mg phosphorus. Other constituents are protein, fat, amino sugars and traces of magnesium. Also available as amino-acid chelated bonemeal which provides 13.5mg calcium in 100mg, plus 7.5mg phosphorus. Usual daily dose of either is up to 6 tablets (i.e. 400-500mg calcium). Often used as an excipient or filler in tablet making.

---

borax, also known as sodium borate; sodium tetraborate; sodium biborate; sodium pyroborate. Provides 11.9mg boron per 100mg borax.

---

boric acid, also known as boracic acid. Provides 17.5mg boron per 100mg boric acid.

---

boron, chemical symbol B. Atomic weight 10.8. Occurs in nature as various compounds at an abundance of 10mg per kg in the earth's crust.

Boron was shown to be an essential element for plants in 1910. There is now evidence that it is needed by animals and man. Human diets provide 2mg per day which is efficiently absorbed and excreted in the urine. Toxic symptoms appear at intakes of 100mg or so. For this reason, the FAO/WHO authorities have now banned boron (as boric acid) as a food additive and preservative.

Medicinal uses have included:

1. external application as a dusting powder or lotion (in the form of boric acid) to treat bacterial and fungal injections;
2. treatment of mouth ulcers, eye infections and as a nasal douche (in the form of a solution of borax).

Toxic effects of boric acid and borax include a red rash with 'weeping skin', vomiting; diarrhoea — characterized by a blue-green colour; depressed blood circulation; profound shock; coma; convulsions. Fatal dose in adults is 15-20g; that in infants 3-6g. Repeated intakes of small amounts can lead to accumulative effects.

In children toxicity can occur by the application of boron-containing dusting powders to broken areas of skin. For this reason, such dusting powders should not contain more than 5 per cent boric acid or borax. Absorption from solutions applied to body cavities and mucous membranes can be significant, so such solutions are not recommended as douches for vagina, bladder, wounds and ulcers.

Boron is distributed throughout the tissues and organs of humans with the highest concentration in the bones and dental enamel. These range from 5 to 15µg per g ash and from 0.5 to 190µg per g dry enamel respectively. Blood plasma boron is high at birth but decreases rapidly within 5 days of birth. After ingestion of boron, the greatest increases occur in spleen, kidney and brain although thyroid levels remain at the same high figures as before.

All foods of plant origin are rich sources of boron but there is little in meat, fish and poultry. Beverages like wine, cider and beer contain significant amounts of the mineral. The mean daily intake in UK diets is 2.8 ± 1.5mg per day.

Deficiency of boron in animals depresses growth. In the absence of vitamin D, boron needs were enhanced. Boron was therefore believed to be associated with calcium, magnesium and phosphorus metabolism. In addition there was an enhanced need for boron during stressful situations.

Postmenopausal women — in human trials, the effects of aluminium, magnesium, and boron on major mineral metabolism in postmenopausal women were studied. A daily supplement of 3mg boron markedly and positively affected the mineral metabolism of seven women consuming a diet low in magnesium and of five women consuming a diet adequate in magnesium. Dietary intake was only 0.25mg daily. Boron supplementation reduced the urinary excretion of calcium and magnesium, particularly with low intakes of magnesium. Phosphorus excretion was reduced in low-magnesium women but not in those with adequate intakes of this mineral when 3mg boron was added to the diet. This extra boron also increased the serum concentrations of female sex hormones, more so in those on low magnesium diets. These beneficial effects of boron in the postmenopausal woman are believed to be due to activation of vitamin D to increase calcium uptake and in the body synthesis of sex hormones. The findings suggest that daily supplementation of the diet with only 3mg boron induces changes in postmenopausal women consistent with the prevention of calcium loss and bone demineralization.

Arthritis — epidemiological studies indicate a relationship between boron intake in the diet and the prevalence of arthritis in various populations. Where boron intake is lowest, there is a high incidence of arthritis (50–70 per cent in Mauritius and Jamaica). Where the diet provides more available boron (0.5-1.5ppm) the incidence of arthritis is 20 per cent (UK, USA, South Africa, Australia, New Zealand). Daily intakes of more than 1.5ppm in boron gives rise to the lowest incidence of arthritis (Israel and limited areas in other countries). Trials indicate that human beings and animals respond well to supplements of 6-9mg boron daily and in a few weeks, reduction of symptoms, in 80-90 per cent of cases has been claimed. This therapeutic dose of 6-9mg boron daily can be reduced to 3mg once symptoms are relieved. When added to the 2mg in the diet, these studies suggest that 3mg supplementation (giving 5mg daily in total) should relieve arthritic symptoms. Extra boron has been found to give harder bones than the normal arthritic femur. In one examination, arthritic femurs had only half the content of boron (29ppm) compared to healthy bone (60ppm).

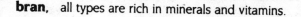

bran, all types are rich in minerals and vitamins.

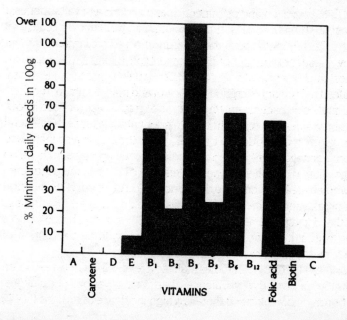

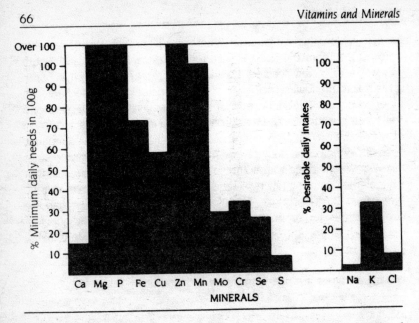

bread, high sodium and chloride is due to added salt in all varieties of bread. White bread contains more calcium than wholemeal because the mineral is added but white bread is inferior in vitamin content.

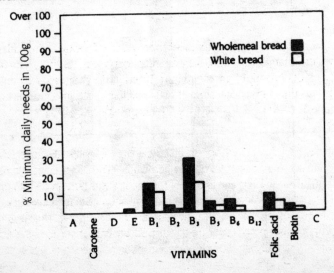

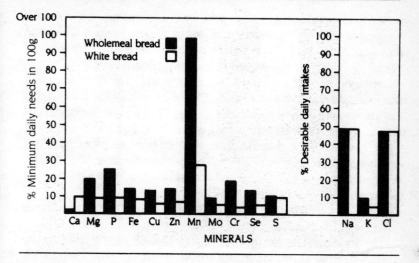

brewer's yeast, Saccharomyces cerevisiae. Dried variety contains following vitamins (in mg per 100g): carotene (trace); thiamine (15.6); riboflavin (4.28); nicotinic acid (37.9); pyridoxine (4.2); pantothenic acid (9.5); biotin (0.08); folic acid (2.4); vitamin C (trace).

Rich source of RNA and DNA which together account for 12 per cent of dried yeast.

Mineral
Fairly low in sodium but excellent provider of potassium, calcium, magnesium, manganese, iron, copper and phosphorus. Supplies significant quantities of chromium and selenium. Dried variety contains (in mg per 100g): sodium 121; potassium 1700; calcium 210; magnesium 231; manganese 0.53; iron 17.3; copper 3.32; phosphorus 1753.

bromine, chemical symbol Br, atomic weight of 79.9. Discovered and isolated in 1826 from salt lakes and sea water. The latter contains 67mg per litre. Although bromine is one of the most abundant and widespread of the recognized trace elements it has not been conclusively shown to perform any essential function in plants, micro-organisms or animals. However, it can replace chloride to support growth of some algae and in chicks it can partially replace chloride. Bromine at trace mineral levels can cause a small significant growth response in chicks and mice fed excessive iodine to produce growth retardation. However, diets deficient in bromine did not cause any reduction of growth in animals and adding bromine later to such diets did not give rise to increased growth rates.

Low blood serium concentrations of bromide in patients receiving haemodialysis have been reported and these levels have been associated with insomnia in these patients. In a double blind trial on haemodialysis patients, quality of sleep improved markedly in those given bromide but not in those receiving chloride. Bromide has been prescribed for many years to promote quality of sleep. The product has now been largely replaced by more effective and less toxic drugs both in the sedative and anti-convulsive fields of therapy.

All animal tissues contain between 50 and 100 times more bromine than iodine except in the thyroid where the reverse is true. The bromine levels of some tissues are affected by illness: e.g. they are elevated in heart disease induced by damage or by uraemia. Dietary intakes of bromine from UK diets have been calculated as 7.5 to 9.3mg per day; from USA diets as 24mg per day and from Finnish diets at 4.2mg per day. Intakes can be increased where organic bromine compounds are used as fumigants for soils and grains. In terms of bromine contents in the diet, growing pigs can tolerate 200µg/g; growing chickens 5000µg/g and growing rats 4800µg/g diet without adverse effects.

---

bronchitis, inflammation of the bronchial tubes. Vitamin A (7500IU daily) helps in therapy by stimulating the mucous membrane of the respiratory tract to resist infection. Vitamin C (500-1000mg daily) increases resistance to bacterial and viral infections.

---

bruises, haemorrhage under the skin due to capillary fragility. Colour changes related to conversion of blood haemoglobin to bile pigments. Excessive bruising prevented by adequate intakes of vitamin C plus bioflavonoids, particularly in those involved in body contact sports.

---

bruxism, grinding of the teeth, often carried on during sleep, that can give rise to dental problems. Has been overcome by increasing intake of calcium pantothenate (100mg) and calcium (300mg) daily.

---

burns, infection and pain of burn area of skin reduced by spray of 3 per cent vitamin C solution (sterile). Healing rate increased by massive doses (up to 10g) of vitamin C orally. Complemented by simultaneous intake of 400IU vitamin E twice daily plus vitamin E cream or ointment (100IU per gram).

---

butter, salted. Good source of fat-soluble vitamins but negligible quantities of water-soluble vitamins present. Provides (in μg per 100g): vitamin A 750; carotene 470; vitamin D 0.76; vitamin E 2000.

Mineral
A high sodium food because of salt added during production. Traces only of the other minerals. Salted, minerals present are (in mg per 100g): sodium 870; potassium 15; calcium 15; magnesium 2; phosphorus 24; iron 0.2; copper 0.03; zinc 0.15; sulphur 9; chloride 1340.

C

C, water-soluble vitamin. Known also as L-ascorbic acid; anti-scorbutic acid; hexuronic acid; cevitaminic acid; L-xyloascorbic acid; ascorbyl palmitate; ascorbyl nicotinate. White, crystalline powder. Isolated from fruits, paprika and adrenal glands by Dr Albert Szent-Gyorgi in 1922 in Hungary. Shown in 1932 by Dr Szent-Gyorgi and Drs W. A. Waugh and C. G. King (USA) that substance cured scurvy.

Best Food Sources in mg per 100g	
Acerola cherry juice	3390
Camu pulp	2994
Rosehip syrup	295
Blackcurrants	200
Guavas	200
Parsley	150
Kale	150
Horseradish	120
Broccoli tops	110
Green peppers	100

Functions

Anti-oxidant
Promotes iron absorption from food
Maintains healthy collagen
Provides resistance to infection
Controls blood cholesterol levels
Makes folic acid active
Produces anti-stress hormones
Produces brain and nerve substances

Recommended Daily Intakes

Should be at least 60mg but see separate entry.

Stability in Foods

Most unstable vitamin
See Losses in Food Processing

Best Food Sources in mg per 100g	
Brussels sprouts	90
Citrus fruits	50-80
Watercress	60
Cabbage	60
Mustard tops	50
All other fruits and vegetables	20-40

Functions

Maintains healthy bones
Maintains healthy teeth
Maintains healthy blood system
Maintains healthy sex organs
As natural anti-histamine

Deficiency Disease is scurvy.

Deficiency Symptoms

Weakness
Lassitude
Muscle and joint pains

Irritability

Bleeding gums
Gingivitis
Loosening of teeth

Haemorrhages in:
  skin
  eyes
  nose

More Needed Daily by:

Those who take:
  aspirin
  contraceptive pill
  antibiotics
  barbiturates
  corticosteroids
  anti-arthritic drugs
Those under stress
The elderly
  athletes
  alcohol drinkers
Anyone undergoing operations
Those with infectious diseases
Anyone with accidental
  wounds
Anyone undergoing dental
  surgery
Diabetics
Those with gastric and
  duodenal ulcers

Therapeutic Uses	*Symptoms of Excess Intake*
Scurvy	Nausea
Iron-deficiency anaemia	Abdominal cramps
Bleeding under the skin	Diarrhoea
Respiratory diseases	These are highly unlikely with
Bleeding gums	daily doses below 3g.
Psychiatric states	Generally regarded as a safe
Colds and influenza	vitamin.
Cancer	
High blood cholesterol levels	
Anti-histamine	
Alcoholism	
Arthritis and leg cramps	

cadmium, chemical symbol Cd. Atomic weight 112.4. It is not an essential nutrient for man and can be toxic after high intakes. Occurs in nature associated with zinc ores, so it is liberated when zinc is extracted. Earth's abundance 0.1 to 0.2mg per kg.

At birth cadmium is absent from the body, but it is absorbed in very small amounts and accumulates over 50 years or so to a body content of 20 to 30mg. More than half of this is found in the liver and kidneys. At a concentration of 22.4mg per 100g it can damage the kidneys. Within the tissues and organs most cadmium is immobilized by complexing with a specific protein called metallothionein. This serves to detoxify cadmium and other toxic minerals by making them unavailable to the tissues and organs. When metallothionein is deficient or saturated, toxic effects of cadmium appear. Excretion is very slow at a level of only 0.01 per cent of body levels daily.

Sources of cadmium include the atmosphere in the vicinity of industrial smelting and plating plants; fertilizers such as superphosphates where 15-21mg per kg may be present; drinking water which can contribute 1.1 μg per litre (soft water provides more than hard since galvanized pipes contain cadmium), vegetables grown on land irrigated by contaminated water or polluted by factory waste; tobacco smoke, up to 5 μg per day, from which cadmium is better absorbed than from food and drink; dental amalgams.

Food sources of cadmium include oysters (3-4 µg per g wet weight); liver and kidneys (1-2 µg per 100g); fruits, vegetables and nuts (0.04-0.08 µg per g); soya beans (1 µg per g) that have been grown on soil heavily fertilized with salvage sludge. Muscle meats and milk are poor sources. Cadmium is lost by food refining and processing, as are the essential trace minerals.

Daily intakes of 55-70 µg per person have been proposed by WHO as tolerable. Calculated intakes have been reported as 60-90 µg per day for young adult female New Zealanders; from 27-64 µg per day in children confined to institutions; as 26 µg per day in daily food intakes of USA individuals; as ranging from 50-150 µg per day amongst various countries.

Competes with zinc, copper and selenium in absorption and metabolism probably by virtue of competition for some protein-binding sites.

Excessive intakes can cause anaemia, probably by antagonizing copper and iron functions in blood formation; high blood-pressure, probably through kidney damage; injurious effects on the reproductive organs in animals; Itai-itai disease (see entry); atherosclerosis. Protection against excessive accumulation of cadmium is possible by adequate intakes of zinc, copper and selenium in the diet. Vitamin C at daily dose levels of 500-100mg protects against cadmium poisoning and helps rid body of mineral.

Acute toxicity effects after eating cadmium include nausea; vomiting abdominal cramps; shock; gastric and intestinal bleeding. After inhalation they are eye irritation; headache; vertigo; cough; constriction of the chest; weakness in the legs; difficulty in breathing; pneumonia.

Chronic toxic effects include yellow pigmentation of the teeth; soreness of the nostrils (cadmium sniffles); loss of smell; emphysema; pain in the back and limbs; bone changes leading to disability; loss of protein in the urine.

Medicinal forms of cadmium include:

1. cadmium sulphide, used in the control of seborrheic dermatitis and dandruff, usually in the form of shampoos. It may cause photosensitization.
2. cadmium salts, used as antihelmintics (to destroy parastic worms in swine and poultry).

---

caesium, alkali metal with the chemical symbol Cs and an atomic weight of 132.91. Occurs in the earth's crust only to the extent of 1ppm. Caesium, like rubidium, has a close physicochemical relationship to potassium. It has similar metabolic actions to rubidium (*see* entry on rubidium).

Like rubidium and potassium, caesium occurs at greater concentration in the red blood cells compared to the blood plasma. Typical levels are 4.82 and 0.74ng per ml respectively. Human organs contain the following amounts (in ng per gram): heart 11.4; kidneys 9.0; lymph nodes 20; testes less than 1; and ovaries 9.0. The mineral content in heart decreases when that organ is diseased or damaged but the significance of these findings are not known.

Most fruit and vegetables are low in caesium with levels falling within 3 and 11ng per g fresh weight. Meats and dairy products have not been examined. These low levels are reflected in total daily intakes of caesium which have been reported as only 6 to 20μg in UK diets and 15μg in those of Italy.

Radioactive caesium, caesium-137, is used in radiotherapy where it decays to barium-137 with emission of beta-rays. Caesium-139, as the chloride, has been used as an agent for imaging lung tumours.

---

calciferol,   D$_2$ vitamin.

---

calcitonin,   also known as thyrocalcitonin. A peptide (chain of amino acids) hormone produced by specific cells of the thyroid gland. It is secreted in response to high blood calcium levels and its action is to reduce blood calcium by inhibiting the rate of calcium release from the bone. Used medically in the treatment of high blood calcium levels and in Paget's disease.

---

calcium,   chemical symbol Ca; atomic weight 40.08. A metallic macro-element present in the skeleton and teeth (1100g) with the remainder (10g) in the nerves, muscles and blood. Calcium in the blood is essential in the process of blood clotting. That in the nerves and in the muscles (including the heart) is necessary for nerve impulse transmission and muscular function.

Best Food Sources in mg per 100g (max.)	
Hard cheeses	1200
Soft cheeses	725
Canned fish	400
Nuts	250
Pulses (beans)	150
White flour (fortified)	140
Cow's milk	120
Root vegetables	80
Eggs	60
Cereals	60
Fruits	60
Wholemeal flour	40
Fish (fresh)	32
Human milk	35

Absorption From Food

Between 20 and 30 per cent of that eaten. Higher figure applies when intakes are low. Absorption more efficient in the presence of:

Vitamin D
Proteins
Lactose (milk sugar)
Stomach acid
Magnesium

Absorption inhibited by:

Phytic acid
Dietary fibre
Phosphate
Saturated fats
Rhubarb (contains oxalic acid)

Daily Losses

Urine — up to 350mg; higher in summer and after the menopause.

Faeces — up to 400mg of which 130mg is from body and 270mg is undissolved from food.

Sweat — only 15mg normally but up to 100mg per hour with heavy work or exercise.

Calcium Regulation

Under control of:

Vitamin D and hormones
Calcitonin
Parathyroid

See separate entries

Oestrogens (female sex hormones)
Thyroid hormone

Excessive losses during and after the menopause.

Functions

Builds and maintains healthy
  bones and teeth
Controls excitability of nerves
  and muscles
Controls conduction of nerve
  impulses
Controls contraction of heart
  and other muscles
Assists in process of blood
  clotting
Controls blood cholesterol
  levels
Assists in absorption of
  vitamin B_{12}

Deficiency Symptoms

Children: Rickets,
characterized by:
  Excessive sweating of the
    head
  Poor ability to sleep
  Constant head movements
  Slowness in sitting, crawling,
    walking
  Bow legs, knock knees and
    pigeon breast
Adults: Osteomalacia, causing
  Bone pain
  Muscle weakness
  Delayed healing of fractures
(Both above conditions similar
to vitamin D deficiency)
Tetany — twitches and
  spasms

Deficiency Causes

Low dietary intake
Lack of vitamin D
Increased intake of uncooked bran, phosphates, animal fats, oxalic
  acid (in rhubarb etc.)
Contraceptive pill
Corticosteroid drugs
Malabsorption due to:
  lack of stomach acid
  coeliac disease
  lactose intolerance
  diuretic drugs
Pregnancy
Breast-feeding

Therapeutic Uses

Rickets
Osteomalacia
Tetany
Osteoporosis
Coeliac disease
Allergy complaints
As detoxifying agent in lead, mercury, aluminium and cadmium poisoning
Depression, anxiety, panic attacks, insomnia, over-activity
Arthritis, muscle and joint pains
Pregnancy
Breast-feeding

Symptoms of Excess Intake

Highly unlikely under normal conditions as body will reject and excrete any calcium that is above its needs.

Probable only if vitamin D intake is also high (See D vitamin entry)

If prolonged, high calcium and vitamin D taken together can cause deposition of calcium in kidneys, heart and other soft tissues.

Recommended Daily Intake — should be between 500 and 1000mg daily but see separate entry.

Calcium Supplements (Calcium in mg per 100mg)

Amino acid chelated calcium (18); bonemeal (40); calcium acetate (25); calcium ascorbate (10.3); calcium carbonate (40); calcium chloride (27.2); calcium glubionate (6.6); calcium gluceptate (8.2); calcium gluconate (8.9); calcium glycerophosphate (19.1); calcium phosphate (38.7); calcium lactate (13); calcium laevulinate (13.1); calcium orotate (20.6); calcium sodium lactate (7.8); calcium tetrahydrogen phosphate (15.9); dibasic calcium phosphate (29.5); dolomite (21.7); tribasic calcium phosphate (38.8).

Under present legislation, white flour has calcium carbonate (chalk) added to it as a source of calcium.

calcium antagonists, also known as calcium blockers, are a group of drugs that appear to function by preventing or slowing the flow of calcium into muscle cells. These cells need calcium to activate contraction of heart and artery muscles. The regulation of calcium movement into heart muscle cells is thus critical to heart muscle tone, resistance and blood-pressure. By blocking the flow of calcium by an antagonistic action, these drugs are valuable in treating angina pectoris, heart failure, high blood-pressure, weak heart muscle, fast heartbeat and coronary artery spasm. Adverse effects of calcium antagonists include transient headache, flushing, lethargy, dizziness, allergic reactions, low blood-pressure, palpitations and occasionally precipitation of anginal pain.

---

calcium pantothenate, calcium salt of pantothenic acid.

---

cancer, any malignant tumour that arises from the abnormal and uncontrolled division of cells that then invade and destroy the surrounding tissues. Malignant growths can be treated with high doses of vitamins in addition to conventional therapy.

Bladder — needs sufficient vitamin C to saturate urinary system to protect against and treat cancer of the bladder. 500mg three times daily is effective. Inositol (1000mg daily) also has inhibiting effect.

Breast — clinical response obtained with 200IU vitamin E three times daily. Simultaneous intake of up to 10g daily vitamin C may complement vitamin E therapy. Dose of C arrived at by increasing intake by 1g each day until diarrhoea occurs. One gram per day less than this is maximum tolerated dose up to maximum of 10g.

Colon — use vitamin C with same regime as in treating breast cancer.

Lung — prevention (particularly in tobacco smokers) and treatment with beta-carotene (4.5mg three times daily).

Skin — preliminary reports suggest 0.05 per cent retinoic acid applied directly to skin areas affected has beneficial effect. Other retinoids may be more effective.

Other cancers — vitamin C therapy as outlined for breast cancer may be beneficial.

Laetrile claimed to be beneficial in all cancers but professional treatment essential.

Mineral

It is important that the diet of anyone suffering from cancer is adequate in all the essential minerals as part of the general approach to nutritional control of the complaint. However, one trace mineral of particular importance in the prevention and perhaps the treatment of cancer is selenium. Epidemiological evidence suggests that the population living in low selenium areas has a higher rate of cancer incidence than a comparable population living in a high selenium area. For example, in the United States where selenium intakes average 50-100µg per person per day the cancer rate is higher than in Bulgaria where the intake is about 250µg per person per day. Within the same country, those with higher blood selenium levels have a lower incidence of cancer than those with low blood selenium levels. Animal experiments have proved that some cancers can actually be cured with selenium supplementation. Selenium appears to function against cancer by:

1. stimulating the immune system that protects against cancer;
2. toughening the cell membrane and making it less prone to attack by cancer-producing antigens.

The quantity of selenium to act as a preventative is at least 200µg per day; for treatment more may be necessary to increase blood levels of selenium, perhaps up to 500µg per day. Daily intakes of 2000µg daily have been taken under medical supervision in the treatment of cancer without any detectable damage to the liver or other side effects.

---

carnitine, constituent of muscles and liver. Synthesis in body dependent on vitamin C. Functions as transporter of fatty acids within body cells prior to using them for energy production.

---

carotenaemia, high blood levels of carotene that may cause yellow coloration of the skin. Completely harmless and removed by reducing intake of carotenes. Eyeballs remain white which distinguishes it from jaundice.

---

carotenoids, coloured pigments widely distributed in animals and plants. More than 100 identified in nature. Includes carotenes designated alpha-, beta-, and gamma-carotene that can give rise to vitamin A. Cryptoxanthin and beta-zeacarotene are also vitamin A precursors. Conversion takes place in intestine and liver.

Richest food sources (in µg per 100g) are: carrots (12000); parsley (7000); spinach (6000); turnip tops (6000); spring greens (4000); sweet potatoes (4000); watercress (3000); broccoli (2500); cantaloupe melons (2000); endives (2000); pumpkin (1500); apricots (1500); lettuce (1000); prunes (1000); tomatoes (600); spring cabbage (500); peaches (500); asparagus (500); ox liver (1540); butter (470); cheese (210); cream (125); cow's milk (22).

Relationship between carotenes and vitamin A is as follows:

1 retinol equivalent = 1 microgram retinol
                       = 6 micrograms beta-carotene
                       = 12 micrograms other carotene precursors
                       = 3.33IU vitamin A activity from retinol
                       = 10IU vitamin A activity from beta-carotene

Beta-carotene is most potent precursor of vitamin A.

Destroyed by high temperatures, oxygen and light particularly with traces of iron and copper. Losses of 40 per cent in boiling water (60mins); 70 per cent in frying (15 mins); freezing and canning and cooking loses 20 per cent; controlled drying of fruits and vegetables causes 20 per cent loss; drying in sun causes virtual complete destruction.

Functions of carotenes are as precursors of vitamin A. No other specific function known.

Deficiency not known to cause any specific disease.

Deficiency symptoms are not known.

Recommended dietary intakes have not been set by any authority. Possible to obtain full daily vitamin A requirements from carotenes alone. Usual diets supply 50 per cent vitamin A needs as vitamin and 50 per cent as carotenes.

Toxicity has not been reported for carotenes. Symptoms of excess are yellowing of skin that is reversible and harmless.

Therapy with beta-carotene claimed to be beneficial in lung cancer in animal tests. Appears to be protective against lung cancer induced by tobacco smoking.

---

cataracts, opacity of the eye lens. Can be induced by deficiency of vitamins B_2 and C and the mineral calcium. May be prevented by vitamin B_2 (10mg daily) vitamin C (500mg daily) and calcium (500mg daily).

---

cathartics, purgatives and laxatives. Prevent absorption of vitamin K and riboflavin.

---

cephalosporins, antibiotics. Prevent absorption of vitamins K, B_{12} and folic acid.

---

cheese, supplies most vitamins and minerals but specially rich in fat-soluble vitamins and calcium.

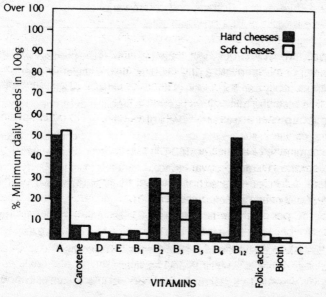

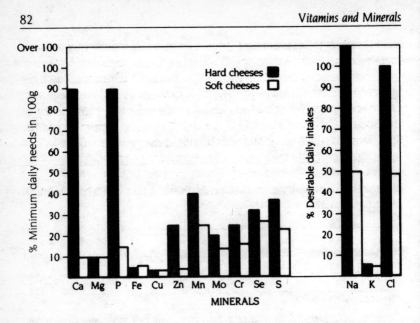

Hard cheeses comprise Cheddar, Danish Blue, Stilton, Camembert and Edam. Soft cheeses are, Cottage and cream varieties.

---

chelation,   from the Greek *chelos*, meaning claw; is the process whereby a mineral is incorporated into a ring structure by the chelating agent. The process is essentially transformation of an inorganic to an organically bound mineral. The resulting mineral chelate has a stability determined by the chelating group. There are three levels of stability:

1. strong chelates such as those formed by the chelating agents ethylenediamine tetra-acetic acid (EDTA) and D-penicillamine which are used in medicine to remove unwanted toxic minerals from the body. Once the chelate is formed it is strong enough to pass through the body unchanged and hence get excreted.

2. weak chelates such as mineral ascorbates, citrates, lactates and gluconates formed from the mineral and sugar-type residues have a stability comparable to mineral salts and are hence easily dissociated;

3. intermediate strength chelates can be either amino acid chelates or orotates. These are strong enough to be absorbed intact but weak enough

for the mineral to be transferred to other groups within the body by normal metabolic processes. Amino acid chelates are true biological chelates since this is how the body absorbs certain minerals, stores them, transports them and utilizes them. Orotates are synthetic derivatives of the mineral with orotic acid and there is scant evidence of their functioning as such within the body.

Chelated minerals that occur naturally include iron in haemoglobin; iron in haemosiderin; iron in ferritin; magnesium in chlorophyll; zinc in insulin; manganese in transmanganin in the blood; copper in haemocyanin (found in the blood of insects, crabs, octopus); calcium in milk; chromium in yeast; selenium in yeast; cobalt in vitamin B_{12}.

chick antidermatitis factor,   pantothenic acid.

chicken, *see* meats.

chilblains,   congestion and swelling of the skin due to cold and attended with severe itching or burning. Can be treated orally with nicotinic acid (25mg) and acetomenaphthone (10mg) per tablet. Complemented by creams containing methylnicotinate (1 per cent) plus other non-vitamin ingredients.

children,   vitamin needs related to weight but requirements for growth must also be accounted for. More likely to have faddy and fickle appetites and have a taste for foods of high calorie intake but low vitamin content. Good diet most important to health but may benefit from low level supplementation of vitamins and minerals.

Studies indicate that deficiency of certain vitamins and minerals may reduce the ability of school children to concentrate, learn and remember knowledge. The findings confirm studies on pre-school children indicating that iron deficiency delayed mental ability and psychomotor development.

For Recommended Dietary Intakes see Table 3.

Table 3: Recommended dietary intakes for children

COUNTRY	AGE (years)	SEX	VIT A µg	VIT D µg	VIT E mg	VIT B₁ mg	VIT B₂ mg	NICOTINIC ACID mg	VIT B₆ mg	FOLIC ACID ** µg	VIT B₁₂ µg	VIT C mg
AUSTRALIA	0-0.5	Both	–	–	–	–	–	–	0.25	–	–	–
	1-2	Both	250	10	–	0.5	0.7	9	0.6	100	0.9	30
	13-14	Both	725	–	–	1.0	1.3	17	1.5	200	2.0	40
	16-17	Both	750	–	–	1.2	1.5	20	2.0	200	2.0	50
NEW ZEALAND	0-0.5	Both	300	7.5	5	0.2	0.4	5	0.4	50	0.3	20
	1-2	Both	300	10	5	0.6	0.7	8	0.6	100	0.3	25
	13-14	Both	725	10	10	0.9	1.4	16	1.6	200	3.0	45
	16-17	Both	750	10	13.5	1.2	1.7	19	2.0	200	3.0	60
USA	0-0.5	Both	420	10	3	0.3	0.6	6	0.3	30	0.5	35
	0.5-1.0	Both	400	10	4	0.5	0.4	8	0.6	45	1.5	35
	1-3	Both	400	10	5	0.7	0.8	9	0.9	100	2.0	45
	4-6	Both	500	10	6	0.9	1.0	11	1.3	200	2.5	45
	7-10	Both	700	10	7	1.2	1.4	16	1.6	300	3.0	45
	11-14	M	1000	10	8	1.4	1.6	18	1.8	400	3.0	50
		F	800	10	8	1.1	1.3	15	1.8	400	3.0	50
	15-18	M	1000	10	10	1.4	1.7	18	2.0	400	3.0	60
		F	800	10	8	1.1	1.3	14	2.0	400	3.0	60
FAO/WHO	0-1.0	Both	300	10	–	0.3	0.5	5.4	–	60	0.3	20
	1-3	Both	250	10	–	0.5	0.8	9.0	–	100	0.9	20
	4-6	Both	300	10	–	0.7	1.1	12.1	–	100	1.5	20
	7-9	Both	400	2.5	–	0.9	1.3	14.5	–	100	1.5	20
	10-12	M	575	2.5	–	1.0	1.6	17.2	–	100	2.0	20
		F	575	2.5	–	0.9	1.4	15.5	–	100	2.0	20
	13-15	M	725	2.5	–	1.2	1.7	19.1	–	200	2.0	30
		F	725	2.5	–	1.0	1.5	16.4	–	200	2.0	30
	16-19	M	750	2.5	–	1.2	1.8	20.3	–	200	2.0	30
		F	750	2.5	–	0.9	1.4	15.2	–	200	2.0	30

	Age	Sex											
UK	0-1	M	450	—	7.5	—	0.3	0.4	5	—	—	—	20
		F	450	—	7.5	—	0.3	0.4	5	—	—	—	20
	1	M	300	—	10	—	0.5	0.6	7	—	—	—	20
		F	300	—	10	—	0.4	0.6	7	—	—	—	20
	2	M	300	—	10	—	0.6	0.7	8	—	—	—	20
		F	300	—	10	—	0.5	0.7	8	—	—	—	20
	3-4	M	300	—	10	—	0.6	0.8	9	—	—	—	20
		F	300	—	10	—	0.6	0.8	9	—	—	—	20
	5-6	M	300	—	10*	—	0.7	0.9	10	—	—	—	20
		F	300	—	10	—	0.7	0.9	10	—	—	—	20
	7-8	M	400	—	10	—	0.8	1.0	11	—	—	—	20
		F	400	—	10	—	0.8	1.0	11	—	—	—	20
	9-11	M	575	—	10	—	0.9	1.2	14	—	—	—	25
		F	575	—	10	—	0.8	1.2	14	—	—	—	25
	12-14	M	725	—	10	—	1.1	1.4	16	—	—	—	25
		F	725	—	10	—	0.9	1.4	16	—	—	—	25
	15-17	M	750	—	10	—	1.2	1.7	19	—	—	—	30
		F	750	—	10	—	0.9	1.7	19	—	—	—	30
CANADA	0-0.5	Both	400	3	10	0.3	0.4	5	0.3	40	0.3	20
	0.5-1.0	Both	400	3	10	0.5	0.6	6	0.4	60	0.3	20
	1-3	Both	400	4	10	0.7	0.8	9	0.8	100	0.4	20
	4-6	Both	500	5	5	0.9	1.1	12	1.3	100	1.5	20
	7-9	M	700	6	2.5	1.1	1.3	14	1.6	100	1.5	30
		F	700	6	2.5	1.0	1.2	13	1.4	100	1.5	30
	10-12	M	800	7	2.5	1.2	1.5	17	1.8	100	3.0	30
		F	800	7	2.5	1.1	1.4	15	1.5	100	3.0	30
	13-15	M	1000	9	2.5	1.4	1.7	19	2.0	200	3.0	30
		F	800	7	2.5	1.1	1.4	15	1.5	200	3.0	30
	16-18	M	1000	10	2.5	1.6	2.0	21	2.0	200	3.0	30
		F	800	6	2.5	1.1	1.3	14	1.5	200	3.0	30

* Supplements of 10μg daily recommended only during winter months for children and adolescents of more than 5 years of age.
** Folic acid intakes not yet recommended, but in adults are 300μg; B₁₂ intakes are 2μg in adults.

Chinese restaurant syndrome,   also known as the Ho Man Kwok syndrome. Symptoms start 15 minutes after eating Chinese food and consist of a numbness at the back of the neck which gradually radiates to both arms and to the back. There is a general weakness and palpitation of the heart. Has been suggested that the monosodium glutamate which occurs naturally in soy sauce may provide a local high concentration of sodium that causes the unpleasant effects. Possibility also that the high glutamic acid content (an amino acid) may contribute to the reaction.

---

chloramphenicol,   antibiotic. Prevents formation of vitamin K by intestinal bacteria.

---

chlorbutol,   anti-nausea agent. Enhances excretion and metabolism of vitamin C.

---

chloride,   chemical symbol Cl. Atomic weight 35.5. Abundance in igneous rock is 0.031 per cent by weight; in sea water 1.9 per cent by weight, primarily as sodium chloride. An essential mineral form of chlorine in plants, animals and man.

Chloride is usually associated with sodium both in the food and in body fluids; high sodium levels are paralleled by high chloride levels and vice versa. In body fluids chloride is negatively charged (anion) and it neutralizes the positively-charged sodium and potassium (cations). Body content of chloride is about 115g. This amount is kept constant by excretion of excess in urine, sweat and the gastrointestinal tract. Most people are in positive chloride balance since intake on adequate diets is more than enough. In parallel with sodium, excessive losses can be caused by heavy sweating and by diarrhoea. In addition, chloride in the form of hydrochloric acid may be lost to a significant degree in persistent vomiting. Normal blood plasma levels of chloride lie between 348 and 376mg per 100ml.

Functions of chloride are:

1. to act as the main anion to sodium and potassium cations in maintenance of body water levels and neutrality;

2. to provide chloride for the production of hydrochloric acid by the stomach.

Food sources of chloride parallel those of sodium. Foods rich in sodium are rich in chloride; poor sources of sodium like fruits, vegetables, nuts and wholegrains are also poor providers of chloride. *See* sodium, and individual foods for contents.

Deficiency of chloride in body fluids is highly unlikely but may parallel excessive sodium losses. No symptoms can be attributed specifically to lack of chloride. The only possible local deficiency of body chloride is in the condition of achlorhydria where the stomach cells fail to produce hydrochloric acid. This is due to a breakdown in the production mechanism, not to lack of chloride.

Supplementary forms of chloride include: sodium chloride — 100mg provides 60.7mg chloride; potassium chloride — 100mg provides 47.6mg chloride. Hydrochloric acid may be taken as betaine hydrochloride; glutamic acid hydrochloride, or dilute hydrochloric acid. *See* hydrochloric acid.

Increased blood plasma levels of chloride are seen in anaemia; heart disease, kidney disease, pregnancy (eclampsia).

Decreased blood plasma levels of chloride are seen in diabetes; fevers; pneumonia.

Urinary excretion of chloride is increased in a diet rich in salt; rickets; liver cirrhosis. It is decreased in chronic kidney disease; early stages of pneumonia; cancer; gastritis.

Excessive dietary levels of chloride are likely only with increased salt and potassium chloride intakes. The toxic effects of both of these are related to the sodium and potassium moieties respectively (*see* sodium *and* potassium). No toxic effects have been attributed to chloride but it has been suggested recently that the high blood-pressure-inducing effect of excessive salt intakes which may be mediated through the hormones renin and aldosterone could be a function of high chloride rather than high sodium in the diet.

---

chlorine dioxide, a food additive used as a bleaching and improving agent for flour. Acceptable level for flour treatment is up to 30mg per kg; from 30-75mg per kg for special purposes. Permitted only as a bleaching or improving agent.

---

cholecalciferol, D_3 vitamin.

---

cholesterol, fatty substance with three essential functions in the body. Constituent of cell membranes particularly the myelin sheath that insulates nerves; precursor of bile acids; precursor of steroid hormones (sex, anti-stress, water balance, metabolic). Production of steroid hormones needs vitamin C and pantothenic acid.

Cholesterol exists in blood and organs as HDL-cholesterol (high density lipoprotein); LDL-cholesterol (low density lipoprotein); VLDL-cholesterol (very low density lipoprotein). High ratio of HDL to LDL and VLDL desirable to protect against atherosclerosis, arteriosclerosis and coronary heart disease. HDL increased by taking PUFA instead of animal fats; by taking 600IU of vitamin E daily.

High *blood cholesterol* levels reduced by taking 500mg vitamin C daily or by taking 3g nicotinic acid daily.

---

cholestyramine, anti-cholesterol agent. Prevents absorption of vitamins A, D, E, K and B_{12}.

---

choline, water-soluble member of the vitamin B complex.

Not a true vitamin as it is synthesized in the liver in limited quantities. Known also as amanitine, lipotropic factor. Active constituent of lecithin. Present in supplements as choline bitartrate, choline chloride, phosphatidyl choline, lecithin. Colourless, crystalline substance.

Therapeutic Uses	Symptoms of Excess Intake
Angina Atherosclerosis Thrombosis Stroke High blood-pressure Alzheimer's disease Senile dementia	None reported apart from occasional mild nausea.

Best Food Sources
in mg per 100g

Lecithin granules	3430
Desiccated liver	2170
Beef heart	1720
Egg-yolk	1700
Lecithin oil	800
Liver	650
Beef steak	600
Wheatgerm	505
Dried brewer's yeast	300
Cereals	240
Nuts	220
Pulses (beans)	120
Citrus fruits	85
Wholemeal bread	80
Greenleaf vegetables	80
Other fruits	44
Root vegetables	40
Milk	30

Functions

As fat-stabilizing agent
As precursor of:
  betaine, needed in
  metabolism; acetylcholine,
  nerve substance
As component of lecithin

Stability in Foods

Very stable

Absorption from Foods

Absorbed better as lecithin
than as choline.

Deficiency Symptoms

Nothing specific but lack can
lead to:
  Fatty liver
  Nerve degeneration
  Senile dementia
  High blood-pressure
  Reduced resistance to
    infection
  Atherosclerosis
  Thrombosis
  Stroke
  High blood cholesterol

Increased Intakes

Needed by:
  Alcoholics
  Diabetics
  Those with conditions in
    Deficiency Symptoms

Recommended Daily Intakes

Difficult to assess because of
body synthesis. Probably
between 500 and 1000mg.

chromium, chemical symbol Cr, atomic weight 52.0. Exists in many forms but trivalent chromium is the only one that can be used by the body. An essential trace element for animals and man.

Body Content

Adult content is between 5.2 and 10.4mg but there is wide geographical variation e.g.

European and	
North Americans	6.00mg
African natives	7.45mg
Middle East	
inhabitants	11.8mg
Far East Inhabitants	12.5mg

Incidence of diabetes and heart disease decreases with increasing chromium levels. Levels decline with age.

On a content of 5mg, 2mg is present in skin; 1.2mg in bone; 0.9mg in muscle and 0.3mg in fat.

Body Turnover

Absorption from the food is very poor and is between 3 and 10 per cent. Only 1 per cent of added chromium (as salts) is absorbed.

When incorporated into yeast, chromium absorption increases to between 10 and 25 per cent.

Excretion is in the faeces and urine where up to 10µg can be lost daily.

Chromium Supplements (in µg per 100µg)

Chromium trichloride or chromic chloride (32.8); chromium acetate (22.7); amino acid chelated chromium (2).

Yeast is an excellent supplement, even more efficient because it contains chromium as GTF. GTF is 50 times as effective as other forms of chromium and is 20 times more readily absorbed. GTF from yeast is 10 times as effective as chromium in foods such as liver, wheatgerm and seafoods.

Best Food Sources in μg per 100g	
Egg yolk	183
Molasses	121
Dried brewer's yeast	117
Beef	57
Hard cheese	56
Liver	55
Fruit juices	47
Wholemeal bread	42
Bran	38
Alcoholic beverages	30
Cereals	30
Honey	29
Wheatgerm	23
Vegetables	21
Fruit	10

Dietary Deficiency

Poor sources include:
  White flour
  Shell fish
  Fish
  Poultry
  Egg white
  Skimmed milk
Hence a diet high in these will not contribute much chromium.

Food refining and processing also remove most of the chromium from the original foodstuffs. Highly refined diets will also lead to deficiency. Wholefood diets contribute adequate amounts.

Functions

Chromium functions as the Glucose Tolerance Factor (GTF) — no other functions are known.

GTF stimulates insulin activity directly by binding to both insulin itself and specific insulin receptors. Chromium alone does not do this.

GTF therefore:
  Controls blood glucose by promoting uptake by muscles and organs.
  Stimulates burning of glucose for energy.
  Controls blood cholesterol levels.
  Reduces fat levels in blood.
  Increases HDL cholesterol.
  Reduces arteriosclerosis in rat experiments.
  Stimulates protein synthesis.
  Stimulates production of essential nerve substances.
  Increases resistance to infection.
  Suppresses hunger symptoms through brain 'satiety centre'.

Effects of Deficiency

Causes condition resembling
  diabetes in experimental rats
Impaired glucose uptake by
  muscles in malnourished
  children
Nervous complaints
Increased blood cholesterol
levels
Formation of arteriosclerotic
  plaques
Increased blood fat levels
May be a factor in heart
  disease
Possibly related to some human
diabetes

Deficiency Causes

Diets high in refined and
  processed foods
Excessive losses from the
  body in some diseases
Prolonged slimming regimes
Pregnancy
Severe malnutrition
Prolonged intravenous feeding
Alcoholism

Recommended Daily Intake

None available but the US
Food and Nutrition Board
suggest a safe and adequate
range of intakes of 50-200µg
chromium daily depending
upon age.

Symptoms of Deficiency

Similar to those of
hypoglycaemia and are:
  Irritability
  Frustration
  Intolerance
  Mental confusion
  Weakness
  Depression
  Learning disabilities
and in addition:
  Alcohol intolerance
  Nervousness
Some symptoms are similar to
early stages of diabetes:
  Frequent passing of urine
  Thirst
  Hunger
  Weight loss
  Itching

Therapeutic Uses

Successful in some child and
  adult diabetes.
Diabetes of pregnancy
Maturity-onset diabetes
Reducing high blood
  cholesterol
Some cases of hypoglycaemia
  (low blood sugar)

Effects of Excess Intake

None have been reported. Low toxicity is the result of very poor absorption. Hexavalent chromium is more toxic but this is never used in supplements or found in foods.

---

cigarette smoking, four main poisons are acetaldehyde, cancer-producing substances (carcinogens), carbon monoxide and nicotine.

Toxic effects of acetaldehyde, carbon monoxide and nicotine neutralized by vitamin B_1, vitamin C and cysteine. Beta-carotene protects against carcinogens.

Heavy smoking can inactivate vitamin B_{12}, inducing pernicious anaemia and eventually blindness. Treat with injections of hydroxocobalamin.

---

cirrhosis, chronic progressive disease of the liver characterized by destruction of liver cells and overgrowth of connective tissue. Complementary vitamin treatment includes high doses of vitamin B complex plus fat-soluble vitamins A, D, E and K to overcome excessive loss due to disease. Choline (up to 3000mg daily) may be needed to prevent fatty infiltration.

---

citrovorum factor, folinic acid.

---

claudication, intermittent. Pains in calves induced by walking and due to narrowing of leg blood vessels. Treated with vitamin E, 400-600IU daily.

---

cobalamin, *see* B_{12} vitamin.

---

cobalt, chemical symbol Co. Atomic weight 58.9. Widely distributed in nature. Abundance in earth's crust 0.001-0.002 per cent. Occurs as cobaltite, linnaeite, smaltite, erythrite.

Essential trace mineral only as a constituent of vitamin B_{12}. Ruminants have a requirement only for cobalt as the micro-organisms in their rumens can incorporate the mineral into vitamin B_{12}. Other animals and man cannot do so and a dietary source of the vitamin is essential for health. Vitamin B_{12} can only be synthesized by micro-organisms.

Body content of cobalt averages 1.1mg. Forty-three per cent of this is stored throughout the muscle tissues; 14 per cent is in the bone; the remainder is mainly distributed throughout the other tissues but mainly in the liver and kidneys. Blood levels vary over a wide range, from 0.007-$0.036\mu g$ cobalt per 100ml whole blood in one study and from 0.17-$1.5\mu g$ cobalt in another. Most of the cobalt of blood is found in the red blood cells rather than in the plasma.

Dietary intakes of cobalt depend upon the amount of mineral in the soil and hence in the plants and animals that thrive on that soil. Children in the USA were found to have diets containing from 0.25-0.69mg cobalt per kg food. In diets of adults, intakes varied from 0.30-1.77mg cobalt per day. Much lower levels are found in the diets of most Japanese who eat only 0.01mg daily. WHO sources recommend a minimum daily intake of $1\mu g$ cobalt to be absorbed.

Food sources that are rich in cobalt include fresh, green, leafy vegetables and some fish; poor sources are cereal and dairy products. Typical values are (in μg per 100g): vegetables 20-60; scallops 225; cod 120; liver 15; kidney 25; muscle meats 12; dairy products 1-3. Some of the cobalt in meat, fish and dairy products is present in their vitamin B_{12} content and the rest is the mineral in some other form. In vegetables and cereals, all is present in some other form.

It has also been used to reduce high blood-pressure because of its action in causing dilatation of blood vessels, but quantities of 50mg oral cobalt chloride daily were required for periods up to 65 days.

In animals high intakes (4-10mg cobalt per kg body weight) can cause anaemia, loss of appetite and low body weight.

Functions of cobalt reside only in its presence in vitamin B_{12}. Many of the vitamin's functions are mediated through the cobalt portion of the molecule and they include synthesis of DNA; production of red blood cells; synthesis of methionine; synthesis of choline; synthesis of creatine. All of these involve transfer of active methyl groups from folic acid (B vitamin) to cobalt and hence to receptor substance. Other functions include maintenance of myelin, the fatty sheath that insulates nerves, and detoxification of cyanide introduced through food and tobacco smoke.

Deficiency of mineral cobalt is unknown but deficiency of vitamin B_{12} causes pernicious anaemia. This anaemia cannot be treated with cobalt — it responds only to injections of the vitamin.

Therapy with cobalt has been used in the past to try and stimulate the bone-marrow to produce more red and white blood cells, but there is no convincing evidence that it helps. *Therapeutic forms* include cobaltous carbonate; cobaltous chloride; cobaltous nitrate. These are usually added to animal feeds.

Food additives containing cobalt are no longer used. Once it was added during the beer-brewing operation to improve the quality of the 'head' of the glass. This practice led to toxicity effects (see below) and the practice is no longer carried out.

Toxic effects of cobalt are highly unlikely with intakes from a normal diet. When used therapeutically in doses of 29.5mg daily side-effects included goitre, hypothyroidism and heart failure. Intakes of up to 17.7mg daily by heavy beer drinkers who drank up to 12 litres of beer (cobalt content about 1.5mg per litre) caused heart disease and death. Protein intake in these people was low; high-protein dietary levels are believed to protect against cobalt toxicity. Other toxic effects of cobalt noted in animals and human beings include overproduction of red cells (polycythaemia vera).

---

cobaltous carbonate, provides 25.9mg cobalt in 100mg carbonate (as hexahydrate). A nutritional factor used in cobalt or vitamin B_{12} deficiency in ruminants.

---

cobaltous chloride, provides 24.7mg cobalt in 100mg chloride (as hexahydrate). A nutritional factor used in cobalt or vitamin B_{12} deficiency in ruminants. Large amounts may lead to death in children. Toxic effects include skin flushing; chest pains; dermatitis; tinnitus (ringing in the ears); nausea; vomiting; nerve deafness; myxoedema; heart failure.

---

cobaltous nitrate, provides 20.0mg cobalt in 100mg nitrate (as hexahydrate). A nutritional factor used in cobalt or vitamin B_{12} deficiency in ruminants. Has been used as a dietary supplement of cobalt in man.

---

cocoa, the powder supplies carotene, vitamin E and some B vitamins but is devoid of vitamin C. Carotene level is 40μg per 100g. Vitamin E content is 3.2mg per 100g. B vitamins present are (in mg per 100g): thiamine 0.16; riboflavin 0.06; nicotinic acid 7.3; pyridoxine 0.07. Folic acid level is 38μg per 100g.

Mineral
Rich source of sodium but even richer in potassium. Excellent provider of all minerals. The powder supplies the following (in mg per 100g): sodium 950; potassium 1500; calcium 130; magnesium 520; phosphorus 660; iron 10.5; copper 3.9; zinc 6.9; chloride 460.

---

coconut, supplies less vitamin E and B vitamins than other nuts but does contain some vitamin C. Desiccated coconut is richer in most vitamins than fresh edible portion. Vitamin E level of edible portion is 1.0mg per 100g; desiccated variety is devoid of vitamin E. B vitamins present are (in mg per 100g) for fresh and desiccated coconut respectively: thiamine 0.03, 0.06; riboflavin 0.02, 0.04; nicotinic acid 1.0, 1.8; pyridoxine 0.04, 0.09; pantothenic acid 0.20, 0.31. Folic acid levels are 26 and 54μg per 100g respectively for fresh and desiccated coconut. Vitamin C content of fresh coconut is 2mg per 100g but there is none in the desiccated variety.

 Coconut milk supplies traces of most vitamins that are in the flesh. Traces only of vitamin E. B vitamins present are (in mg per 100g): thiamine, and riboflavin, traces only; nicotinic acid 0.2; pyridoxine 0.03; pantothenic acid 0.05. No folic acid or biotin have been detected. Vitamin C level is 2mg per 100g.

Mineral
Should be regarded as a good provider of potassium, magnesium, phosphorus, iron, copper and zinc. A low sodium food, the desiccated variety is richer in all minerals than the fresh nut. Mineral contents are for fresh and desiccated respectively (in mg per 100g): sodium 17, 28; potassium 440, 750; calcium 13, 22; magnesium 52, 90; phosphorus 94,

160; iron 2.1, 3.6; copper 0.32, 0.55; zinc 0.5, (desiccated not measured); sulphur 44, 76; chloride 110, 220. Milk provides more calcium but less of other minerals.

---

cod liver oil, rich source of fat-soluble vitamins but completely devoid of water-soluble variety. Provides (in mg per 100g): vitamin A 18.0; vitamin D 0.21; vitamin E 20.0.

Contains also polyunsaturated fatty acids known as Eicosapentaenoic Acid (EPA) 9.0 per cent and Docosahexaenoic Acid (DHA) 8.0 per cent that have essential roles in body metabolism. Total polyunsaturated fatty acids present at level of 23g per 100g oil.

Mineral
Contains the following minerals, in trace amounts only: sodium; potassium; calcium; magnesium; phosphorus; iron; copper; zinc; sulphur; chloride.

---

coenzyme Q_{10}, a vitamin-like substance that is found in all cells of the body but is particularly rich in heart muscle, nervous tissue and blood. There are at least ten types of coenzyme Q designated coenzyme Q_0 to coenzyme Q_{10} but the human variety is coenzyme Q_{10}. The coenzyme is present in the diet, mainly as coenzyme Q_{10} from meats but it is also made within the body. The body makes coenzyme Q_{10} exclusively. In the early days of research, the substance was available only from the heart, liver and kidney but it is now manufactured in large quantities using a bacterial fermentation.

Coenzyme Q_{10} functions essentially in the transfer of oxygen and energy between the blood and body cells and between components of those cells. The cell cannot function effectively without coenzyme Q_{10} and when it is deficient, the work-rate of muscle cells is adversely affected. Low levels of coenzyme Q_{10} have been found in heart cells of those suffering from heart problems and heart failure; in the nervous tissue and brain cells of those with mental problems and in the white blood cells of those who suffer infections. Treatment with oral coenzyme Q_{10} in all these cases studied has improved the individual's condition.

Intracellular levels of coenzyme Q_{10} have also been found to be reduced as a person grows older and its deficiency appears to be related to ageing effects. Clinical trials have indicated that some anti-ageing criteria improve tremendously with coenzyme Q_{10} therapy. One aspect of ageing, namely gum deterioration, has been shown to be halted by taking extra oral coenzyme Q_{10}

All the trials carried out indicate that a daily intake of 30mg coenzyme Q_{10}, preferably taken in three divided doses of 10mg each, is sufficient to give a beneficial effect in these cases. A similar dose can also have a prophylactic effect against the conditions induced by a lack of coenyzme Q_{10}.

Coenzyme Q_{10} is fat-soluble and in structure is somewhere between vitamin E and vitamin K. Hence, not surprisingly, its function overlaps to some extent with these two vitamins.

---

coffee, all types of coffee are devoid of carotene and vitamin E. Rich source of nicotinic acid.

Ground, roasted variety supplies 0.20mg riboflavin per 100g and 10.0mg nicotinic acid per 100g. The quantity of nicotinic acid increases during the roasting process because it is liberated from a bound form. A dark roasted variety may contain 30 to 40mg nicotinic acid per 100g. No other vitamins have been measured.

Infused ground coffee supplies much lower quantities of the above vitamins. Riboflavin content is 0.01mg per 100g. Nicotinic acid content is 0.7mg per 100g.

Instant coffee (in dried form) is a very rich source of nicotinic acid at between 24.9 and 41.5mg per 100g. Riboflavin content is 0.11mg per 100g. Also contains pyridoxine (0.03mg per 100g) and pantothenic acid (0.4mg per 100g).

Decaffeinated coffee (in dried form) provides similar vitamin levels to ground, roasted variety. Instant decaffeinated coffee has similar vitamin levels to instant coffee.

Mineral
Fairly low in sodium but very rich in potassium, calcium, magnesium, phosphorus, iron, copper and sulphur. As a drink, all concentrations are reduced. The instant variety is richer in all minerals than ground coffee because it is concentrated.

Ground, roasted variety (in mg per 100g): sodium 74, potassium 2020; calcium

130; magnesium 240, phosphorus 160; iron 4.1; copper 0.82; sulphur 110; chloride 24.

Infused ground coffee (in mg per 100g): sodium trace; potassium 66; calcium 2; magnesium 6; phosphorus 2; iron trace; copper trace; chloride trace.

Instant variety (in mg per 100g): sodium 41; potassium 4000; calcium 160; magnesium 390; phosphorus 350; iron 4.4; copper 0.05; zinc 0.5; chloride 50.

---

colchicine, used to treat gout. Prevents absorption of vitamins A and B_{12}.

---

cold, viral infection of the upper respiratory tract. Also know as coryza, rhinitis, cold in the head.

Increase vitamin A intake during period of illness. Treat with vitamin C at intake of 1 gram every 4 hours until relief is obtained, then gradually reduce over one week to 1 gram per day then 500mg maintenance dose.

Mineral

Symptoms have been relieved by sucking lozenges containing 23mg zinc, as a zinc gluconate, per lozenge every two wakeful hours. In the trial, 20 per cent of those with colds for less than three days lost their cold symptoms within 24 hours; none sucking a placebo lozenge did. After a week, 86 per cent of those with colds who had taken zinc recovered; half of those taking placebo lozenges still had symptoms. Zinc tablets that are swallowed do not have any beneficial effect in relieving cold symptoms so it is possible that the mineral has a direct action on the cold viruses in the mouth, nose and throat which stops their multiplication.

---

cold sores, caused by a herpes virus. They begin as small tender lumps on the lips, tongue, roof of the mouth, gums or cheek, usually preceded by a tingling or itching sensation. Lumps usually develop into painful ulcerations that form a scab in about a week. Healing takes between ten days and three weeks. Cold sores may be prevented or treated with supplementary zinc. Studies indicate that 25-50mg of elemental zinc daily is needed for therapy. Complementary vitamin C (500mg daily) may also help. Zinc creams applied directly to a developed cold sore have been claimed to accelerate healing. The mineral apparently blocks reproduction of the virus, allowing natural healing to proceed. *See also* cold.

---

colitis, chronic, inflammatory and ulcerative disease of the colon. Drug treatment should be supplemented with high potency multivitamin preparation plus extra vitamin C and B_6 when on corticosteroids.

---

collagen, main protein of connective tissues (skin, joints, vital organs) throughout body. Starting material for production of gelatin. Rate of wound healing depends upon rate of production of collagen, itself dependent on vitamin C.

Vitamin C (500 to 1000mg daily) often given routinely to patients undergoing surgery and those recovering from accidental injury to accelerate healing process.

---

colon cancer, *see* cancer.

---

colouring agents, for those used in vitamin tablets and capsules manufactured in the UK, *see* E Numbers.

---

constipation, stubborn cases may respond to vitamin B_1 (10mg daily). Complete vitamin B complex sometimes used to stimulate intestinal bacteria growth to relieve constipation, particularly after antibiotic treatment.

---

contraceptives, barrier types, such as condoms or diaphragms, with or without contraceptive creams or jellies, have no known effect on vitamin or mineral requirements.

---

contraceptives, coil or IUD (intra-uterine device). Excessive bleeding controlled by bioflavonoids (1000mg daily) *or* vitamin E (100IU every other day).

---

contraceptives, oral. Consist of synthetic oestrogens and progestogens that can increase requirements for certain vitamins. Supplementary vitamin B_6 (25-50mg), vitamin B_{12} (5μg), folic acid (200μg), vitamin E (100IU) and vitamin C (100mg) needed daily plus the minerals zinc (15mg) and manganese (5mg). High dose (1000mg and above) vitamin C improves the bio-availability of the oestrogenic ingredient of the Pill causing higher blood levels. Hence supplementary vitamin C should always be taken at a separate meal or time of day to that of the contraceptive pill.

---

convalescence, stage of post-illness often characterized by mild deficiency of vitamins induced by low food intake and by medicinal drugs. Supplement with all-round multivitamin preparation plus extra vitamin C (500-1000mg) in illnesses of infection and in post-operative period.

---

copper, chemical symbol Cu, from the latin cuprum. Atomic weight 63.5. An essential trace element for man, animals and many plants.

Best Food Sources in mg per 100g		Non-food Sources
Liver	8.0	Much of the copper we receive does not arise in the original food we eat. It comes from:
Shell fish	7.6	
Dried brewer's yeast	3.3	Processing and storage of food
Olives	1.6	
Nuts	1.4	Pesticides and fungicides left behind in the food
Pulses (beans)	0.8	
Cereals	0.7	Copper containers
Meat, fish and poultry	0.3	Copper pipes that carry water — especially the soft varieties
Wholemeal bread	0.3	
Dried fruits	0.3	Copper kettles

Body Content

An adult contains between 75 and 150mg. Half of this is contained in the skeleton and muscles. A further 10 per cent is in the liver with significant amounts in brain, kidney and heart. As adult ages, liver copper decreases and that in the brain increases to the same concentration but the significance of this is not known.

Babies have liver copper concentrations ten times those in adult livers. This acts as a store since milk is not a rich source of the trace mineral.

Recommended Dietary Intakes

Should be at least 2mg daily which is met by most diets.

Therapeutic Uses

Treating deficiency symptoms
As supplement in treating those with deficiency
Anaemia (rare)
Rheumatoid arthritis
Intra-uterine device in contraception

Excretion

The copper stored in the liver is normally incorporated into bile from where it is secreted into the intestine and hence excreted into the faeces.

Medicinal Sources

Expectorant cough mixtures
Cough suppressant preparations
Decongestant preparations
Anti-algae solutions in swimming pools

Deficiency Symptoms

In babies:
  Failure to thrive
  Pale skin
  Diarrhoea
  Depigmentation of hair and skin
  Prominent dilated veins in skin

In adults:
  Anaemia
  Water retention
  Irritability
  Brittle bones
  Hair depigmentation
  Poor hair texture
  Loss of sense of taste

Functions	Deficiency
Co-factor for many enzymes e.g. natural colouring pigments that form in skin and hair. Those needed for skin healing Those that protect against toxic agents Those concerned with nerve impulses in the brain Blood formation, when it aids iron absorption and incorporation into haemaglobin In formation of healthy bones In developing resistance to infection	Has been noted in: Malnourished children Malabsorption problems Infantile anaemia Premature babies Children with Menke's syndrome (unable to absorb copper) Those living on highly refined diets Anyone with prolonged diarrhoea Those taking excessive amounts of zinc, cadmium, fluoride or molybdenum Those on high phytic acid diets (see separate entry)

Symptoms of Excess Intake

Although toxicity of copper is generally low, acute high concentration poisoning can occur giving rise to:
    Nausea; vomiting; abdominal pain; diarrhoea; diffuse muscle pains. Abnormal mental states leading to coma and death.

An inability to rid the body of copper can also occur in two hereditary diseases: Wilsons disease and Indian childhood cirrhosis. Both need medical treatment to dispose of the excess copper.

Copper Supplements (in mg per 100mg)

Copper amino acid chelate (2); copper gluconate (14); copper sulphate (25.4).

copper bangles, traditional preventative and curative therapy for arthritis when worn on the wrist or ankle. Generally believed that copper dissolves in the acid secretion of skin and is then absorbed in a form that can be utilized in the body. Blood levels of copper in arthritis are usually high but mineral is in a non-utilizable form. Confirmation that this hypothesis is true has come from studies indicating that fat-soluble copper salicylate (aspirin) complexes are absorbed through the skin. They are strikingly effective in reducing the inflammation of artificially-induced arthritis in animals and of the clinical condition in man.

corticosteroids, hormones produced by the adrenal glands from cholesterol. These plus synthetic analogues (called steroid drugs) used extensively in medicine at relatively high levels. Adversely affect certain vitamins. Increase requirements of vitamins B_6 and C and probably D. Needs are B_6 (25-50mg daily in both sexes), C (500-1000mg daily) and D (400IU daily). Zinc (15mg daily) also needed.

cortisol, a natural corticosteroid. *See* corticosteroids.

cortisone, a natural corticosteroid. *See* corticosteroids.

coryza, cold in the head. *See* cold.

co-trimoxazole, antibacterial agent. Impairs folic acid utilization.

cramps, leg. When induced by exercise is called intermittent claudication. Nocturnal (night-time) cramps treated with vitamin E (200IU daytime, 200IU before sleep) plus vitamin C (500mg daily). Cramps due to restless leg syndrome treated with vitamin E (400IU daily).

cream, shows seasonal variations in fat-soluble vitamins. Water-soluble constant levels are (in mg per 100g): thiamine 0.03; riboflavin 0.12; nicotinic acid 0.64; pyridoxine 0.03; folic acid 0.004; pantothenic acid 0.30; biotin 0.0014; vitamin C 1.2; vitamin B_{12} 0.2µg.

Summer single (light) cream provides (per 100g): vitamin A 0.2mg; carotene 0.125mg; vitamin E 0.5mg; vitamin D 0.165µg. *Winter single (light) cream* provides (per 100g): vitamin A 0.145mg; carotene 0.07mg; vitamin E 0.4mg; vitamin D 0.081µg. Double (heavy) cream contains approximately twice the quantity of fat-soluble vitamins as single cream.

Mineral

A low sodium food supplying good quantities of calcium, phosphorus and potassium with useful amounts of the trace minerals.

Single cream provides (in mg per 100g): sodium 42; potassium 120; calcium 79; magnesium 6; phosphorus 44; iron 0.31; copper 0.20; zinc 0.26; chloride 72.

Double cream provides (in mg per 100g): sodium 27; potassium 79; calcium 50; magnesium 4; phosphorus 21; iron 0.20; copper 0.13; zinc 0.17; chloride 46.

Whipping variety provides (in mg per 100g): sodium 34; potassium 100; calcium 63; magnesium 5; phosphorus 27; iron 0.25; copper 0.16; zinc 0.21; chloride 58.

Sterilized, canned variety (in mg per 100g): sodium 56; potassium 120; calcium 80; magnesium 6; phosphorus 44; iron 0.30; copper 0.20; zinc 0.26; chloride 140.

---

cream of magnesia, an aqueous suspension of hydrated magnesium oxide containing the equivalent of 7.45-8.35 per cent of magnesium hydroxide. Ten ml contains the equivalent of 550mg of magnesium oxide providing 300mg magnesium.

---

cretinism, also known as congenital hypothyroidism, juvenile hypothyroidism; a syndrome of dwarfism, mental retardation and coarseness of the skin due to lack of thyroid hormone from birth. May affect as many as 20 per cent of the population in isolated areas of Nepal, the

Andes, Zaire and New Guinea. Iodine deficiency during foetal or early life may lead to cretinism in the child.

Cretins are often associated with particular areas where iodine is deficient in the soil and water supply. Infants afflicted have a characteristic look: the tongue is enlarged, lips are thickened, mouth stays open and drooling. Face is usually broad and the nose flat. Feet and hands puffy with hands spade-shaped. The child is dull, apathetic, has low body temperature and suffers from constipation and other gastrointestinal complaints. It may be large at birth but as age progresses they have defective development and often stay as dwarfs when they develop into adults. Mentally they range from mildly backward to severely retarded. If diagnosed early enough, iodine or thyroid hormone treatment reverses the condition and in most communities the condition is soon recognized. Only in the more remote areas is it prevalent.

As well as lack of iodine in prenatal or early life, other causes of cretinism are iodide transport defect; failure to convert iodides to the hormones; defective synthesis of thyroglobulin; absent or undeveloped thyroid; failure to respond to thyroid hormones at the cellular level; failure of the gland to respond to thyroid-stimulating hormone (TSH). In all causes, the only treatment is to give oral thyroid hormone, usually thyroxine.

Crohn's disease, generalized inflammatory disease of the small intestine and lower intestinal tract. Also known as regional enteritis. Drug treatment complemented by high potency multivitamin supplementation. Extra vitamin C and B_6 also recommended when on corticosteroids.

---

cyanocobalamin, B_{12} vitamin.

---

cycloserine, antibiotic. Reduces availability of folic acid.

---

cystic fibrosis, inherited disease usually starting in infancy and typified by chronic infection of respiratory system, pancreatic insufficiency and susceptibility to heat. Infection needs increased vitamin C intake (up to 1000mg daily); pancreatic insufficiency leads to fat malabsorption so increased intakes of vitamin A (7500IU), vitamin D (400IU), vitamin E (250IU) needed daily preferably water-solubilized.

---

cysts, cystic disease of the breast, a benign condition, is the most common disease of the female breast occurring in about 5 per cent of middle-aged women. Pain or premenstrual breast discomfort is a frequent symptom and cyst may be tender but more often condition has no symptoms. Discovery usually by palpation.

Once malignancy has been discounted treatment, apart from surgery, may be two-fold:

1. 600IU vitamin E daily for eight weeks should give clinical response;

2. oil of evening primrose, 3000mg daily divided into three doses.

D

D, fat-soluble vitamin. Occurs naturally as cholecalciferol (D_3) found only in foods of animal origin and as ergocalciferol (D_2) produced by the action of light on yeast. Isolated in 1930 from cod liver oil by Dr E. Mallanby. Known as the Sunshine Vitamin.

1 microgram is equivalent to 40 international units (IU).

Best Food Sources in µg per 100g	
Cod liver oil	210.00
Kippers	210.00
Mackerel	17.50
Canned Salmon	12.50
Sardines	7.50
Tuna	5.80
Eggs	1.75
Milk	0.03

Non-food Source

Substantial amounts are produced in the skin by the action of sunlight.

Three hours of summer sun on the face produces 10µg vitamin D. Winter light produces 1µg. Whole body exposure needs less time.

Functions

Only as 1, 25-dihydroxy vitamin D which is produced by the liver and kidneys from dietary or skin vitamin D. The active form 1, 25-dihydroxy D: Promotes absorption of calcium and phosphate from the food; Causes release of calcium from the bone.

Deficiency Disease

Is rickets in children
Osteomalacia in adults
In both there is softening of the bones due to lack of calcium phosphate.

Deficiency Symptoms

Children:
  Unnatural limb posture
  Excessive sweating of head
  Delayed ability to stand
  Knock knees or bow legs
Adults:
  Bone pain
  Muscular weakness
  Muscular spasms
  Brittle bones — easily
    broken

Deficiency Causes

Lack of meat, poultry, fish and dairy products in diet, lack of exposure to sunshine.

When sun exposure is sufficient, dietary sources are not required.

Therapeutic Uses

Rickets
Osteomalacia
Osteoporosis
Rheumatoid arthritis

Symptoms of Excess Intake

The most toxic of the vitamins
Loss of appetite
Nausea
Vomiting
Constant thirst
Head pains
Child becomes thin, irritable
  and depressed

Recommended Daily Intakes

Should be at least 10μg (400IU) but see separate entry. Supplement should not exceed 10μg daily.

Stability in Foods

Very stable but see Losses in Food Processing

deafness,   may be due to otosclerosis, a disease where the bones of the middle ear become fused and unable to vibrate and so transmit sound. Particularly in elderly where it may be related to long-term vitamin A deficiency. Cannot be cured by vitamin therapy but adequate intakes throughout life may prevent it.

---

decubitus ulcer,   *see* bedsores.

---

deficiency,   lack of sufficient vitamin intake. For example: four stages of vitamin deficiency identified in volunteers deprived of B_1:

1. no obvious changes in first 5-10 days but vitamin stores depleted;
2. altered cell metabolism after 10-60 days;
3. clinical defects after 30-180 days with non-specific symptoms like weight loss, appetite loss, malaise, insomnia, increased irritability;
4. anatomical defects from 180 days on leading to specific signs of gross deficiency that if untreated may lead to death.

Can be caused by poor nutrition; poor cooking methods; overprocessing and over-refining of foods; habits like smoking tobacco and drinking alcohol; stress; medicinal drugs; contraceptive pill; malabsorption; inefficient utilization.

---

deficiency causes,   there are many factors that can give rise to mild vitamin deficiency and most individuals are prone to the influence of one or more.

Apathy —is often a feature of people living alone, particularly those who have lost a spouse and those who no longer have a family to look after. There is little incentive to prepare adequate meals which are often monotonous and less and less nourishing. Impaired digestion may be associated with the apathy and this further lowers the nutritional status. Often seen in the elderly, middle-aged bachelor or spinster living in a one-room apartment with poor cooking facilities or in teenagers and students living alone for the first time.

Dental problems — poor dentition due to loss of teeth or dental decay can make eating uncomfortable, leading to aversion to foods such as salads, meat and vegetables. An ill-balanced diet results which can lead to poor nutrition, particularly in the elderly.

Excessive losses — water-soluble vitamins tend to be excreted in the urine and sweat. Physical exertion can thus lead to excessive excretion of vitamins. Hot climates may have a similar effect.

Foods fads — often occur in the young when foods of high calorie intake but low vitamin content are popular and make up the main part of the diet, e.g. high-sugar foods, soft drinks, confectionery, potato snacks, sweets, cakes. Old people too are not immune from similar nutritional fads. Food fads of pregnancy are well known and very variable but it has been suggested they may be satisfying a demand by the woman for specific nutrients.

Food taboos — often are religious in origin but may also stem from public health ideas, e.g. avoiding meat prone to parasitic infection. Complete avoidance of food as in fasting may be beneficial as an occasional habit but extensive fasting can be harmful. Water-soluble vitamins may be depleted and body protein is known to be broken down as well as body fat.

Specific foods that are nutritionally sound are avoided because of superstitious belief, completely unfounded, that they do harm. Many such beliefs abound in Africa. In Bolivia, any food containing animal blood is believed to make children mute; in Pakistan buffalo milk is believed to make a person physically strong but mentally dull. Most affected are pregnant women who often suffer nutritionally from such beliefs at a period when their diet should be sound. Sometimes because they are pregnant they are denied certain foods acceptable to them in other circumstances, so they suffer twice over.

Individual requirements — minimum daily requirements of vitamins are based on average intakes of a population or are an extension of animal studies applied to humans. Experiments indicate that animals of the same species can vary one from another in their vitamin requirements as much as five-fold. It is likely that human beings vary also so that two people on a similar diet can show wide variation in blood levels of vitamins which may also reflect requirements.

Infections — are more likely in those suffering from malnutrition and particularly amongst children. Infections can also aggravate malnutrition (e.g. by reducing the appetite) and in turn malnutrition weakens resistance to infection. Infections most likely to occur in malnourished children are bacterial (e.g. tuberculosis), viral (measles, which can be a killing disease in malnutrition) and parasitic. Deficiencies of vitamins A and C are most likely to predispose to infections. Keratomalacia, the end stage of vitamin A deficiency resulting in blindness, is often aggravated by a concurrent infection in children. Vitamin deficiency may lower resistance to infection by a reduced antibody formation; reduced activity of bacterial- and viral-engulfing white blood cells (phagocytes); decreased levels of protective enzymes (e.g. lysozyme in tears) and reduced integrity of the skin and mucous membranes, the wet surfaces of the body.

Infections can precipitate gross deficiencies of vitamins in those on a poor diet and even mild deficiencies in those on an adequate diet. For example, children with meningococcal meningitis, diarrhoea, tuberculosis, measles and other acute infections can develop vitamin A deficiency severe enough to cause them to develop keratomalacia and eventually blindness. Fever can cause symptoms of scurvy, due to vitamin C deficiency, in children even when there are apparently adequate intakes of the vitamin. Gross signs of thiamine deficiency can be precipitated in borderline cases following infections; diarrhoea and beriberi results.

Lactation — little is known about precise vitamin requirements in the woman who is breast-feeding her child and ignorance is reflected in the varying figures suggested by different authorities. All agree, however, that increased vitamin intakes during this period are desirable.

Suggested vitamin intakes are given in Table 4.

Table 4: Suggested vitamin intakes during lactation

	Australia	Canada	New Zealand	UK	USA	WHO/FAO
Vitamin A µg	1200	1400	1200	750	1200	1200
Vitamin D µg	10	5.0	10	10	10	10
Vitamin E mg	—	8.0	13.5	—	11	—
Vitamin C mg	60	60	60	60	100	60
Thiamine mg	1.3	1.5	1.3	1.1	1.6	1.1
Riboflavin mg	1.7	1.7	2.5	1.8	1.7	1.7
Nicotinic acid mg	22	25	21	21	18	18.2
Pyridoxine mg	3.5	2.6	2.5	—	2.5	—
Folic acid µg	300	250	400	300	500	500
Vitamin B_{12} µg	2.5	3.5	4.0	2	4.0	4.5

Malabsorption — usually affects the fat-soluble vitamins but pernicious anaemia is due solely to an inability to absorb the water-soluble vitamin B_{12}.

Diseases such as sprue, idiopathic steatorrhoea, pancreatic diseases, lack of bile production, etc. can cause generalized malabsorption of fats which include the fat-soluble vitamins and so can give rise to deficiency. Lack of intrinsic factor, needed to complex with vitamin B_{12} as a prerequisite for absorption, prevents the assimilation of the vitamin.

Malabsorption problems are medical conditions that are the province of the medical doctor and unsuitable for self-treatment.

Medicinal drugs — most common vitamin deficiency is that of B complex during antibiotic therapy. Essential to supplement with whole of vitamin B complex for any antibiotic taken for more than three days. Pyridoxine is particularly vulnerable during drug therapy but especially with corticosteroids, oral contraceptives, isoniazid and penicillamine. *See* individual drugs.

Other food nutrients — may affect the needs for certain vitamins. For example, high polyunsaturated fatty acid intake (as in vegetable oils) requires high vitamin E levels to accompany it; thiamine intake is increased when high carbohydrate levels are part of the diet; high protein intake requires more pyridoxine to be taken at the same time, as well as extra riboflavin. Less riboflavin is retained when protein intake is low.

Leucine is an amino acid that in high concentration requires extra nicotinic acid. Millet is a food with high leucine content and is a significant part of the diet in India but nicotinic acid intake does not always parallel that of the seed and deficiency of the vitamin can be induced.

Avidin is a protein unique to raw egg-white that combines with and inactivates biotin. Cooking the egg-white destroys avidin and so prevents the inactivation of the vitamin.

Some raw fish contain an enzyme thiaminase that destroys thiamine. Where raw fish is part of the staple diet, as in the Far East, thiamine deficiency can be induced. Some bacteria, e.g. Bacillus thiaminolyticus, can break down thiamine. Some 3 per cent of Japanese are afflicted with this infective organism and show signs of mild thiamine deficiency.

Other vitamins — excessive intakes of one vitamin may induce deficiency of another. Occurs mainly in animal experimentation but one established case in humans is where an excess of folic acid can cause a deficiency of vitamin B_{12}. In lambs, rickets can be induced in animals with a just-adequate intake of vitamin D by feeding high levels of carotene.

A deficiency of one vitamin can also induce a deficiency of another, e.g. vitamin C is needed to convert folic acid to its active form folinic acid. In the absence of vitamin C, folic acid cannot be activated and anaemia results. High intakes of folic acid in humans can mask a deficiency of vitamin B_{12}. Lack of folic acid gives rise to an anaemia similar to that caused by lack of vitamin B_{12}. However, vitamin B_{12} deficiency also causes nerve degeneration in the spinal column. If only the anaemia is being monitored, treatment with folic acid of B_{12} deficiency may appear to cure the anaemia. The nerve degeneration is not affected and progresses until it becomes irreversible. Hence the importance of diagnosing whether anaemia is due to folic acid or vitamin B_{12} deficiency, because the two vitamins function together in the production of normal red blood cells.

Parasitic infections — produce specifically vitamin B_{12} deficiency. The parasite responsible is fish tape-worm which utilizes dietary vitamin B_{12}, making it unavailable for absorption.

Poor diet — a poor selection of foods coupled with bad cooking methods, over-processing and over-refining can give rise to deficiency of vitamins. *See* losses in food processing.

Poor digestion — can be caused by defective mastication of the food in the mouth; reduction of volume and acidity of gastric secretions; reduction of digestive enzymes in pancreatic, liver and intestinal secretions and reduction of bile secretion. Vitamins are liberated as food is digested so when this is inefficient, they do not become available for absorption.

Physical activity — increases the need for certain vitamins, particularly those concerned with stress (the vitamin B complex), energy requirements (thiamine) and muscle action (vitamins C and E). If increased levels are not supplied, mild deficiency can result. Recommended dietary allowances for men (20 to 26 years) in three different countries are given in Table 5. *See also* athletes.

Pregnancy — many studies indicate marked reductions in blood levels of vitamin A, nicotinic acid, pyridoxine, vitamin B_{12}, folic acid and vitamin C in pregnant women.

Most comprehensive studies were on pyridoxine and it has been concluded that pregnant women need 10mg of the vitamin daily to maintain normal metabolic functions compared with only 2mg in non-pregnant women.

Folic acid is the most common deficiency. Recommended intakes during pregnancy are given in Table 6.

Table 5: Recommended vitamin requirements for men aged 20-26 years.

		UK	West Germany	USSR
Thiamine	Sedentary	1.0	1.7	1.8
mg	Moderately active	1.2	2.2	2.0
	Active	1.3	2.5	2.5
	Very active	1.3	2.9	3.0
Riboflavin	Sedentary	1.6	1.8	2.0
mg	Moderately active	1.6	1.8	2.5
	Active	1.6	1.8	3.0
	Very active	1.6	1.8	3.5
Nicotinic	Sedentary	18	14	12
acid mg	Moderately active	18	16	15
	Active	18	18	20
	Very active	18	20	25
Vitamin C	Sedentary	30	75	60
mg	Moderately active	30	75	70
	Active	30	75	100
	Very active	30	75	120

Table 6: Recommended vitamin requirements during pregnancy.

	Australia	Canada	New Zealand	UK	USA	WHO/ FAO
Vitamin A μg	750	900	750	750	1000	750
Vitamin D μg	10	5.0	10	10	10	10
Vitamin E mg	—	7.0	13.5	—	10	—
Vitamin C mg	60	50	60	60	80	60
Thiamine mg	1.2	1.2	1.2	1.0	1.4	1.0
Riboflavin mg	1.5	1.5	2.5	1.6	1.5	1.5
Nicotinic acid mg	19	15	18	18	15	16.8
Pyridoxine mg	2.6	2.0	2.5	—	2.6	—
Folic acid μg	400	250	500	300	800	600
Vitamin B_{12} μg	3.0	4.0	4.0	2	4.0	5.0

Rapid growth — the growing child needs vitamins for the growth process as well as for normal metabolism. Most studies have been carried out in animal husbandry when it was established that optimum levels of vitamins rather than adequate intakes were required to ensure maximum growth. However, most authorities agree that the need in children is relatively higher than that in adults when worked out on a body-weight or food-intake basis.

Slimming diets — when undertaken without professional advice reduced food and calorie intake may not supply the minimum requirements of vitamins. These are required for health irrespective of calories in the diet apart perhaps from thiamine. A reduction of calories from 2500 to 1000 per day which most slimming diets supply is hence likely also to reduce the vitamin intake by a similar factor. If 2500 calories are supplying barely the minimum needs of vitamins, deficiency must result if calories are reduced to 1000. All slimming regimes should include a good all-round multivitamin-multimineral preparation daily as insurance against deficiency. This may also prevent the tiredness often associated with slimming diets.

Stress — any stressful situation increases the requirements of some vitamins, notably the B group, C and E. If increased amounts are not taken in the diet mild deficiency may result. Quantities required may be 2, 3 or even 5 times the normal intakes. *See also* stress; athletes.

---

deficiency groups,   it is now recognized by some authorities (including the UK) that certain sectors of the population may be at risk of being deficient in vitamins and minerals and would benefit from supplementation. In most cases, a general all-round multivitamin-multimineral preparation supplying the minimum daily requirements is sufficient when taken regularly. For the reasons for lowered intake in these groups, *see* deficiency causes.

Groups at risk of deficiency are:

1. pregnant women, *see* deficiency causes: Pregnancy.
2. nursing women, *see* deficiency causes: Lactation.
3. women of child-bearing age who may need supplementary iron. Simultaneous supplementation with vitamin C will ensure efficient absorption of the mineral in the proportion 100mg vitamin to 10mg iron.
4. those who embark on a weight-reducing diet without professional advice. *See* deficiency causes: Slimming diets.
5. those who eat nutritionally inadequate snacks or foods which may have

been overcooked or kept for long periods, thus losing most of their content of the more labile vitamins. *See* deficiency causes: Poor diet.

6. children and adolescents in winter and housebound adults who may not get sufficient vitamin D from sunlight falling on the skin. In the absence of sufficient dietary vitamin D, that produced in the skin becomes the main source of supply of the vitamin.

7. children and adolescents who, because of fads, do not have a properly balanced diet. *See* deficiency causes: Food fads.

8. those convalescing from an illness who have leeway to make up in their nutrition. Deficiency of vitamins in convalescents is caused by: (a) low intake of food during illness; (b) effect of medicinal drugs: (c) infection, if it is present. *See* deficiency causes: Infections; Medicinal drugs.

9. the elderly and others who, through various disabilities or apathy, fail to prepare balanced meals. *See* deficiency causes: Apathy; Dental problems; Poor digestion.

10. those who live alone and often do not trouble to prepare fresh or adequate meals.

11. athletes in training and those in physically active occupations. *See* athletes; deficiency causes: Physical activity.

---

deficiency symptoms, specific symptoms and signs exist for most of the vitamin deficiencies, particularly when the vitamin level is seriously reduced and at this stage is the province of the medical practitioner. However, mild abnormalities that could be associated with a less serious deficiency of a vitamin are now being recognized in certain sectors of the population. In this respect, certain areas of the body provide useful information and, with proper interpretation, coupled usually with physical examination and medical history, can indicate poor nutrition. The more obvious areas are the skin, the mouth and the eyes but some symptoms of the gastro-intestinal tract and the nerves can become apparent to the individual affected. Changes in the blood, the blood vessels, the heart, the bones and the reproductive system associated with vitamin deficiency require more sophisticated diagnostic techniques that are best left to the medical practitioner.

The skin — much of what is known about the effects of vitamin deficiencies has come from animal studies and these do not always translate to the human being, but skin problems can often respond to vitamin A.

Vitamin A — hard, stippled skin, known as toad skin, has been attributed to vitamin deficiency but it may also be attributed in part to polyunsaturated fatty acid deficiency. Small, raised lesions that are hard and deeply pigmented have been suggested as due to vitamin A deficiency. Many minor skin irritations and those like eczema, acne and psoriasis often respond to vitamin A treatment, both topical and oral, which suggest that they are due, at least in part, to vitamin A deficiency.

Vitamin E — wounds that fail to heal or scar tissue that is consistently painful or striae that will not disappear may be associated with vitamin E deficiency.

Vitamin K — purple patches under the skin (known as purpura) may reflect a prothrombin deficiency which in turn may result from lack of vitamin K.

Vitamin C — small effusions of blood beneath the skin, known as petechiae, scattered in a diffuse manner over various skin areas are characteristic of vitamin C deficiency. Hardened pimples that appear over hair follicles particularly on the calves and buttocks may indicate vitamin C deficiency. The hairs either fail to erupt or take on a spiral shape.

Pyridoxine — deficiency causes scaly, dry skin and excessive looseness and hence loss of body hair. Excessive secretion of the sebaceous glands, known as seborrhoea, is seen about the eyes, nose, lips and mouth, sometimes extending to the eyebrows and ears. Redness of the moist surfaces of the body is also a sign of pyridoxine deficiency. Scaly, pigmented dermatitis sometimes occurs around the neck, forearms, elbows and thigh.

Riboflavin — typical skin lesions include cracking of the lips and angles of the mouth, known as cheilosis; seborrhoea of the nose and lips; scrotal and vaginal dermatitis; mouth and tongue ulcers.

Nicotinic acid — gross deficiency causes pellagra where the initial change is a temporary redness like sunburn. This clears to produce a more severe coloration in the form of deep red spots that coalesce to form a dark red or purple eruption followed by scaling and loss of skin. Face, neck, hands and feet are most affected, sometimes with concomitant oedema and ulceration. Usually clearly defined rough patches on hand termed 'pellagrous glove'.

Pantothenic acid — in animals, deficiency symptoms are greying of hair and ulceration of the skin but no evidence that human beings show similar signs. 'Burning feet' syndrome on soles of feet may be nervous rather than skin deficiency symptom. Some skin lesions like those noted with riboflavin deficiency have responded to pantothenic acid therapy suggesting they are more likely due to multivitamin lack.

Biotin — a localized, scaly, shedding dermatitis is a symptom of deficiency in infants.

The mouth — lesions of the mouth include those of the lips and are accepted as specific in some cases for certain deficiencies.

Riboflavin — a sore tongue with cracking of the lips and angles of the mouth, sometimes accompanied by intractable mouth ulceration are features of deficiency. The tongue is magenta-coloured with deep fissures and raised pimples (papillae).

Nicotinic acid — the tongue is swollen and the red colour of raw beef. Deficiency produces inflammation of the gums, inflammation of the mouth and an inflamed tongue.

Pyridoxine — deficiency characterized by cracking of the lips and corners of the mouth; inflammation of the tongue. Symptoms may be due to generalized B complex deficiency rather than specifically pyridoxine.

Vitamin B_{12} — the smooth, sore tongue associated with deficiency is almost diagnostic since it is usually a feature of pernicious anaemia.

Vitamin C — in a severe deficiency there are bleeding gums, inflamed gums and a loosening of the teeth. Small localized haemorrhages appear in the mouth.

Biotin — in infants suffering from the specific dermatitis associated with deficiency there is also rawness of the surface of the mouth.

The Gastro-intestinal tract — can be affected by vitamin B complex deficiency at any level.

Thiamine — deficiency characterized by diarrhoea, accompanied by abdominal distension and stomach pains.

Nicotinic acid — deficiency invariably gives rise to diarrhoea.

Pantothenic acid — paralysis of parts of the intestinal tract including post-operative paralytic ileus may be associated with deficiency. Symptoms are abdominal distress and distension, sometimes with the inability to pass motions.

The eye — deficiencies can affect both sight and eye tissues.

Vitamin A — specific symptom of deficiency is night blindness characterized by poor adaptation of the eye to low-intensity light conditions. Eye tissue is also thickened and dry, particularly that of the sclera (white of the eye) and conjunctiva (mucous membranes).

Riboflavin — white of the eye (sclera) develops prominent redness due to blood vessels; conjunctivitis (inflammation of the mucous membranes) is common in the lower lid; feeling of grittiness in the eye; constant watering and failing vision are symptoms of deficiency.

Thiamine — most common symptom of deficiency in eye is dimness of vision not associated with a specific lesion of the eye. Other ocular signs include involuntary rhythmic movement of the eyeballs, known as nystagmus; eye muscle fatigue; paralysis of the eye with loss of visual acuity (acuteness or clearness).

Nicotinic acid — symptoms are very similar to those associated with thiamine deficiency suggesting they are multivitamin-deficient in origin.

Vitamin C — haemorrhages inside the eye often appear before those on the skin.

Vitamin K — when lacking in the newborn, often induces haemorrhages in the retina.

The Central Nervous System — deficiency of most of the B vitamins causes symptoms associated with the nerves.

Thiamine — gross deficiency causes mental confusion leading to coma. Milder deficiency gives rise to nystagmus (involuntary rhythmic movement of the eyeballs) and sometimes mental confusion. Other mental symptoms include narration of fictitious experiences (confabulation) and polyneuritis (nerve inflammation). Nervous consequences include foot and wrist drop when motor nerves are involved.

Pyridoxine — in infants deficiency has been found to produce convulsions due to inadequate level of GABA (gamma aminobutyric acid) in brain. In adults most usual symptom is generalized inflammation of the nerves (peripheral neuritis) characterized by tingling, numbness, burning pain and loss of vibratory sensation.

Nicotinic acid — early signs are peripheral neuritis (see above) and encephalopathy (brain disease or inflammation). Later symptoms are due to progressive dementia characterized by apprehension, confusion, derangement and maniacal outbursts.

Vitamin B_{12} — symptoms of deficiency are pins and needles in feet and hands, weakness in the limbs, leg stiffness, unsteadiness, lethargy and fatigue. Delirium and confusion are seen in advanced cases. Tactile (touch) sensation is impaired and reflexes are depressed.

Folic acid — only mental deficiency symptom is psychosis characterized by mental derangement in which the patient is confused and lacks ability to describe events and is unaware of symptoms.

The blood — various vitamins when deficient give rise to anaemias of different types. Symptoms of all anaemias are similar and include paleness, tiredness, lethargy, breathlessness, weakness, vertigo, headache, tinnitus (constant noises in the head), spots before the eyes, drowsiness, irritability, amenorrhoea, loss of libido and sometimes low-grade fever. Occasionally gastro-intestinal complaints and even heart failure may develop.

Particular type of anaemia requires blood and sometimes bone-marrow examination for correct diagnosis and must be left to medical practitioner.

Hypochromic anaemia — characterized by red blood cells depleted of haemoglobin. May be caused by deficiency of pyridoxine or riboflavin. Sometimes complicated by small red blood cells also when it is known as microcytic hypochromic anaemia.

Megaloblastic anaemia — characterized by excessive numbers of immature red cells in the blood that cannot function as oxygen-carriers. May be caused by deficiency of folic acid or vitamin B_{12}.

Iron-deficiency anaemia — characterized by inability to produce haemoglobin because of lack of iron. If vitamin C is deficient, iron cannot be absorbed or incorporated into haemoglobin. Vitamin C deficiency also causes haemorrhage so this too may contribute to the anaemia.

Haemolytic anaemia — characterized by unstable red blood cells that burst readily and have a short life. May be caused by vitamin E deficiency in infants and adults.

The heart and blood vessels — thiamine deficiency in later stages causes severely weakened heart muscles leading to circulatory failure. The heart is grossly enlarged. Vitamin B_6 deficiency may give rise to massive deposition of fats in the heart and blood vessels, known as atherosclerosis.

The bones — changes in the bones due to vitamin deficiency can usually be detected by X-ray diagnosis and clinical diagnosis only. Some changes, such as those produced by deficiency in vitamin A, riboflavin, pyridoxine and pantothenic acid, have been noted only in animals.

Vitamin C — deficiency produces irregular calcification but this is obvious only from X-ray examinations.

Vitamin D — deficiency in infants causes rickets, the most obvious signs of which are restlessness and inability to sleep; retarded ability to sit, crawl or walk; retarded closure and hardening of the skull bones due to lack of mineralization. The long bones fail to ossify and are unable to stand the weight of the child so that they bend, leading to bow-legs and knock-knees. Pigeon-breast deformity is sometimes obvious. These changes are detected earlier in X-ray examination.

Deficiency of vitamin D in adults leads to osteomalacia, different to rickets because in the adult disease the bones are pre-formed. Demineralization occurs rather than a failure to mineralize the bones. Bones affected are spine, pelvis and lower extremities. As bones soften, the legs may become bowed, the vertebrae shortens (reducing the height) and the pelvic bones flatten.

The reproductive system — vitamin deficiencies in most animal species induce changes in the reproductive organs and process. In the females foetal abnormalities sometimes resulting in abortion are symptoms of deficiency. No exact parallel in human beings but there are scattered reports that vitamin B_{12} or vitamin E deficiency can produce sterility in males and miscarriage in females, reversible by appropriate vitamin therapy.

---

deficiency tests,   deficiencies in vitamins are usually determined from blood tests but these are normally taken only in conjunction with clinical signs before a medical diagnosis of deficiency is accepted. Hair analysis cannot indicate the vitamin status of an individual but it does give a clue to possible mineral deficiencies. Tests for vitamin deficiency are as follows:

Vitamin A — the level of this and of carotene can be determined in the blood but neither measurement is a good indication of body status of these vitamins, since there is considerable storage of each in the body. Normal vitamin A concentration is between 15 and 60µg per 100ml blood serum; that of carotene is between 8 and 40µg per 100ml blood serum.

Vitamin D — the best diagnostic procedure to determine vitamin D deficiency is to estimate 25-hydroxycholecalciferol in the blood but it is a specialized assay. Radiographic examination is a good way to detect rickets and osteomalacia in individuals, particularly X-ray pictures of the ends of the long bones. A third test is to measure the blood concentration of the enzyme alkaline phosphatase — high levels may indicate rickets even before the X-ray changes prove it but this test is not specific.

Vitamin E — there are three tests that can indicate a possible vitamin E deficiency; first, the measurement of blood serum tocopherol levels is simple and a reliable index of the circulating vitamin. Normal values lie between 1.0 and 3.0mg per 100ml blood serum.

The second test involves measuring the creatine content of the patients' urines. Usually this is absent from urine but when vitamin E is deficient, creatine appears in the urine. Creatine, usually excreted as creatinine, comes from the muscles and excess amount in the urine is indicative of muscle breakdown which is a function of vitamin E deficiency.

The third test involves measuring the fragility of the red blood cells in the presence of hydrogen peroxide. Normal red blood cells are resistant to hydrogen peroxide but when they are vitamin E-deficient they readily burst in the presence of the peroxide. Such tests are carried out on isolated blood.

Vitamin K — this is impossible to measure directly in the blood but an indication of vitamin K status comes from assay of the levels of the clotting factors of the blood. The usual test is to measure prothrombin time which gives a reasonable estimation of the vitamin K present. This test is also used to monitor the effect of the vitamin K antagonists like warfarin on the clotting of the blood when the drugs are being taken regularly.

Vitamin C — possible deficiency can be indicated by a combination of blood plasma levels and the extent of urinary excretion of the vitamin. White blood cell levels of vitamin C are a better indication of blood levels than those of plasma but the technique is time-consuming and is used more in research than as a standard technique. Normal blood levels of vitamin C are from 0.4 to 1.5mg per 100ml but white blood cells contain from 25 to 38mg per 100ml. A level of below 7mg per 100ml white blood cells indicates a high risk of scurvy.

Normally only 13 to 15mg of vitamin C is excreted daily in the urine; less than this indicates a possible deficiency. Confirmation usually comes from a saturation test. Multiple small doses of the vitamin are given over a period of time. Four to six hours after these, the urine level of the vitamin is measured. If the individual is suffering from vitamin C deficiency urine levels will not rise because the body saturates its tissues before excreting any. Hence the appearance of greater-than-normal amounts of the vitamin in the urine suggests the body is saturated and hence there is no deficiency. If none is excreted, vitamin C intakes are increased until the vitamin appears in the urine. An individual can easily determine if he or she needs vitamin

C by carrying out the above test on himself. A dose of 300mg every 4 to 6 hours is taken in water. Vitamin C is assessed in the urine by adding a dye to a sample of the urine. If the dye is decolorized vitamin C is present. A suitable dye is 2, 4-dinitrophenyl hydrazine, available impregnated into paper dipsticks. A mass screening test involves introducing a harmless blue dye, 2, 6-dichlorophenolindophenol, onto the tongue or just beneath the surface of the gum. The time taken for the dye to decolorize reflects the vitamin C status of the body — the longer the time the more chance of deficiency of the vitamin. The test is simply a preliminary one and must be confirmed by other means before a diagnosis can be made of true vitamin C deficiency.

Thiamine — can be measured directly in the blood and urine or indirectly by assaying an enzyme dependent on the vitamin for activity. Blood plasma levels are very low under normal conditions at concentration between 0.5 and 1.3μg per 100ml. Measurement of the vitamin excreted in a 24-hour urine sample is a reliable indication of thiamine deficiency. It can be improved in sensitivity by measuring urinary excretion after taking an oral dose of the vitamin. If this stays low, there is a good chance that the individual is lacking thiamine.

Riboflavin — the usual criteria for determining if a patient is deficient in riboflavin are the medical history, clinical examination and response to therapy with the vitamin. Red blood cell determinations are not easy because the normal level is very low, between 20 and 28μg per 100ml. For this reason an enzyme, glutathione reductase, that requires riboflavin, is usually assayed to indicate riboflavin levels.

Pyridoxine — the amount of pyridoxal phosphate present in the blood before and after an oral dose of the vitamin can be indicative of deficiency of the vitamin. Normal levels are at least 5μg per 100ml. A second test involves measuring xanthurenic acid in the urine. Normally this is less than 25mg per day but if an oral dose of the amino acid tryptophane is given to an individual who is deficient in pyridoxine, xanthurenic acid is excreted at levels greater than 50mg per day. Pyridoxine is necessary to convert xanthurenic acid further in body metabolism, so in the absence of the vitamin this compound builds up and is readily excreted.

Nicotinic acid — blood measurements are not reliable because no test is sufficiently sensitive or specific. Assay is usually carried out by measuring the ratio of methyl nicotinic derivatives to creatinine in the urine.

Vitamin B$_{12}$ — blood levels can be measured directly using the fact that some bacteria need the vitamin for normal growth. The extent of growth of the micro-organism indicates the amount of vitamin B$_{12}$ present in a sample of blood. Normal blood levels are 0.015 to 0.03μg per 100ml blood plasma. Levels below 0.01μg per 100ml are indicative of vitamin B$_{12}$ deficiency.

The more usual test for deficiency involves radio-activity labelled B$_{12}$ to measure its absorption. This is described under Schilling Test.

Folic acid — a diagnosis of deficiency is usually assessed on the basis of a macrocytic anaemia (in the absence of B$_{12}$ deficiency), a megaloblastic bone marrow and leucopenia (low white blood cell count). Blood serum levels can be measured but are difficult and time-consuming on a routine basis. Normal values are 0.5 to 2.0μg per 100ml in serum; 16 to 64μg per 100ml red blood cells. When the amino acid histidine is given orally, the quantity of formimino-glutamic acid (FIGLU) in the urine is increased dramatically in folic acid deficiency. This test is usually carried out in conjunction with the other tests mentioned above.

Pantothenic acid — measurement of the pantothenic acid level in the blood alone is usually indicative of deficiency of this vitamin. Confirmation usually comes from measuring coenzyme A activity which contains and is dependent on pantothenic acid levels.

---

dehydroretinol, A$_2$ vitamin.

---

delta tocopherol, *see* E vitamin.

---

dental caries, a gradual disintegration and dissolution of tooth enamel and dentin that eventually affects the pulp. Results from interaction of three factors: a susceptible tooth surface; acid-forming bacteria; high sugar concentration. Increased intakes of selenium, usually in areas where soil selenium is high, can also induce dental caries in children.

Signs and symptoms include sensitivity to heat and cold; discomfort after eating sugar-based foods; a darkened area between teeth; softened enamel or dentin which becomes obvious on dental examination.

Prevention is a combination of good dental hygiene with adequate intakes of fluoride and calcium. Supplementary fluoride level depends upon concentration of the mineral in the drinking water but a daily total intake up to 1.0mg should be aimed for. Dietary calcium intakes of between 500 and 700mg per day are necessary in children; in adults 800-1000mg calcium may help prevent caries. Children who live in areas of high soil content of molybdenum have low incidence of dental caries so this trace mineral too may prevent the condition developing.

---

deodorant,   vitamin E included as antioxidant to retard degradation of oxygen-containing components of sweat.

---

deoxyribonucleic acids,   DNA. Nucleic acids, constituents of all cells, essential for synthesis of protein and transmission of hereditary characteristics to offspring. The basis of life's processes, lack of DNA production has profound effects on health, first sign of which is megaloblastic anaemia, and process of ageing.

Vitamins essential for DNA synthesis are A, folic acid, B_6, B_{12}, E and choline. Abnormal DNA metabolism may be related to cancer.

---

depression,   mild variety can be related to vitamin B_6 deficiency induced by drugs, contraceptive pill or premenstrual tension (PMT). Treated with 25 to 50mg B_6 daily or 50 to 100mg from day 10 of one menstrual cycle to day 3 of the next when due to PMT or contraceptive pill. When associated with drugs need at least 25mg B_6 daily.

---

dermatitis,   inflammation of the skin characterized by redness, oozing, crusting, scaling and sometimes blisters. May be related to lack of vitamin B complex, vitamin A or polyunsaturated fatty acids. Treated with whole B complex at high potency; vitamin A, both oral and topical; PUFA orally, especially safflower oil or oil of evening primrose.

---

desiccated liver, concentrated beef liver powder which has been dried in vacuum at a low temperature to conserve original nutrient value of the liver.

Vitamins present (in mg per 100g) are: vitamin A (20mg); thiamine (1.0); riboflavin (9.57); pyridoxine (2.31); nicotinic acid (44.9); pantothenic acid (24.1); folic acid (1.09); vitamin B_{12} (0.363); biotin (0.109); vitamin C (75.9); vitamin E (1.39); carotene (5.08).

---

dextriferron, iron dextrin injection, provides 100mg iron in 5ml dextriferron solution. May be injected directly into bloodstream. Toxic effects include flushing, nausea, unpleasant taste, headache, abdominal pain and transient diarrhoea. Allergic reactions have been reported. Normally used when oral treatment is ineffective. Total dose of iron in this form over whole treatment should not exceed 2g.

---

diabetes insipidus, a disorder induced by lack of production of vasopressin, causing excessive thirst and the production of large volumes of very dilute urine (up to 30 litres per day).

---

diabetes mellitus, associated with high blood sugar level that persists long after meals because of lack of hormone insulin. Long-term consequences are arteriosclerosis, heart disease, gangrene, blindness that may be related to specific vitamin deficiencies. Increased requirements for vitamin B_6 (25mg), C (500mg), E (400IU), A (7500IU) (because diabetics cannot produce it from carotenes), daily.

Mineral

Diabetics tend to lose more zinc in their urine than non-diabetics, suggesting that simple replacement of this by diet or by supplementation can be beneficial. Chromium also tends to be low in the blood of diabetics. This trace mineral is an essential component of glucose tolerance factor which controls blood sugar. Supplementation with this mineral, preferably in the organic form (i.e. in yeast or amino-acid chelated) can also be beneficial. Studies in people suffering from diabetic neuropathy have indicated that their blood magnesium levels are significantly lower than those of people who are not diabetics. Those with the most advanced and severe retinopathy had the lowest blood magnesium levels of all. The significance of these observations is not known but every diabetic should ensure adequate intakes of all three minerals.

diarrhoea, specifically associated with severe deficiency of nicotinamide but may respond to supplementation with whole vitamin B complex.

dicoumarol, anti-coagulant drug. Acts by inhibiting action of vitamin K.

digestive tract, gastrointestinal tract. Stomach and intestines where digestion of food and absorption of nutrients takes place.

Nicotinamide (at doses up to 3000mg daily) has been used to treat malabsorption diseases of the intestine such as sprue. Folic acid deficiency can destroy lining cells of the small intestine and impair absorption process. Lack of pantothenic acid can cause abdominal distension. Supplementary vitamin can reduce post-operative distension and nausea including effects of paralytic ileus. Thiamine promotes good digestion and better functioning of the digestive tract. Improves muscles of the tract and can cure stubborn cases of constipation.

Vitamin C, when taken with aspirin, can prevent gastric bleeding induced by the drug. Gastric ulcers can be prevented by high doses of vitamin E (up to 600IU daily). Better results with vitamin A which at high doses (150 000IU daily for four weeks) has been used to treat gastric ulcers. Indications that prevention of stomach cancer may benefit from vitamin A supplementation.

disease resistance, depends on efficiency of development of immune response which requires adequate protein, vitamins and minerals. *See* immune system.

diuretic drugs, substances that promote the excretion of water and electrolytes by the kidneys. They are used in the treatment of congestive heart failure; liver, kidney or lung diseases that give rise to salt and water retention leading to oedema. The disease process in these conditions is not usually affected by the removal of excess water but the oedema is relieved. Diuretics are used to counter salt and water retention induced by other drug treatments; to enhance the effects of drugs given to reduce high blood-pressure; to treat drug overdosage or poisoning to enhance excretion of the toxic materials. The groups of diuretics are:

1. thiazides which inhibit sodium and chloride reabsorption in the kidney and hence promote excretion of these minerals. As a side-effect they also cause excretion of potassium to such an extent that supplementation with the mineral becomes essential; lowered excretion of uric acid which builds up in the joints to cause gout.

2. frusemide type, which act by stimulating excretion of sodium, potassium and chloride by the kidney, thus increasing water loss. Side-effects as for thiazides.

3. mercurial drugs, which act by inhibiting sodium reabsorption but at different sites in the kidney to other diuretics. Also promote potassium excretion necessitating supplementation with the mineral.

4. aldosterone inhibitors, which function by preventing the action of natural aldosterone. These are potassium-sparing diuretics, decreasing its excretion but promoting that of sodium and chloride. Normally used in conjunction with (1), (2) and (3) above, where they counteract the potassium-losing effects of these diuretics.

5. carbonic anhydrase inhibitors, which act by decreasing the rate of carbonic acid formation and hence acid production. Kidney secretion of acids and reabsorption of bicarbonate and sodium are thereby inhibited. Normally used in conjunction with other diuretics to compensate for increased potassium loss.

6. some diuretics that diminish the excretion of potassium and hence are used with other diuretics to counter their potassium-depleting effects.

7. caffeine, which is a weak diuretic and is found in coffee, tea and other beverages.

8. herbal diuretics which are milder than synthetic drug varieties and are less likely to cause potassium loss.

In addition to potassium loss induced by some of the above diuretics, calcium, magnesium and zinc excretion may also increase under their influence.

dolomite, mixed calcium and magnesium carbonates. Provides 21.7mg calcium and 13.0mg magnesium in 100mg. Usual supplementary dose is 3-6 tablets daily, providing 295 or 591mg calcium and 177 or 354mg magnesium. Taken in the evening, four tablets have been claimed to help induce sleep. Also available as amino-acid chelated dolomite tablets which are claimed to be better absorbed.

drinking chocolate, useful source of some vitamins. Figures are for the dry form. Vitamin E content is 0.9mg per 100g. B vitamins present are (in mg per 100g): thiamine 0.06; riboflavin 0.04; nicotinic acid 1.1; pyridoxine 0.02. Folic acid level is 10µg per 100g. Devoid of vitamin C.

Mineral
High sodium, potassium, magnesium, phosphorus and iron levels. Good source of copper and zinc. Figures are for the dried form (in mg per 100g): sodium 250; potassium 410; calcium 33; magnesium 150; phosphorus 190; iron 2.4; copper 1.1; zinc 1.9; chloride 130.

drinking water, can vary from soft through various grades of hardness. Extent of hardness usually reflects the amount of calcium carbonate in the water but some authorities express water in terms of total dissolved mineral content. Technically a water is regarded as hard if it contains more than 75mg of dissolved solids per litre.

Adults drink on average about 2 litres of water daily and more than half this can be tap water. This quantity in a hard-water area can therefore supply a significant proportion of the daily requirements of minerals — more than 10 per cent of calcium, magnesium, copper, iron and zinc, but all in the ionized inorganic form. A typical daily intake from hard tap water would be (in mg per day): calcium 250; magnesium 50; iron 3; silicon 20; zinc 2; copper 1; fluorine 1 or more; sulphur 0.05; iodine 0.04; chromium 0.01; lithium 0.01; arsenic, lead and mercury — all traces. The benefits of hard water over soft water are from epidemiological studies: lowered mortality rates from cardiovascular disease; a protective effect of calcium in preventing absorption of toxic trace minerals; lower rates of sudden heart failure because of the protective action of the magnesium content; a possible connection between low magnesium rates in tap water and sudden unexpected infant-death syndrome; lower death rates from coronary heart disease related to high silicon content of hard water.

Waters containing significant amounts of fluoride appear also to protect against calcification of the aorta as well as dental caries; iodine from water may contribute up to 20 per cent of daily requirements of the mineral; areas where tap water contains 2.6mg chromium per litre had higher incidence of coronary heart disease than those where the chromium content was 8.6mg per litre; areas where lithium content of tap water is high (8mg per litre) have been reported to have a less aggressive and less competitive population than those where lithium level is low. Other epidemiological studies indicate that in hard water areas there are lower cardiovascular mortality rates, decreased incidence of gastric and duodenal ulcers. Smaller number of admissions for mental diseases and a lower rate of violent behaviour are reported in areas where the drinking water contains 100mg per litre lithium. So many minerals are present in hard water that it is likely that its protective action against heart disease is a result of all being presented together in meaningful amounts. No one has determined with certainty that any one is more significant than another.

Soft water can contain more toxic trace minerals than hard water because it tends to dissolve them from pumping machinery and pipes. All water can be contaminated by industrial effluents like cadmium and mercury or with nitrates from heavily fertilized agricultural land. Water containing high levels of nitrates or nitrites should not be used to make up bottle feeds for babies, since these minerals increase the risk of methaemoglobinaemia, a disease where the blood has a decreased capacity to transport oxygen.

Some waters are so hard that they are partially softened at source before being fed into domestic and industrial water supplies. Domestic softening of water has many advantages for household functions, but the water should be kept separate from that used for drinking. The reasons are twofold:
1. hard water is more conducive to health;
2. the act of softening water with ion exchange resins exchanges the desirable calcium ions for the less desirable sodium ions. Softened water

will therefore have an increased sodium content.

---

drugs, may increase requirements for certain vitamins; may cause malabsorption of vitamins; may interfere with utilization and activation of vitamins. See individual drugs.

---

dry skin, increase intake of vitamin A (7500IU daily) and PUFA (safflower oil, wheatgerm oil or oil of evening primrose up to 3g daily) and lecithin (up to 6 capsules daily). Treat affected area with vitamin E cream.

E

E, tocopherol from 'tokos' birth and 'phero' to bear.

Fat-soluble vitamin. Known as d-alpha tocopherol (natural) and available in supplements as d-alpha tocopheryl acetate and d-alpha tocopheryl succinate. Also available as synthetic dl-alpha tocopherol. Natural forms also include d-beta tocopherol, d-gamma tocopherol, and d-delta tocopherol, all less active than d-alpha tocopherol. All four natural types found in food.

Best Food Sources in mg per 100g		Functions
Wheatgerm oil	190.0	Antioxidant
Soyabean oil	87.0	Reduces oxygen needs of muscles
Maize oil	66.0	Anti-blood clotting agent
Safflower oil	49.0	Blood vessel dilator
Sunflower oil	27.0	Maintains healthy blood vessels
Peanut oil	22.0	

Recommended Daily Intakes

Should be at least 30mg but see separate entry.

Stability in Foods

Unstable. See Losses in Food Processing.

Best Food Sources
in mg per 100g

Cod liver oil	20.0
Roasted peanuts	12.0
Potato crisps	11.0
Shrimps	6.6
Olive oil	4.6
Greenleaf vegetables	2.3
Pulses	1.7
Tomatoes	1.4
Meats	0.6
Fruits	0.5
Root vegetables	0.1

Functions

Protects polyunsaturated oils
Protects amino acids
Protects vitamin A
Prevents thrombosis
Prevents atherosclerosis
Prevents thrombophlebitis
Increases 'safe' cholesterol
Acts with selenium
Promotes ability of white
   blood cells to resist
   infection

Deficiency Symptoms

In children:
   Irritability
   Water retention
   Haemolytic anaemia
In adults:
   Lack of vitality
   Lethargy
   Apathy
   Lack of concentration
   Irritability
   Decreased sexual interest
   Muscle weakness

Symptoms of Excess Intake

Nausea
Diarrhoea
Muscle weakness
Transient increase in blood-
   pressure
Palpitations
Blood-pressure increase is rare
   and does not occur in those
   already taking heart drugs

Therapeutic Uses	Deficiency Causes
Intermittent claudication	Malabsorption of fats
Cerebral thrombosis	Consistent use of liquid paraffin
Coronary thrombosis	Gastric or intestinal surgery
Atherosclerosis	Alcoholism
Arteriosclerosis	Cirrhosis of the liver
Varicose veins	Obstructive jaundice
Thrombophlebitis	Cystic fibrosis
Menstrual problems	Coeliac disease (gluten sensitivity)
Low fertility	Excessive intake of polyunsaturated oils lacking the vitamin
Skin ulcers	Excessive oxygen (as in oxygen tents)
Diabetic gangrene	
Nerve, joint and muscular complaints	
Haemolytic anaemia of the new-born	
Thalassaemia	
Sickle-cell anaemia	
Cystic breast disease	
Oxygen excess in premature babies	
Direct application to:	
Scar tissue	
Stretch marks	
Sunburn	
Burns	
Scalds	

E numbers, most vitamin preparations in tablet and capsule forms are classed under UK labelling regulations as foods. Hence label information must include a list of all ingredients in descending order of weight. Those ingredients that are not active are referred to as excipients or bulking agents or fillers plus lubricants, emulsifiers, preservatives, colouring agents and processing aids. The substances used and approved for use in tablets and capsules are given here. (E numbers are only used in the UK and Europe.)

In addition, acceptable daily intake (ADI) is given for each substance.

This is expressed as mg per kg body weight and is the amount of the additive that can be taken daily in the diet, even over a lifetime, without risk, as evaluated by the Joint FAO/WHO Expert Committee on Food Additives. CI refers to the official Colour Index Number.

E100 — Curcumin, also known as Natural Yellow 3 and CI 75300. Natural orange-yellow colour whose main colouring is turmeric. ADI is up to 0.1mg per kg body weight.

E101 — Riboflavin, also known as vitamin B_2 and lactoflavin. Used as orange-yellow colouring agent. ADI is up to 0.5mg per kg body weight.

E102 — Tartrazine, also known as Food Yellow 4, FD and C Yellow 5, CI 19140. Synthetic, yellow powder, one of the coal-tar dyes. Used as colouring agent. ADI is up to 7.5mg per kg body weight.

May cause allergic reaction in susceptible people, particularly those also sensitive to aspirin. Adverse effects include acute bronchospasm, urticaria, rhinitis, blurred vision, oedema and purple patches on the skin.

E104 — Quinoline Yellow, also known as Food Yellow 13, CI 47005. Synthetic, yellow colouring agent, one of the coal-tar dyes. ADI is up to 0.5mg per kg body weight.

E110 — Sunset Yellow FCF, also known as Orange Yellow 5, FD and C Yellow 6, Food Yellow 3, CI 15985. Synthetic, yellow colouring agent, one of the coal-tar dyes. ADI is up to 5.0mg per kg body weight.

E120 — Cochineal, also known as Carmine, Carminic acid, Natural Red 4, CI 75470. Natural red colour extracted from the insect Coccus cacti L. ADI is up to 2.5mg per kg body weight.

E122 — Carmoisine, also known as Azorubine, Food Red 3, CI 14720. Synthetic red to bluish-red colour, one of the azo dyes. ADI is up to 1.25mg per kg body weight.

E123 — Amaranth, also known as Food Red 9, CI 16185. Synthetic bluish-red colour, one of the coal-tar dyes. In the UK is used widely in liquid vitamin C preparations but is prohibited in the USA and some European countries. ADI is up to 0.75mg per kg body weight.

Incompatible with anti-infective cetrimide.

E124 — Ponceau 4R, also known as cochineal red 4A, Food Red 7, CI 16255. Synthetic red to dark red colour, one of the coal-tar dyes. ADI is up to 0.125mg per kg body weight.

May cause hypersensitivity in those susceptible to tartrazine.

E127 — Erythrosine BS, also known as Food Red 14, FD and C Red No.

3, CI 45430. Synthetic yellowish-pink to bright bluish-red colour, one of the coal-tar dyes. ADI is up to 2.5mg per kg body weight.

Contains iodine sufficient to raise protein-bound iodine to hyperthyroid values. Can cause phototoxicity.

E131 — Patent Blue V, also known as Food Blue 5, CI 42051. Synthetic bright, greenish-blue colour, one of the coal-tar dyes. ADI not been allocated.

Allergic reactions include redness of skin, itching and urticaria. More severe are shock, breathing problems, nausea, tremor and low blood-pressure.

E132 — Indigo carmine, also known as Indigotine, FD and C Blue No. 2, Food Blue 1, CI 73015. Synthetic blue colour, one of the coal-tar dyes. ADI is up to 5mg per kg body weight.

May cause nausea, vomiting, high blood-pressure, skin rashes, itching and breathing problems.

E140 — Chlorophyll, also known as Natural Green 3, CI 75810. Natural green colour extracted from plants. ADI is not limited.

E141 — Copper chlorophyll, also known as Natural Green 3, CI 75810. Blue-green powder that is a complex of the mineral copper with chlorophyll. ADI is up to 15mg per kg body weight.

E142 — Green S, also known as Acid Brilliant Green BS, Lissamine Green, Food Green 4, CI 44090. Synthetic, greenish-blue colour, one of the coal-tar dyes. ADI has not been allocated.

E150 — Caramel, also known as Natural Brown 10. Produced by the action of heat and chemicals on sugars. Brown to black colour. ADI is up to 100mg per kg body weight.

E151 — Black PN, also known as Brilliant Black BN, Food Black 1, CI 28440. Synthetic black colour, one of the coal-tar dyes. ADI is up to 1mg per kg body weight.

Causes intestinal cysts in pigs fed dye for 90 days but not yet studied in human beings.

E153 — Carbon black, also known as vegetable carbon. Black colour produced from combustion of vegetables. ADI has not been allocated.

E160 — Carotenoids. Natural yellow to orange colours, some with vitamin A activity. ADI has not been allocated.

E160*a* — Alpha, beta and gamma-carotene, also known as Natural Yellow 26, CI 75130.

E160*b* — Annatto, also known as Bixin, Norbixin, Natural Orange No. 4, CI 75120. Natural yellow-orange to red colour. ADI is up to 1.25mg per kg body weight.

E160*c* — Capsanthin, also known as Capsorubin. Red colouring agent from paprika. ADI has not been allocated.

E160*d* — Lycopene, also known as Natural Yellow 27, CI 75125. Natural carotenoid red colour from tomatoes. ADI has not been allocated.

E160*e* — Beta-Apo-8′-carotenal, also known as Food Orange No. 6, CI 40820. Natural orange to yellowish-red colour. ADI is up to 5mg per kg body weight.

E160*f* — Ethyl ester of beta-apo-8′-carotenal, also known as Food Orange 7, CI 40825. Natural yellow to orange colour. ADI is up to 5mg per kg body weight that also includes beta-apo-8′-carotenal and beta-carotene.

E161 — Xanthophylls, natural colouring agents that occur as range of colours from yellow to orange to red. All obtained from plants, mainly leaves. Individual xanthophylls are designated below.

E161*a* — Flavoxanthin, natural yellow colour. ADI not allocated.

E161*b* — Lutein, natural yellow-reddish colour. ADI not allocated.

E161*c* — Cryptoxanthin, natural yellow colour. ADI not allocated.

E161*d* — Rubixanthin, natural yellow colour. ADI not allocated.

E161*e* — Violaxanthin, natural yellow colour. ADI not allocated.

E161*f* — Rhodoxanthin, natural yellow colour. ADI not allocated.

E161*g* — Canthaxanthin, natural orange colour. Known also as Food Orange 8 and CI 40850. ADI is up to 0.25mg per kg body weight.

E162 — Beetroot red, known also as Betamin. Red colour obtained from beetroots. ADI is not specified.

E163 — Anthocyanins, water-soluble vegetable colours in various shades of red, violet or blue. ADI not allocated.

E170 — Calcium carbonate, known also as chalk. Used as firming agent and release agent in vitamin tablets. Dietary calcium supplement. ADI is not limited.

E171 — Titanium dioxide, known also as Pigment White 6 and CI 77891. Natural pigment used as white colouring agent in vitamin tablets and capsules. ADI is not limited.

E172 — Iron oxides and hydroxides, known also as CI 77472, 77499, 77489, 77491. Natural pigments giving yellow, red, brown or black colours, depending on mixtures of the oxides and hydroxides. ADI is up to 0.5mg per kg body weight.

E173 — Aluminium, known also as CI 77000. A surface colouring matter giving silvery finish to surface of pills and tablets. ADI not allocated.

E174 — Silver. A lustrous white metal used in the form of silver leaf. Has been used as surface colouring matter in vitamin pills, dragees and sugar-coated confectionery. ADI is not allocated.

E175 — Gold, known also as CI 77480. Soft, yellow metal used in the form of gold leaf as surface colouring agent on some vitamin pills. ADI not allocated as use is very limited and is not considered a hazard.

E180 — Pigment Rubin, known also as Lithal Rubin BK and CI 15850. Synthetic reddish pigment, used as calcium salt. ADI not allocated.

E200 — Sorbic acid. Functions as preservative in vitamin tablets and capsules. In capsules usually confined to gelatin shell. Occurs naturally in certain fruits but can also be made by synthetic chemical methods. ADI is up to 25mg per kg body weight.

E201 — Sodium sorbate, sodium salt of sorbic acid. *See* E200.

E202 — Potassium sorbate, potassium salt of sorbic acid. *See* E200.

E203 — Calcium sorbate, calcium salt of sorbic acid. *See* E200.

E210 — Benzoic acid. Functions as preservative in tablets and capsules. Occurs naturally but can be made by chemical methods. ADI is up to 5mg per kg body weight.

Allergic reactions including asthma, urticaria and oedema have been reported with benzoic acid. Large doses may produce gastric irritation.

E211 — Sodium benzoate, sodium salt of benzoic acid. *See* E210.

E212 — Potassium benzoate, potassium salt of benzoic acid. *See* E210.

E213 — Calcium benzoate, calcium salt of benzoic acid. *See* E210.

E214 — Ethyl 4-hydroxybenzoate, known also as Ethyl parahydroxy-benzoate, ethyl ester of p-hydroxybenzoic acid, ethyl parabens, ethyl parasept. Preservative in tablets and capsules acting against moulds, fungi, yeasts and some bacteria. ADI is up to 10mg per kg body weight.

Adverse effects are hypersensitivity reactions in some people, mainly affecting the skin.

E215 — Ethyl 4-hydroxybenzoate, sodium salt. Known also as sodium ethyl p-hydroxybenzoate. *See* E214.

E216 — Propyl 4-hydroxybenzoate, known also as n-Propyl p-hydroxy-benzoate Nipasol M, propyl parabens, propyl parasept. *See* E214.

E217 — Propyl 4-hydroxybenzoate, sodium salt. Also known as sodium n-propyl p-hydroxybenzoate. *See* E214.

E218 — Methyl 4-hydroxybenzoate, also known as methyl p-hydroxybenzoate, methyl parabens, methyl parasept. *See* E214.

E219 — Methyl 4-hydroxybenzoate, sodium salt. Also known as sodium methyl p-hydroxybenzoate. *See* E214.

E220 — Sulphur dioxide. Used as preservative, improving agent and bleaching agent. Preservative for gelatine in vitamin capsules. ADI is up to 0.7mg per kg body weight.

E221 — Sodium sulphite. *See* E220.

E222 — Sodium hydrogen sulphite, also known as sodium bisulphite, and sodium sulphite. *See* E220.

E223 — Sodium metabisulphite. *See* E220.

E224 — Potassium metasulphite, also known as potassium disulphite, potassium pyrosulphite. *See* E220.

E226 — Calcium sulphite. *See* E220.

E227 — Calcium hydrogen sulphite also known as calcium bisulphite. *See* E220.

E300 — L-Ascorbic acid, known also as vitamin C. Used as antioxidant, vitamin, improving agent for flour, meat-colour preservative. ADI is not limited.

E301 — Sodium-L-ascorbate, sodium salt of ascorbic acid, known also as vitamin C. *See* E300.

E302 — Calcium-L-ascorbate, calcium salt of ascorbic acid, known also as vitamin C. *See* E300.

E304 — 6-0-Palmitoyl-L-ascorbic acid also known as Ascorbyl palmitate, vitamin C palmitate. Used as vitamin C, E300, but has advantage of being fat-soluble. ADI is up to 1.25mg per kg body weight.

E306 — Extracts of natural origin rich in tocopherols (vitamin E). Used as antioxidant, vitamin. ADI is up to 2mg per kg body weight as food additive.

E307 — Synthetic alpha-tocopherol, known also as DL-alpha-tocopherol, vitamin E. Used as antioxidant, vitamin. ADI is up to 2mg per kg body weight as food additive.

E308 — Synthetic gamma-tocopherol, known also as DL-gamma-tocopherol, vitamin E. Used as antioxidant, vitamin. ADI is up to 2mg per kg body weight as food additive.

E309 — Synthetic delta-tocopherol, known also as DL-delta-tocopherol, vitamin E. Used an antioxidant, vitamin E. ADI is up to 2mg per kg body weight as food additive.

E320 — Butylated hydroxyanisole, known also as BHA, 3-tertiary-butyl-4-hydroxyanisole. Used as antioxidant. ADI is up to 0.5mg per kg body weight (also include BHT or sum of both). Hypersensitivity reactions have occurred following application of BHA to the skin.

E321 — Butylated hydroxytoluene, known also as BHT, 2, 6-tertiary-butyl-p-cresol. Used as antioxidant. ADI is up to 0.5mg per kg body weight (also includes BHA or sum of both).

Hypersensitivity reactions have occurred following application of BHT to the skin.

E322 — Lecithins. A complex mixture of phosphatides derived from soybeans, other vegetable matter and of animal origin. Used as emsulifier, antioxidant. ADI is not limited.

E400 — Alginic acid. Obtained from brown seaweeds. Used in tablets as natural disintegrant causing quick dispersion of tablet after swallowing. Also acts as tablet binder. ADI is up to 50mg per kg body weight.

E401 — Sodium alginate, sodium salt of alginic acid. *See* E400.

E402 — Potassium alginate, potassium salt of alginic acid. *See* E400.

E403 — Ammonium alginate, ammonium salt of alginic acid. *See* E400.

E404 — Calcium alginate, calcium salt of alginic acid. *See* E400.

E405 — Propane-1, 2-diol alginate, known also as propylene glycol alginate, alginate ester. *See* E400.

E406 — Agar, known also as Agar-agar. Natural disintegrating agent and binder for tablets, derived from certain seaweeds. ADI is not limited.

Adverse effects of large amounts are flatulence, distension and intestinal obstruction.

E407 — Carregeenan, known also as carrageen, Irish Moss. Natural disintegrating agent and binder for tablets, derived from certain seaweeds. ADI is up to 75mg per kg body weight.

When intact, carrageenan is generally regarded as safe up to the above limit. Degraded carrageenan can cause liver damage, stomach ulcers, colonic irritation and immunological effects.

E410 — Locust bean gum, known also as carob gum, made from ground endosperms of Ceratonia siliqua seeds. Natural disintegrating agent and binder in tablets. ADI is not specified.

E412 — Guar gum known also as Jaguar gum, guar flour, made from ground endosperms of Cyamopsis psoraloides. Natural disintegrating agent and binder in tablets. ADI is not specified.

Adverse effects of large quantities are flatulence, nausea and vomiting. Possible intestinal obstruction.

E413 — Tragacanth, a gum exudate obtained from the tree Astragalus gummifer. Used as disintegrating agent and binder in tablets. ADI has not been allocated.

Adverse effects are rare but confined to those after inhalation and consist of allergic responses. Contact dermatitis has been reported from use on the skin. Has been used as bulk laxative.

E414 — Acacia gum, also known as Gum Arabic. Air-dried gummy exudate from the tree Acacia senegal. Used as granulating and binding agent in tablets. Functions as demulcent in lozenges and pastilles where it provides slow disintegration. ADI is not limited.

Hypersensitivity reactions have occurred rarely after inhalation or ingestion of acacia.

E415 — Xanthan gum, a gum produced in fermentations of Xanthomonas campestris. Also known as Corn Sugar Gum. Used as granulating agent and binder in tablets. ADI is up to 10mg per kg body weight.

E420 — Sorbitol, also known as Sorbitol Syrup. Used as a sweetener in chewable vitamin tablets and capsules. Occurs naturally in some fruits but can also be synthesized chemically from glucose. ADI is not specified.

Excessive amounts of sorbitol may cause flatulence, abdominal distension and diarrhoea when taken orally.

E421 — Mannitol, also known as Manna Sugar. Used as a sweetener in chewable vitamin tablets and capsules. Occurs naturally and is similar to sorbitol. ADI is up to 50mg per kg body weight.

When given by mouth, mannitol may cause diarrhoea, nausea and vomiting.

E440*a* — Pectin, also includes Amidated Pectin (E440b). Obtained from the inner portion of the rind of citrus fruits or from apple pomace. Used as binder and filler in tablets. ADI is not specified.

Large amounts may temporarily increase flatulence and distension, sometimes causing intestinal obstruction. Oesophogeal obstruction may be caused if pectin is swallowed dry.

E460 — Microcrystalline cellulose, prepared from wood cellulose. Also known as alpha-cellulose, powdered cellulose. Used as a binder, filler, disintegrant and lubricant in tablets, particularly when calorie-free preparation is needed. ADI is not specified. Intakes of up to 30g have been tolerated by man.

E461 — Methylcellulose, a chemically-modified cellulose. Used as bulking agent and binder in tablets. ADI is up to 25mg per kg body weight.

Large amounts may temporarily increase flatulence and distension. Intestinal obstruction has been reported and when taken in the dry form, methylcellulose may give rise to obstruction in the oesophagus.

E463 — Hydroxypropylcellulose, a chemically-modified cellulose. *See* E461.

E464 — Hydroxyproplymethylcellulose, a chemically-modified cellulose. *See* E461.

E465 — Ethylmethylcellulose, methylethylcellulose. *See* E461.

E466 — Carboxymethylcellulose, sodium salt. A chemically-modified cellulose. *See* E461.

Other E numbers refer to additives that may legally be added to foods but are not used in tablets and capsules containing vitamins.

None of the additives used in preparing tablets and capsules affect in any way the potencies of the vitamins in those preparations.

The following tablet and capsule additives are used at present but their E numbers are only proposed and unlikely to be effective before 1986:

101a — Riboflavin-5'-phosphate. *See* E101.

107 — Yellow 2G; Acid Light Yellow 2G; Acid Yellow 17; CI Food Yellow 5; CI No. 18965. Synthetic coal-tar dye, soluble in water. Permitted for use in foodstuffs and cosmetics. ADI is not known.

128 — Red 2G; Acid Red 1; Food Red 10; Ext. D and C Red No. 11; Geranine 2G; CI No. 18050. Synthetic coal-tar dye, soluble in water. ADI is up to 6μg per kg body weight.

133 — Brilliant Blue FCF; Blue EGS; CI Food Blue 2; CI Acid Blue 9; Patent Blue AC; FD and C Blue No. 1; CI No. 42090. Synthetic coal-tar dye. Has been used to produce green hues with tartrazine. ADI is up to 12.5mg per kg body weight, established after repeated subcutaneous injections in animals.

154 — Brown FK; CI Food Brown 1; Chocolate Brown FK. A mixture of synthetic azo dyes. Experiments on bacteria suggest that two of the constituents are mutagenic, i.e., causing cell changes.

155 — Chocolate Brown HT; CI Food Brown 3; CI No. 20285. Synthetic coal-tar dye. ADI is up to 250μg per kg body weight.

375 — Nicotinic acid, one of the B vitamins.

516 — Calcium sulphate; gypsum; terra alba. Mineral used as filler in tablet-making. ADI is unlimited.

542 — Edible Bone Phosphate. Used as filler in tablet-making. ADI is unlimited.

551 — Silicon dioxide: Colloidal silicon dioxide; Colloidal silica. Used as an anti-caking agent in tablet-making. ADI is unlimited.

570 — Stearic acid. Used as lubricant in tablet-making and as a coating for pills and tablets. Naturally occurring fatty acid occurring in all animal fats and vegetable oils. ADI is unlimited.

572 — Magnesium stearate. Used as a lubricant in tablet-making. ADI is unlimited.

901 — Beeswax; White Wax; Yellow Wax; Cera Alba; Cera Flava. The wax obtained by melting with hot water the walls of the honeycomb of the bee and removing the foreign matter. Used as an ingredient in some soft-gelatin capsules. White variety is bleached yellow beeswax.

Causes occasional allergic dermatitis in beekeepers but no reports of toxic effects in the minute amounts used in soft-gelatin capsules.

904 — Shellac, Lacca. Obtained by purifying the resinous secretion of the insect Laccifer lacca Kerr (Coccidae). Used as a coating for pills and tablets. No adverse effects reported from small amounts used in tablets.

---

eczema,   acute or chronic non-contagious itching, inflammatory disease of the skin. Can be due to EFA (essential fatty acids) deficiency, but more specifically that of gamma linolenic acid (GLA).

Infantile eczema may due to lack of GLA in cow's milk. Treat with oral oil of evening primrose (1500 to 3000mg daily).

Atopic eczema due to allergic reaction. Shown to respond to oral oil of evening primrose (up to 3000mg daily).

Other vitamin treatment includes vitamin A (7500IU), vitamin C (up to 1000mg) and high potency vitamin B complex including inositol (500mg daily).

Mineral
Some cases respond to oral zinc therapy. Usual dose is 50mg elemental zinc three times daily that can be reduced to 25mg of the mineral three

times daily as condition responds. More effective if taken in conjunction with daily vitamin C (1000mg) and essential fatty acids in the form of safflower oil or oil of evening primrose capsules (three 500mg strength daily). Response can be slow. perhaps needing several months for complete remission.

---

eggs, a moderate source of all vitamins except vitamin C. Egg-white is devoid of all fat-soluble vitamins. The vitamin B complex occurs mainly in the yolk. Good source of all the essential minerals.

Vitamins remaining after the various cooking methods for eggs are also shown. Vitamins not mentioned show zero loss.

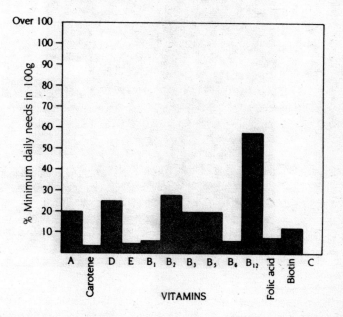

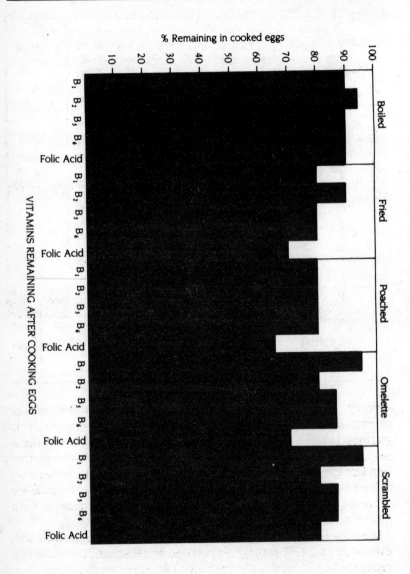

% Remaining in cooked eggs

VITAMINS REMAINING AFTER COOKING EGGS

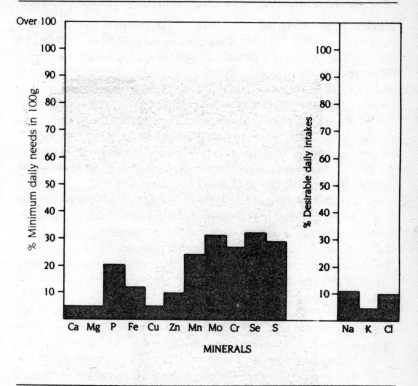

elderly, largest single group of population prone to mild deficiency of vitamins, particularly B complex C and K. Reasons include aversion to salads and meat because of poor dentition; reluctance for physical or emotional reasons to shop frequently for a variety of food; loss of marital partner with less care in preparing food because of apathy; undue reliance on refined carbohydrates and simple beverages as staple diet; dependence on restaurant or institutional cooking; inefficient absorption of food micronutrients.

Most elderly persons will benefit from daily multivitamin supplement with extra vitamin C (250-500mg) plus choline as phosphatidyl choline (3-6 capsules daily) or lecithin (5-15g) daily to improve mental activity.

electrolytes,   electrically charged atoms or groups of atoms that exist in aqueous solution. They are known as ions and are divided into anions and cations. *Anions* are negatively charged (so-called because under the influence of an electric current they migrate towards the anode or positive end). Examples are Chloride (Cl^-); phosphate ($PO4^-$); bicarbonate (HCO_3^-) sulphate (SO_4^-). *Cations* are positiyely charged (because under the influence of an electric current they migrate towards the cathode or negative end). Examples are sodium (Na^+); potassium (K^+); calcium (Ca^{++}); magnesium (Mg^{++}). All metals may be regarded as cations when they are present as salts in solution within the body. Hydrogen when positively charged (H^+) confers acidity in solution.

The principle cation inside body cells is potassium (K^+) but magnesium (Mg^{++}) is also present. In fluids that bathe the cells (extracellular fluids) the principle cation is sodium (Na^+), but a small amount of calcium (Ca^{++}) is also present. Because ions can move freely across cell membranes, the maintenance of potassium inside and sodium outside cells is an energy-requiring process. (*See* sodium pump.) Maintaining this balance is very important to ensure the correct volume of water inside and outside body cells. Imbalance can lead to dehydration or conversely oedema (water retention). All positively charged cations are neutralized by an equal number of negatively charged anions so that the acidity of the fluid of body cells is maintained near neutral.

The transmission of nerve impulses and the contraction of muscles depend upon the correct electrolyte equilibrium at the cell membrane. Whenever a nerve or muscle is active there is a charge of impulse which allows sodium and calcium to enter the appropriate cell; at the same time potassium and magnesium move out of the cell. Once the impulse has passed the ionic pump comes into play to restore the original equilibrium.

The nerves (called motor nerves) that actually stimulate muscle contraction are dependent on the correct calcium-magnesium ionic ratio in the blood. When calcium is lacking these nerves become over-susceptible to stimuli. The result is a condition called tetany, characterized by spasm and twitching of the muscles, particularly those of the face, hands and feet.

Functions of electrolytes are: maintenance of water balance in the body (*see* sodium *and* potassium); maintenance of nerve-impulse transmission; maintenance of smooth muscle contraction; maintenance of acid-alkali (or base) balance of the body (*see* acid-base balance); participation in some enzymatic and hormonal reactions.

The presence of an electrical charge (either positive or negative) on a mineral changes its fundamental properties. *Sodium* (Na) as a pure metal is highly reactive being violently decomposed by water, producing caustic soda and hydrogen which can ignite spontaneously. As the cation sodium (Na^+) it is perfectly stable in water and exists as such in salt solutions and within the body.

Potassium (K) also reacts violently with water, producing caustic potash and hydrogen. As the cation potassion (K^+) it is perfectly stable and exists as such in the body.

Calcium (Ca) reacts with water but less violently than sodium and potassium do. As the cation calcium (Ca^{++}) with two positive charges it is present to a small extent in body fluids as a stable substance necessary for nerve-impulse transmission, muscle contraction and clotting of the blood.

Magnesium (Mg) as the pure metal reacts only very slowly with water and is far more stable than sodium, potassium and magnesium. Heat causes spontaneous ignition with a blinding light which is why it was once used in flash photography. As the cation (Mg^{++}) it carries two positive charges which stabilize the mineral for its functions within the body.

Phosphorus (P) is a very reactive substance that ignites spontaneously at temperatures above 30°C. As the free metal it is highly toxic, causing gastrointestinal irritation, liver damage, skin eruptions, circulatory collapse, coma, convulsions and death with as little as 50mg. On the skin it causes severe burns. When combined with oxygen to form phosphate (PO_4) and in its anionic form phosphate ($PO_4^{\equiv}$) it is innocuous and performs its functions within the body, as insoluble calcium phosphate in the bones and teeth and as ionic phosphate in body fluids.

Chlorine (Cl) is a highly dangerous, yellow gas with a suffocating odour. As a charged atom chloride (Cl^-) it comprises half of common salt and acts within the body as an important anion that neutralizes the cations sodium and potassium.

---

embolism,   obstruction or occlusion of a blood vessel, especially an artery, by a transported clot. Treatment, *see* blood clot.

---

endurance,   increased by vitamin E. Optimum daily intake of 100-150IU for training period of 1.5-2.0 hours; 250-300IU for training period of 3-4 hours.

In racehorses, daily intakes of 5000-10000IU vitamin E have increased performance and calmed nervous animals.

---

enteritis,   regional. Crohn's disease.

---

epilepsy,   convulsive seizures. Large amounts of folic acid may neutralize action of anti-convulsive drugs, particularly phenytoin.

---

etretinate,   vitamin A-related, synthetic derivative of retinoic acid used in treating psoriasis and other skin disorders by oral route.

Side-effects include dryness of mucous membranes and hair loss. Teratogenic (causing abnormal foetus), so pregnancy must be avoided during use. Strict medical use only.

---

exophthalmia,   abnormal extrusion of the eyeball; pop-eyes. Symptom of Grave's disease due to excessive production of thyroid hormones.

---

extrinsic factor, B_{12} vitamin.

---

eyes,   sight process depends upon adequate vitamin A (2500IU daily). Bloodshot eyes prevented by vitamin B_2 (10mg daily). Heavy smoking causes tobacco amblyopia (reduced vision) due to inactivation of vitamin B_{12}.

F

farnoquinone, K_2 vitamin.

fatigue, mental or physical tiredness that may follow prolonged or intense activity; tiredness that cannot be associated with any measurable medical cause. Can produce tearfulness, depression and irritability — the 'housewife syndrome'. Early sign of deficiency of pantothenic acid; of thiamine; of vitamin C; of vitamin E. May be associated with generalized mild deficiency of vitamins. Treat with multivitamin preparation. If no improvement after one month seek medical advice.

Mineral
Studies indicate that in the absence of any other cause fatigue may be associated with mild deficiency of magnesium and potassium. Supplementation with these minerals is more likely to help in cases of tiredness due to muscle fatigue. Studies indicate that taking extra quantities of magnesium (500mg daily) and potassium (1500mg) daily overcame waking tiredness in a high proportion of individuals suffering from chronic fatigue. Potassium was found to be best taken as increased intakes of fresh fruit and vegetables along with dried fruit and vegetable and fruit juices as part of the diet rather than as tablets. Fatigue caused by lack of iron is associated usually with anaemia. *See* anaemia.

fats, complexes of fatty acids, both polyunsaturated and saturated, and glycerine. Hard fats usually contain mainly saturated and mono-unsaturated fatty acids (e.g. fats of animal origin); oils usually contain mainly poly-unsaturated with some mono-unsaturated fatty acids (e.g. vegetable oils).

Hard margarines are mainly saturated and monosaturated fatty acids; soft margarines contain more polyunsaturated fatty acids.

All fats and oils of whatever origin provide 9 k calories per gram. Dietary fats in Western world provide about 40 per cent of total calorie intake. Most authorities now recommend reduction to between 25 and 35 per cent of total calorie intake. Some suggest replacement of saturated fats in diet to polyunsaturated variety by switching from animal fats to vegetable oils. High polyunsaturated fat intake requires increased vitamin E concomitantly.

High blood fats can be reduced with vitamin E (400IU) and vitamin C (500mg) and soya lecithin granules (15g) daily. Lecithin provides 120 kilocalories in 15g that must be counted against fat intake. High blood fats associated with high fat intake regarded as increasing chances of developing cancer, gout, coronary thrombosis, stroke and complications of diabetes. *See* polyunsaturated fatty acids.

---

fatty acids,   metabolism dependent on vitamin B_2; vitamin C (via carnitine in muscle cells). *See* fats and polyunsaturated fatty acids.

---

fertility,   measured in men by number and mobility of spermatozoa in semen. No definite association in men between infertility and vitamin deficiency but some evidence that vitamins A, B_{12} and E needed for normal sperm production. These vitamins definitely required by many species of animals for reproduction. No strong evidence that vitamin E can help infertile human females but 200IU daily has prevented miscarriage in those prone to it. Vitamin B_{12} can also help some women unable to conceive.

---

fish,   *white variety* includes cod, haddock, Atlantic halibut, lemon sole, plaice, saithe and whiting. Traces only of fat-soluble vitamins and negligible vitamin C. Good source of vitamin B_{12} with moderate amounts of the rest of the B complex.

Fatty variety includes eel, herring, bloater, kipper, mackerel, pilchard, salmon, sardines, sprats, trout, tuna and whitebait. Higher potencies of the fat-soluble vitamins than in white fish but similar quantities of the vitamin B complex. Negligible vitamin C present.

All types of fish provide only moderate amounts of the essential minerals. Vitamins left after cooking fish in various ways are also shown.

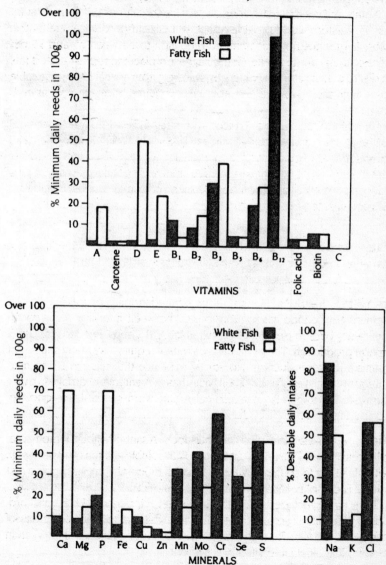

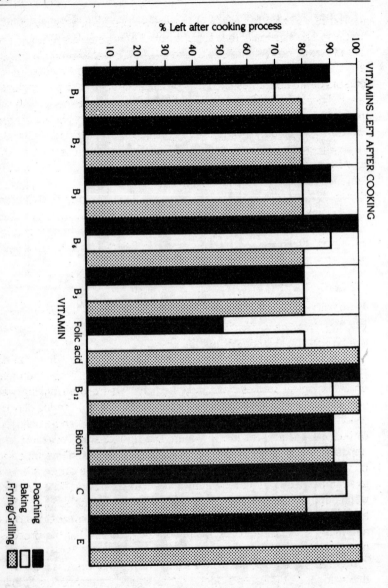

% Left after cooking process

VITAMINS LEFT AFTER COOKING

VITAMIN

Poaching
Baking
Frying/Grilling

fish oils, fish body oils as well as fish liver oils are rich sources of PUFA but also two especially that are not found in vegetable seed oils. These are EPA (eicosapentaenoic acid) and DHA (docosahexaenoic acid). Both are members of an essential fatty acid family that function as precursors of the hormones known as prostaglandins. These prostaglandins are believed to inhibit formation of blood clots in the circulatory system; reduce blood fat levels; increase HDL-cholesterol levels and reduce risk of heart disease and stroke. They effectively thin the blood. Daily intake of ½-1 lb of oily fish (such as mackerel or herring) supplies sufficient EPA and DHA for protective effect. Cod liver oil will supply them but too risky because of vitamins A and D content.

Supplements now available that provide EPA (180mg) and DHA (120mg) per capsule that doubles usual daily intake. Preventative therapy requires up to 3 capsules daily (900mg total EPA and DHA). For those with angina or who have suffered heart attacks or stroke, five daily is sufficient (1500mg total EPA and DHA) to help prevent further attacks.

---

fluoridation, is the addition of fluoride to a waste water supply that lacks the trace element in order to raise its concentration to a level that will reduce the incidence of dental caries.

It has been known since 1916 that fluoride in drinking water can help prevent dental caries in the teeth of growing children. Since then many epidemiological studies have indicated that where the drinking water contains at least 1mg fluoride per litre water (1 ppm) the incidence of childhood dental caries is lower than in comparable areas where only traces of fluoride are present in the water. The fluorides are believed to be deposited on the enamel surface of developing teeth and this appears to be where they exert their anti-cariogenic action. These observations led to a campaign by various local authorities in the UK to add fluoride to their water supply if this was deficient in fluoride. Western European countries have not accepted fluoridation with the same enthusiasm as Great Britain and many states of the USA, mainly on the grounds that the process is neither safe nor essential.

There seems little doubt from various studies that there is a decline in the incidence of children's dental caries where water previously low in fluorine has had fluoride added to it. What is in doubt is how much this action has contributed to dental health in view of: improvement in dental-health awareness amongst the population as a whole; the knowledge that prevention is possible; better health education; application of fluoridated gel to the teeth of children; mouth rinses containing fluoride; better dental care by the dentist; widespread use of fluoridated toothpaste. Fluoride is now generally accepted as an anti-cariogeniç agent — controversy rages over the best way to ensure an adequate intake.

One objection to fluoridation is the possibility of supplying too much fluoride to children and some cases of fluorosis have been noted in those drinking treated water. A more serious objection was raised in the USA where a 5 per cent increase in cancer death-rate in some 20 cities with fluoridated water has not been seriously challenged by fluoridation supporters. The only hard fact to arise from fluoridation of water is that if there are any benefits to be gained, these are confined to a lower incidence of dental caries in children.

Fluorides used to fluoridate drinking water include: hydrofluorosilicic acid; sodium fluoride; sodium silicofluoride.

---

fluorine,   chemical symbol F. Atomic weight 19.0. It is a halogen that occurs as fluoride in the earth's crust at an abundance of 65mg per 100g. Most important natural sources are fluorite, cryolite and florapatite. It is an essential trace element for animals and man.

It was first detected in the animal body by Gay-Lussac in 1805. As fluoride, fluorine is now known to be present in trace amounts in the bones, teeth, thyroid gland and skin of animal and human tissues. When eaten in the food or obtained by drinking water, ingested fluorides are all present as negatively charged atoms (anions) so there is no barrier to absorption. They are rapidly absorbed and distributed in a manner similar to that of chlorides and like these, fluorides tend to stay in the extra-cellular fluid. Much of the fluorides find their way to the skeleton (e.g. in animal studies 60 per cent ended up in the bone after 2 hours), and any excess is efficiently excreted via the urine. Some is also deposited in the teeth but whereas sufficient is protective to the teeth, excess can be harmful. Blood levels of fluoride are between 14 and 19μg per 100ml, of which 15-20 per cent is ionic. The mineral does not appear to cross the barrier from blood plasma to breast milk, so increasing maternal intakes during lactation is unlikely to provide more for the baby. More fluoride is retained by the body during childhood than in the adult state.

Food sources of fluoride are widespread and drinking water supplies appreciable amounts. Few quantitative analyses of individual foods for the mineral are available, but the UK Ministry of Agriculture, Fisheries and Food has published the following average intakes (in mg per day): cereals 0.15; meat 0.05; fish 0.08; fats 0.03; fruits and sugars 0.04; root vegetables 0.04; other vegetables 0.02; milk 0.09, and beverages (not including fluoride from the water source) 1.33.

Total dietary intake is thus estimated at 1.82mg fluoride per day. To this must be added the amount contained in the water supply. Assuming an intake of 1.1 litres daily, unfluoridated water will supply an extra 0.11-0.21mg; fluoridated water will supply 1.1mg extra fluoride. The richest source of dietary fluoride is tea, particularly the China variety which contains up to 10mg fluoride in 100g dried leaves. Six cups of this daily will provide about 3mg fluoride from the infused dried leaves alone. Indian tea will provide about half this quantity.

Functions of fluoride are not known with certainty, but it appears to confer strength and stability to bones and teeth, probably by forming insoluble fluoro-phosphates; it acts as an anti-cariogenic agent in the developing teeth of children, probably by reducing the solubility of tooth minerals or by discouraging the growth of acid-producing bacteria in the mouth; it may play a part in preventing osteoporosis in the elderly.

Deficiency in animals causes anaemia in mice; infertility in mice; stunted growth in rats and chicks; lack of skeletal development in rats and chicks. In human beings, deficiency gives rise to dental caries in children; osteoporosis in elderly adults (possibly) where it may be associated with low calcium intakes.

Signs of deficiency are probably confined to the appearance of caries in the teeth of children. *See* dental caries.

Therapy of deficiency can be: fluoridation of drinking water supplies, *see* fluoridation; use of fluoride toothpaste; oral fluoride tablets; direct application to teeth of fluoride gel; mouth rinses with fluoride solutions. All have been claimed to be effective in reducing the incidence of dental caries in children.

Therapy: sodium fluoride has been used to treat osteoporosis; Paget's disease; bone pain; otosclerosis. (See entries under specific complaint.)

Excessive intakes of fluoride causes fluorosis.

In cattle and sheep excessive intakes may be taken when they graze on land contaminated with fluoride-containing dust. Both teeth and skeleton are affected. Signs are first seen in the teeth of young, growing animals as white mottled patches and a rough enamel surface. In adult animals the surfaces of the large bones and lower jaw become thickened and the bone density thickens with extra calcification. Sometimes bony outgrowths appear. Weakness and reduced milk yield are also signs of excessive fluoride intake in dairy animals.

In man, the first and most obvious sign is mottling of the teeth caused when the chalky-white irregular patches on the surface of the enamel become infiltrated by yellow or brown staining. Severe fluorosis weakens the enamel, resulting in surface pitting. All teeth may be affected but fluorosis is seen on the incisors of the upper jaw. Dental fluorosis does not mean that skeletal fluorosis is present, but the latter can occur with extremely high intakes of fluoride taken over long periods.

When the water supply contains more than 10mg fluoride per litre of water (10 ppm) or when excessive amounts of fluoride are inhaled as in smelting aluminium, fluorosis affects more than the teeth. Appetite is depressed; there is increased density (sclerosis) of the bones of the spine, pelvis and limbs; the supple ligaments of the spine become calcified; resulting in the so-called 'poker back'; calcium is deposited in muscles and tendons; nerve disturbances following the changes in the spinal column can appear. All of these changes are classed as osteosclerosis.

Treatment of fluorosis is to reduce the intake of dietary fluoride.

Recommended dietary intake of fluoride is suggested as 1mg per day in adults by the West German authorities. The Dental Health Committee of the British Dental Association has recommended intakes of fluoride (in mg per day) as: 2 weeks to 2 yrs 0.25; 2-4 yrs 0.5; 4-16 yrs 1.0. This advice applies where water fluoride levels are below 0.3mg per litre. When the water fluoride level is between 0.3 and 0.7mg per litre, no supplements should be given until age 2 years, after which doses are halved.

The ideal drinking water supply is regarded as 1mg per litre, which would supply between 1 and 2mg fluoride daily. Whilst this may be suitable for growing children who drink milk, which has very little fluoride content, it is additive for those who drink tea which is rich in the mineral.

fluorosis, excessive deposition of fluoride in the teeth causing mottling. Can also apply to large amounts of fluoride deposited in bone. *See* fluorine.

folacin, folic acid.

folates, group of folic-acid-related compounds that occurs in foods only some of which show vitamin activity.

folic acid, water-soluble vitamin, member of the vitamin B complex. Also known as vitamin Bc; vitamin M; pteroyl glutamic acid, PGA; liver lactobacillus casei factor; folacin. Anti-anaemia vitamin. Yellow-orange crystalline powder.

Isolated in 1939 from liver then in 1940 found to be growth factor for bacteria. In 1945 Dr Tom Spies demonstrated it cured anaemia of pregnancy. Active form is folinic acid produced from folic acid with the aid of vitamin C in the liver.

Best Food Sources µg per 100g	
Dried brewer's yeast	2400
Soya flour	430
Wheatgerm	310
Wheat bran	260
Nuts	110
Pig's liver	110
Greenleaf vegetables	90
Wholegrains	80
Pulses (beans)	80
Pig's kidney	42
Wholemeal bread	39
Citrus fruits	37
Eggs	30
Brown rice	29

Functions

Needed for metabolism of RNA (ribonucleic acids) and DNA (deoxy-ribonucleic acids) in the body cell protein synthesis.
Blood formation
Genetic code transmission
Builds up resistance to infection in new-born and infants

Stability in Foods

Destroyed by light and air
See Losses in Food Processing

Deficiency Symptoms

Weakness
Fatigue
Breathlessness
Irritability
Sleeplessness
Forgetfulness
Mental confusion

Deficiency Causes

Pregnancy
Contraceptive pill
Old age
Many drugs

Deficiency Consequences

Possible spina bifida
Premature birth
Toxaemia of pregnancy
Premature separation of
  placenta from uterus
Habitual abortion

Recommended Daily Intakes

Should be at least 400µg but
see separate entry

Therapeutic Uses

Preventing deficiency
  consequences
Megaloblastic anaemia
Schizophrenia
Mental deterioration
Psychosis
Malabsorption diseases
  e.g. sprue

Symptoms of Excess Intake
(more than 15mg daily)

Loss of appetite
Nausea
Flatulence
Abdominal distension
Sleep disturbances

No problems with lower
intakes

folinic acid,   active form of folic acid produced under the influence of
vitamin C in the liver.

food preservatives,   vitamins C and E are only recognized natural food
preservatives but bioflavonoids have some function.

food sources,   in a study carried out in 1980 under the auspices of the Ministry of Agriculture, Fisheries and Food, the contributions of various food items in the British diet to intakes of specified vitamins and minerals were calculated. They are shown thus:

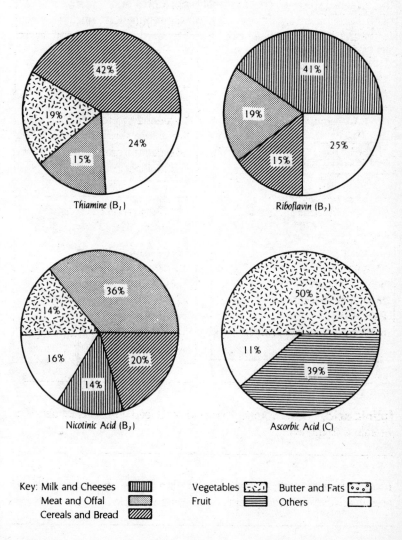

Thiamine (B₁)

Riboflavin (B₂)

Nicotinic Acid (B₃)

Ascorbic Acid (C)

Key: Milk and Cheeses   Vegetables   Butter and Fats
       Meat and Offal   Fruit   Others
       Cereals and Bread

Mineral
A balanced diet will provide trace minerals from all food items and a major study has indicated the contributions made by such ingredients to the daily requirements. These average intakes of trace minerals were obtained from the 'total diet study' by chemical analysis of food. Representative amounts of 68 foods (based on National Food Survey information to include sweets, water and soft drinks) were obtained, prepared, cooked then analysed. The results are as shown in Table 7.

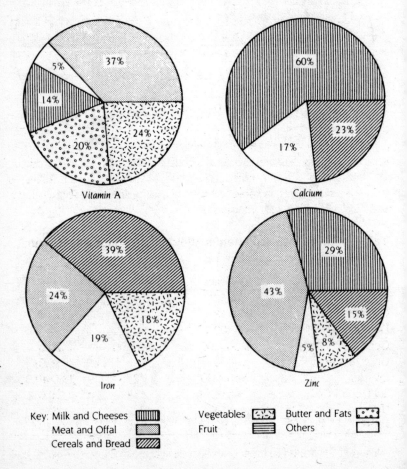

Vitamin A

Calcium

Iron

Zinc

Key: Milk and Cheeses | Vegetables | Butter and Fats
Meat and Offal | Fruit | Others
Cereals and Bread

Table 7: Trace minerals obtained from an average balanced diet

Foodstuffs	Zinc (mg)	Copper (mg)	Iodine (μg)	Selenium (mg)	Manganese (mg)	Fluoride (mg)
Cereals	1.8	0.38	31	30	1.42	0.16
Meat and eggs	3.5	0.37	36	12	0.08	0.05
Fish	0.1	0.03	15	10	0.01	0.07
Milk	1.5	0.04	92	4	0.04	0.03
Fats/dairy products	0.9	0.02	17	1	0.16	0.03
Root vegetables	0.6	0.16	15	1	0.22	0.02
Other vegetables	0.3	0.10	8	1	0.17	0.01
Fruit and sugar products	0.4	0.20	25	1	0.20	0.04
Beverages	0.3	0.17	16	0	2.92	1.41
TOTAL	9.4	1.47	255	60	5.22	1.82

fortification of foods, falls into three categories as far as vitamin addition is concerned:

1. Restoring original vitamin content. In the countries where this is carried out on white flour, restoration is statutory at present but the extent of adding vitamins varies. The recommended additions for white wheat flour (in mg per kg flour) are given in Table 8. Where rice is the staple diet of a country, this also is fortified with vitamins.

Table 8: Recommended vitamin additions to white wheat flour

Country	Thiamine	Riboflavin	Nicotinic acid
Brazil	4.50	2.50	—
Canada	4.18	2.42	30.5
Denmark	5.00	5.00	—
Germany	3.00-4.00	1.50-5.00	20.0
Great Britain	2.40	—	16.0
Sweden	2.60-4.00	1.20	23.0-40.0
Switzerland	4.18	2.53	50.0
USA	4.18	2.42-2.53	30.5
USSR	4.00	4.00	20.0

Vitamin C is added to most brands of dehydrated potato to restore that lost during the drying process but this restoration is not obligatory.

Vitamin E is added to some vegetable oils to replace that lost during the refining process. Many cooked cereals have thiamine, riboflavin and nicotinic acid added to them to replace those vitamins lost during refining and processing but this is not obligatory.

2. Enrichment, where the vitamin is added to give concentrations greater than in the original food. Examples are the addition of vitamin C to fruit juices and drinks; the addition of vitamin A to liquid milk; the addition of all vitamins to dried milk.

3. Vitaminization — adding vitamins to a food that does not normally contain them. The process is carried out to ensure that the foods are equal in vitamin content to those for which they are being substituted. One example is margarine, which is produced by hardening of vegetable oils (hard type) or by blending of vegetable oils with partially hardened oils (soft type). As produced margarines are devoid of vitamins A and D so these are added to give the margarine similar content of these vitamins to that of butter. Sometimes vitamin E and polyunsaturated fats are added to increase the intake of these essential nutrients. Addition of vitamins A and D in the UK is statutory; that of other vitamins is not obligatory.

The substitution of expensive animal proteins by cheaper protein is likely to require extensive vitaminization since soya protein is highly refined and processed. To make the two sources of protein equivalent, most vitamins must be added but particularly vitamin B_{12} since this is completely lacking in soya protein.

---

frost bite,   injury to the skin induced by extreme cold and characterized by redness, swelling and pain that can reach deep tissues. In cold climates vitamin C (425mg daily) can help prevent frost bite by maintaining skin temperature.

---

fruit juices,   include apple, blackcurrant, grape, grapefruit, lemon, lime, orange and pineapple.

As well as being a refreshing drink, fruit juices of all varieties (fresh, reconstituted or frozen) should be regarded as moderate providers of carotene, vitamin E and the vitamin B complex. Vitamin C content can vary depending upon how much has been added since the vitamin is lost during the production process. Only in freshly squeezed juices is the full content retained.

Blackcurrant juice is particularly high in vitamin C level.

All fruit juices are low sodium drinks and supply excellent intakes of potassium along with useful quantities of trace minerals.

Vegetables juices tend to provide more carotene (e.g. carrot) than fruit juices but contents of other vitamins are similar. Whilst vegetable juices also provide excellent potassium levels, they are often salted to improve taste so sodium levels can be increased.

---

fruits,   bananas, apples, pears and melons. *See* separate entries.

---

fruits — citrus,   include oranges, lemons, limes, mandarins, tangerines and pineapples.

Supply some carotene, vitamin E and the vitamin B complex but most

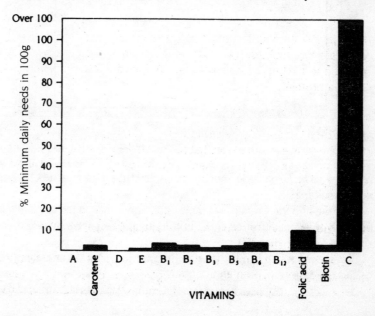

important contribution is their vitamin C content. Should be regarded as low sodium foods that provide high intakes of potassium with useful quantities of the trace minerals.

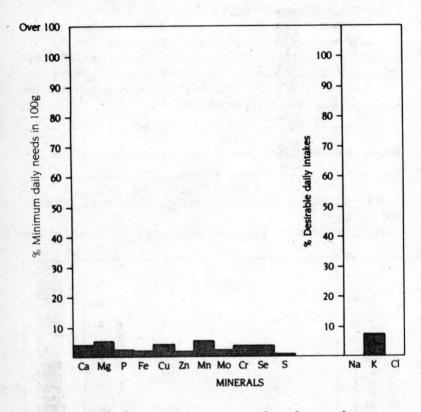

fruits — dried, include apricots, currants, dates, figs, peaches, prunes, raisins, sultanas.

Carotene and the vitamin B complex are higher than in the original fruit because of a concentration effect but drying process destroys vitamin E and most of the vitamin C.

All are low sodium foods that are also excellent sources of potassium, calcium, magnesium, iron and copper.

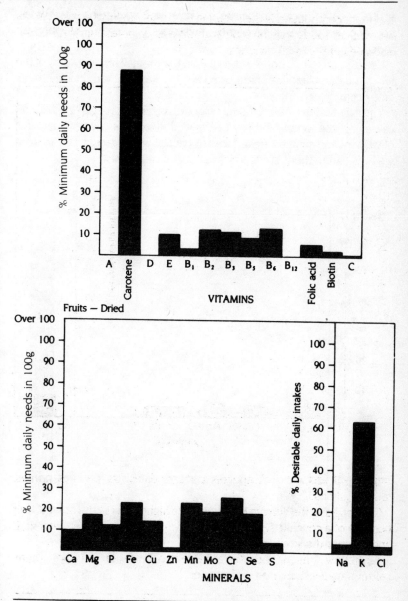

fruits — soft, include bilberries, blackberries, blackcurrants, cranberries, gooseberries, grapes, loganberries, mulberries, passion fruit, raspberries, redcurrants, strawberries.

Useful sources of carotene and vitamin E with small amounts only of the vitamin B complex. Important providers of vitamin C with blackcurrants an extremely rich source.

Virtually sodium free, all supply good dietary intakes of potassium, calcium, phosphorus and iron. When stewed all varieties lose small amounts of vitamins and minerals are reduced by dilution and sugar but if the stewing water is eaten, there are little losses of micronutrients.

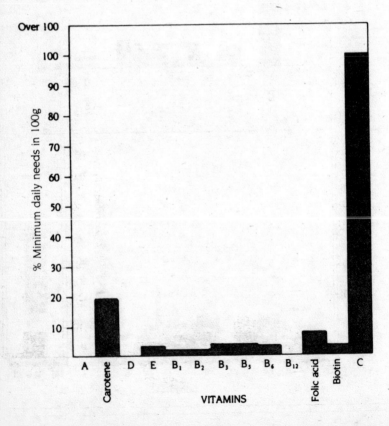

fruits — those with stones, these include apricots, avocados, cherries, damsons, greengages, nectarines, olives, peaches, plums.

A good source of carotene with useful levels of the vitamin B complex and C. Canning causes some loss of vitamins but they can be recovered in part from the syrup. Stewing results in small losses.

All are low sodium foods that are excellent sources of potassium, calcium, magnesium, iron and copper. Canning and stewing give small, mainly recoverable losses of all minerals.

All figures refer to edible part only.

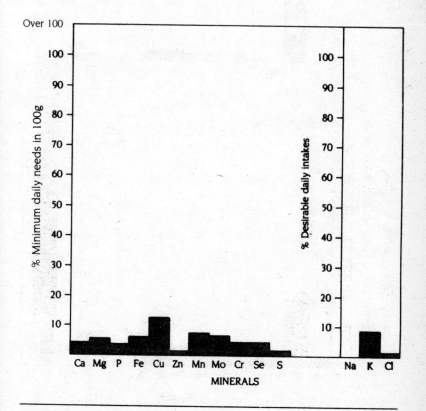

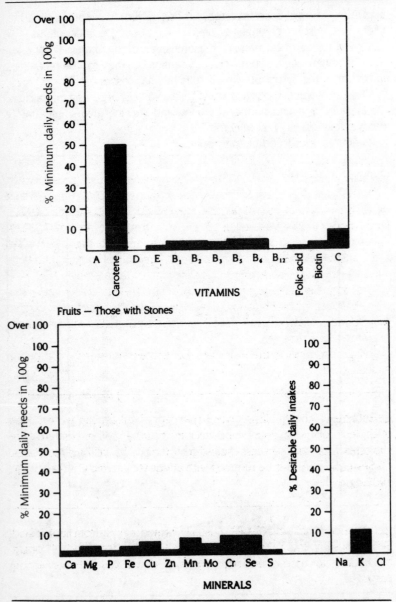

Fruits — Those with Stones

G

gallium, chemical symbol Ga, atomic weight 69.72. Gallium is found in all human tissue, albeit at very low concentrations. Typical values are (in μg per g fresh tissue): brain 0.0006; kidney 0.0003; liver 0.0007; lung 0.005; lymph nodes 0.007; muscle 0.0003; testis 0.0009 and ovary 0.002. When gallium at the level in drinking water of 5μg per ml was fed to mice for life, there was some evidence of slight toxicity. It significantly, but not markedly, suppressed growth and reduced the lifespan of females.

Radioactive gallium-67 is used in diagnostic medicine to identify suspected hidden areas of inflammation. When given to mice, the radioactive material accumulated in the bones but there were significant differences between the sexes.

Gallium can bind to the iron transport protein transferrin, competing against iron.

gallstones, cholelithiasis. Over 80 per cent of gallstones are composed of cholesterol, bile pigments and calcium; a further 10 per cent are pure cholesterol. Caused by excess cholesterol in the bile crystallizing into stones. Cholesterol in bile can be reduced with adequate vitamin C intake (up to 1000mg daily).

gammalinolenic acid (GLA), usually formed in body from linoleic acid. Substantial amounts found only in oil of evening primrose, the oil of borage, blackcurrant and gooseberry seeds but some in spirulina. *See* oil of evening primrose.

gamma tocopherol,   *see* E vitamin.

---

gangrene,   death of a tissue due to failure of arterial blood supply. Late complication of diabetes. May be prevented with adequate intakes of vitamin E throughout life (200-400IU daily). Has been treated with higher intakes of the vitamin (1200IU daily).

   Medical advice essential in diabetes because insulin requirements may be reduced at this level of vitamin supplementation.

---

gastrointestinal tract,   digestive tract.

---

gelatin,   provides traces only of all B vitamins except B_{12}.

---

geophagia,   also known as clay eating. The habit of eating clay is common in rural areas of the United States, in the Middle East and in some areas of Africa. The practice is considered normal during pregnancy in many places throughout the world, usually amongst communities in the lower economic strata, and is believed to supply calcium. Clay is eaten for its mineral content; to relieve hunger; to relieve gastrointestinal discomfort; to overcome diarrhoea; to detoxify harmful minerals. Amongst people on poor diets, clay eating can provide substantial quantities of essential minerals. There is no evidence that the practice causes ill-effects, but once diets are improved, the habit usually stops. It has been associated also with an attempt to cure iron deficiency by some researchers; others believe that geophagia causes malabsorption of iron inducing anaemia. Zinc too is supplied in clay, but the chelating effect of clay on zinc may make it unavailable and at the same time immobilize zinc from other dietary sources.

---

germanium,   also known as ekasilicon, has the chemical symbol Ge with an atomic weight of 75.29. Widely distributed in nature, its abundance in the earth's crust is 0.0007 per cent. Despite its situation in the periodic table within the range of biologically active trace elements, there is no evidence that germanium is essential in mammalian nutrition. Germananates have a low order of toxicity in rats and mice. Almost all of 125 samples of foods commonly eaten contained detectable germanium but only 4 contained more than $2\mu g/g$ food and 15 others provided between 1 and $2\mu g/g$. It is present in the bran of wholewheat flour but cannot be detected in white flour. Vegetables, seeds, meats and dairy products all provide similar quantities of germanium at levels between 0.15 and $0.45\mu g/g$ fresh weight. Richer sources of the mineral (in μg per gram) are the following medicinal herbs: garlic (754); comfrey (152); aloe (77); chlorella (76); ginseng (250-320); sushi (262); sanzukon (257); waternut (239); boxthorn seed (124); wisteria gall (108); pearl barley (50).

Germanium is naturally present in all human tissues and organs with kidney and testis (9.0 and $0.5\mu g/g$) as the richest sources. Rats and mice given extra germanium ($5\mu g$ per ml drinking water) for life experienced reduced lifespan and increased incidence of fatty degeneration of the liver suggesting slight toxicity on lifelong high dose intake. Germanium depressed chromium levels in liver, lungs, heart, kidneys and spleen of rats and increased copper levels in the liver when high intakes were given for life. In plants, germanium supplementation can delay boron deficiency signs suggesting a sparing effect on this essential mineral.

Little is known about the metabolism of germanium that is eaten from the diet. Doses of sodium germanate given orally are absorbed rapidly and almost completely from the gastrointestinal tract within a few hours and excreted largely in the urine during the next 4-7 days. In human trials of a 1.5mg dose of germanium given orally, 1.4mg appeared in the urine and 0.1mg was excreted in the faeces. Western diets tend to provide about $200-500\mu g$ germanium daily.

The following conditions have been reported to respond favourably to germanium at doses that are therapeutic rather than nutritional: arthritis, angina pectoris, myocardial infarct (heart attack), stroke, Raynauds disease; Candida albicans infection, burns, cancer pain (where it is alleged to have an analgesic effect) and some types of cancer. These reports are in the main anecdotal or taken from physicians' case histories rather than double blind, crossover, controlled clinical trials. It is generally believed by its supporters to function by boosting the action of oxygen in generating energy and the life-force i.e. the flow of energy from organ to organ in the body.

Germanium maintains homoeostasis in the body and so is claimed to reduce high blood pressure to normal, lower high blood cholesterol levels, protect against demineralization in osteoporosis, normalize haemoglobin production and reduce the development of hypoxia (lack of oxygen supply to tissue and organs). It is alleged to exert a positive effect on the immune system by normalizing antibody production in cases of allergy. It is possible to demonstrate dose-dependent antiviral, antibacterial and antitumour activity. One way in which it appears to function in this respect is by stimulating interferon production by the body cells. In addition, germanium joins other antioxidants like vitamins C and E, beta-carotene and minerals zinc and selenium in protecting the body against harmful free radicals, pollutants and environmental stresses of all kinds.

The analgesic effect of germanium is seen with very high doses, i.e. 3 to 4 grams, which should only be taken under medical supervision. Ongoing trials in Japan include tests of its analgesic qualities in terminal cancers (where it is claimed to enhance the activity of morphine) and even in treating cancers such as those of the lung, brain and gastrointestinal system. Childhood leukaemias, lymphomas and obstetric cancers are also under active study with germanium as a therapeutic agent.

The conventional animal safety tests indicate that germanium is a highly safe compound at doses equivalent to grams in a human being. It is not entirely free of side-effects in the therapy of human complaints, however. Daily dose of 2.1 grams of the mineral (in the form of biscarboxyethyl germanium sesquioxide) caused initial minor complaints in some post-operative patients but the problems disappeared within three weeks. One clinic reported a 2-3 per cent incidence of minor skin eruptions which resolved themselves in a few weeks. Mild diarrhoea has been reported on high doses but no life-threatening side-effects have so far been reported. Doses of germanium for therapeutic purposes can vary from 10mg to 2 grams daily. Despite reports of its lack of toxicity, however, high doses of germanium (i.e. exceeding 50mg) should not be taken without medical supervision.

---

gingivitis,   inflammation of the gums. Has been treated with very high doses of vitamin A (500000IU) and vitamin E (30IU) daily by injection for six days; then 50000IU vitamin A three times daily with 200IU vitamin E twice daily for three weeks orally. Complete cure claimed with no relapses.

glandular fever,   also known as infective mononucleosis. Caused by Epstein-Barr virus, one of the herpes type, and characterized by high fever, sore throat and swelling of the lymph glands.

Supplements should include high intake of vitamin C (up to 1500mg daily); high potency vitamin B complex and amino acid L-lysine, 1500mg daily.

glaucoma,   disease of the eye characterized by increased pressure within eyeball causing restricted field of vision, coloured halo about lights, lessening of visual power eventually resulting in blindness. Ensure adequate daily intakes of vitamin A (7500IU) and riboflavin (10mg) for good sight. In addition pressure may be reduced with vitamin C (500mg per kg body weight) taken daily over several months.

glossitis,   inflammation of the tongue. Symptom of vitamin B_{12} and riboflavin deficiency. When due to other causes may respond to nicotinamide at doses up to 300mg daily.

gluconates,   complexes of minerals with glucose-like residues that are better absorbed than conventional mineral salts. The glucose-like residue is gluconic acid, a natural substance that the body makes and is able to utilize for energy purposes. This enables the minerals combined with it to pass from the intestine into the bloodstream at a more efficient rate so that less of the mineral is wasted by non-absorption. Gluconates are under body control like any other type of mineral supplement so excessive amounts are not absorbed — the body simply takes what it needs. A full daily complement of mineral needs as gluconates would supply only ten calories.

A recent comprehensive report prepared for the Food and Drug Administration of the United States Government has concluded that mineral gluconates are safe and effective mineral supplements. They were found to be superior to mineral salts in the amounts absorbed from the diet.

Potassium gluconate is of particular interest because it was found that it had less tendency than potassium chloride to cause small bowel ulceration when presented in tablet form.

Gluconates available include calcium, magnesium, iron, zinc, manganese, potassium and copper (see individual mineral for potencies).

---

glucose tolerance factor,   usually abbreviated to GTF, is the only active form of chromium known to function in the body. It is present in foods and can be synthesized in the body from trivalent chromium, nicotinic acid and certain amino acids. It is a complex whose exact structure is not known, so only natural source material is available.

Its history goes back to 1929 when yeast extracts were found to potentiate the action of the hormone insulin. This action was attributed to the vitamins in yeast, and interest waned until 1955 when rats fed on torula yeast were found to develop diabetes and liver degeneration. No known nutrients were able to reverse these conditions so the existence of a new dietary agent, GTF, was postulated. In the early 1960s GTF was identified as a complex of trivalent chromium, nicotinic acid and protein-like material. Animals fed diets deficient in the complex developed a diabetes-like condition.

In the mid-1960s many adults and elderly people with glucose intolerance (a factor in diabetes) were found to improve on a supplement of 150-250µg chromium daily in the form of chromic chloride. Similar benefits were noted in malnourished children in Jordan, Nigeria and Turkey, but not from Egypt. This suggested that children in Egypt, unlike the others, did not lack chromium. Many experiments and observations then led to the conclusions that:

1.   simple chromium salts did not meet the criteria of an essential element;
2.   chromium salts did not cross the placental barrier;
3.   chromium salts supplementation in man always took several days or weeks to be noticeable;
4.   chromium salts did not equilibrate with body pool of organic chromium;
5.   calculations of chromium balance in man indicated a very wide deficit when the absorption rate for chromic chloride was assumed to be the same as for food chromium. For example, if food chromium were absorbed at the same rate as chromic chloride, its calculated dietary intake of 50-100µg per day would lead to only 0.25-0.5µg in the urine. The usual daily excretion

via this route is 7-10µg, suggesting that more food-origin chromium is absorbed and more excreted.

Chromium in the form of brewer's yeast is better absorbed, can be transported across the placenta, is quickly distributed to the tissues and has a faster action in reducing blood sugar than does chromic chloride in rat experiments. Studies in isolating the factor thus yielded GTF, albeit in a crude form.

GTF is far superior to chromium salts as a therapeutic or supplementary form of chromium. Attempts to synthesize it from chromium, nicotinic acid and amino acids have not been successful. Twenty-five per cent of the chromium of GTF in brewer's yeast is absorbed compared with 1 per cent of chromium salts. Yeast can be enriched with chromium by adding the mineral salt to growing yeast, removing the excess chromium salt and drying the yeast. In this way yeast is available containing up to 60µg chromium per g of yeast, all of it presented as GTF. Although precise quantitative assessment of GTF is difficult, the following foods are known to be rich in it (all in descending order of biological activity): dried brewer's yeast; black pepper; calves' liver; cheese; wheatgerm. Moderate sources are: wholemeal bread; cornflakes; white bread; spaghetti; beef; wholewheat grain; butter; rye bread; margarine; oysters; chilli peppers; wheat bran; shrimp. Poorer, but nonetheless useful, sources are: lobster; mushrooms; chicken leg; haddock; beer; egg-white; chicken breast; skimmed milk.

The toxicity of GTF is low. Studies suggest that human beings can tolerate up to 1mg per kg body weight or 60mg in the average adult. The corresponding figure for chromium salts is 18mg.

---

glutamic acid,   amino acid, usually supplied by the food but can be synthesized within the body. Precursor of gamma-aminobutyric acid (GABA), a natural calming agent produced by the central nervous system. Vitamin B_6 essential for GABA synthesis, lack of which causes convulsions in infants.

---

glutethimide,   hypnotic drug. Prevents absorption of folic acid and prevents conversion of vitamin D to 25-hydroxy vitamin D.

---

glycerophosphates,   introduced into medicine on the grounds that lecithin contains phosphorus in the form of glycerophosphate and therefore these compounds would be more easily assimilated into body tissues and particularly the brain. No evidence to support this but glycerophosphates were widely used in the past and are still used as general tonics rather than as suppliers of phosphorus.

---

goitre,   a swelling of the neck due to enlargement of the thyroid gland — the gland enlarges in an attempt to increase the output of hormone.

Endemic is goitre due to lack of iodine in the soil and hence in the diet.

Sporadic is due usually to simple overgrowth of the gland or to a tumour.

Exophthalmic is when the swelling is associated with overactivity of the gland. *See* hyperthyroidism. The condition may also be due to increased intake of certain foods. *See* goitrogens.

Goitres are particularly apt to occur at puberty and during pregnancy.

Endemic goitre occurs mainly in three types of terrain:

1.   mountainous areas of Europe, Asia, North and South America, the Alps, Himalayas, Andes, Rockies, Cameroon mountains, Highlands of New Guinea;

2.   on alluvial plains once covered by glaciers, e.g., the area around the Great Lakes of North America, some areas of New Zealand;

3.   in isolated localities where the water originates in limestone, e.g., Derbyshire and the Cotswolds of England. Simple goitres in non-endemic areas also occur, e.g., in Glasgow where iodine intake was found to be only 60 per cent of the norm.

Treatment of endemic goitre with iodine has been known since the mid-eighteenth century, but it was not until 1920 that American researchers D. Marine and O. P. Kimball demonstrated unequivocally that sodium iodide reduced the incidence of goitre in children. Confirmation of the presence of thyroxine in the thyroid gland came from E. C. Kendall and A. E. Osterberg of the USA in 1919; that of triiodothyronine came from J. Gross and R. Pitt-Rivers of the UK in 1952.

Endemic goitre responds to iodide therapy. Simple goitre in non-endemic areas rarely requires treatment. Iodides are unlikely to cause it to shrink. Only if the goitre becomes disfiguring is thyroxine used. If this is unsuccessful surgery is usually considered. When the goitre is due to intakes of goitrogenic foods, these should be discontinued.

---

goitrogens, substances found in some foods that inhibit formation of hormones by the thyroid gland. They occur principally in the seeds of cabbage, mustard and rape and also in cabbage leaves, kale and turnips. The active substances are glucosinolates and thiocyanates which prevent the synthesis of thyroxine and reduce the amount of iodine in the thyroid gland respectively. There is no strong evidence that these foods cause goitre in man — probably because not enough is eaten. It is possible in farm animals who have large intakes of these foods and some of the goitrogens may find their way into the milk but not enough to cause goitre in the humans who drink it. Ground-nuts, cassava and soya beans are also goitrogenic but the active principles are not known. Cooking methods tend to destroy goitrogens.

---

gold, chemical symbol Au from the Latin *aurum*. Its atomic weight is 196.97 making it one of the heaviest metals. Occurrence in the earth's crust is only $0.005\mu g$ per g.

Foods contain gold at levels of only a few nanograms per gram. A daily intake from the diet is probably less than $7\mu g$. Despite these very low intakes, gold is present in all human tissue and blood. Typical values are (in ng per g fresh weight): heart 0.0338; lung 0.72–1.6; brain grey matter 0.024; brain white matter 0.04; cerebrospinal fluid 0.0062; whole blood 0.055; blood serum 0.08. Normal hair values range from 0.036 to $0.15\mu g$ per g. Cancer patients were found to have elevated hair gold levels of $1.5\mu g$ per g. Pregnancy apparently increases gold in blood with levels of 13mg per ml compared to 3.4mg per ml in non-pregnant women. When gold is given by injection, most of it appears in the urine but some is excreted in the faeces.

Radioactive gold has been used to treat tumours.

---

gold salts, gold thioglucose; sodium aurothiomalate; sodium aurothiosulphate. All are used in treating rheumatoid arthritis. Ineffective in osteoarthritis. Given by deep intramuscular injection, either in aqueous solution or in oil suspension. Toxic effects include mouth ulceration; itching; urticaria; eczema; seborrheic dermatitis; alopecia; inflamed gums; gastritis; colitis. Skin reactions are the most common. Blood abnormalities and kidney damage may also occur..

---

gout, a recurrent acute arthritis of toe and finger joints which results from deposition in the joints and tendons of crystals of sodium urate (uric acid). Has been treated with orotic acid (4g daily for six days) which dissolves uric acid crystals and removes pain and swelling.

Grave's disease, *see* hyperthyroidism.

---

grey hair, caused by loss of natural pigment. In animals development of grey hair is symptom of pantothenic acid and/or biotin deficiency. No hard evidence that these vitamins prevent greying of hair in man but cases on record where they have restored natural colour. PABA deficiency in animals causes premature greying of hair. Colour restored with oral PABA but no hard evidence that it does so in man.

---

growth, depends on adequate supply of protein, fats, carbohydrates and calories. Transformation of these into growing tissues requires adequate thiamine, riboflavin, pantothenic acid, biotin, vitamin B_{12} and vitamin A during pre-natal and post-natal growth.

---

gum disease, also known as periodontal disease, characterized by a progressive inflammation and infection of the gum tissue and underlying jaw-bone. Believed to be due to residual food, bacteria and tartar deposits that collect in the tiny crevices between the gums and the necks of the teeth. As the bacterial infection spreads deeper into the tissue surrounding the jaw-tooth connection, the gums recede until teeth loosen and fall out. Resistance to gum disease may be increased with correct diet. Extra calcium has been shown to reduce the onset of the complaint and in some cases reverse it. Typical intakes were 500mg calcium twice daily. Found to be important at the same time to maintain low dietary phosphorus:calcium ratio. Ideal ratio is 1:1 but most popular foods have a high ratio, e.g., meat 20:1; refined cereals 6:1; potatoes 5:1. Soft drinks are high in phosphorus. Bonemeal has 1:2 ratio but since much phosphorus is supplied in other foods, the ideal calcium supplement for periodontal disease is that with no phosphorus. Dolomite, amino-acid chelated calcium, calcium gluconate, calcium lactate and calcium orotate are all suitable.

---

gums, *see* gingivitis.

H

haemorrhoids, commonly known as piles, characterized by dilated veins of the rectum. Treated with high intakes of bioflavonoids (lemon bioflavonoid complex plus rutin — up to 1000mg daily) plus vitamin C (500mg daily).

hair analysis, assay of a sample of hair for its mineral content. After preparation and dissolution of the hair, the resulting liquid is measured for minerals using atomic absorption spectroscopy; neutron activation analysis or electron microprobe analysis allowing accurate determinations of many trace minerals at concentrations down to $0.1\mu g$ per gram and less in some cases. Hair analysis offers certain advantages over the more usual blood and urine analysis for minerals. These are:

1. hair provides a better assessment of normal trace mineral concentrations because these reflect average levels over the period of growth;

2. hair allows long-term variations in trace mineral concentrations to be assessed. As hair grows, it reflects body status of minerals during the period of growth so if long hair is subdivided into lengths, measurement will show the variation in mineral content over those periods. The technique has been used to determine mineral status during pregnancy.

3. hair is an inert, chemically homogeneous substance that is a permanent record of the minerals in it. Once a mineral has been deposited in hair it stays there.

4. the concentrations of most trace elements are higher in hair than those in blood and most tissues of the body. Chromium levels are 50 times higher in hair than in blood; cobalt levels are 100 times higher.

5.   hair provides a record of past as well as recent trace-mineral levels. Body status can therefore be measured in retrospect.

6.   collection of hair is painless, is not an invasive technique, can be carried out by unqualified persons and the product can be kept indefinitely without deterioration.

Against the value of hair analysis are the objections that:

1.   there is a possibility of variations across the scalp. Any variation can be minimized by taking hair always from the same part of the head, usually the short hair at the back.

2.   procedures for washing and preparing the hair sample before analysis can differ amongst those carrying out the assays. The washing stage can be with solvents or with detergents but studies suggest that the two are compatible and the problem is not serious.

3.   hair may have been treated with bleach or dye which can leach out trace elements. Shampooing and conditioning do not have this effect.

4.   zinc and selenium are used extensively in hair shampoos, colouring agents and conditioners and these may be absorbed into the hair. There is no clear evidence that this happens.

5.   there is no correlation between concentrations of trace elements in hair and in blood. This is not surprising in view of the differing time-scales that each type of assay reflects. Comparative hair analyses carried out by the same procedures by the same analyst on the same individual over a particular time-scale could give useful information about body changes in mineral status.

Interpretation of hair analysis is not straightforward and should be left to an expert. It has been suggested that hair examination in this way is of more use in determining toxic minerals and the significance of levels of essential minerals is debatable. There do appear to be correlations between low levels of hair copper and high levels of hair zinc with higher blood-pressure in man. There is strong positive correlation between some toxic elements in hair and the incidence of high blood-pressure in children. Low hair-zinc levels are known to be associated with dwarfism. It has also been claimed that certain patterns are emerging, for example that:

1.   schizophrenics have high calcium, low iron, high copper and low zinc levels in their hair;

2.   arthritics have high lead, low iron and low copper levels in their hair. Sometimes they show low manganese and a high calcium level that may

depress magnesium concentration.

3. diabetics often have low chromium, low manganese and low zinc with excessively high calcium levels in their hair. The significance of these findings has not yet been worked out. They cannot be regarded as diagnostic of these conditions without accompanying biochemical analyses and clinical signs.

For most individuals it is safe to treat low levels of essential minerals in hair with a change in diet or supplements to supply those minerals that are low. Essential minerals that are present in high quantity may then be reduced to normal levels. High levels of toxic minerals should be treated by a qualified practitioner who will assess their significance by carrying out other tests. High calcium intakes combined with vitamin C and pectin is one combination that may help remove small amounts of toxic trace minerals.

Hashimoto's disease, also known as Hashimoto's thyroiditis; Hashimoto's struma; chronic lymphatic thyroiditis; auto-immune thyroiditis. The most common cause of hypothyroidism. More prevalent in women (8 times as often as in men) and usually between the ages of 30 and 50 yrs. It is an auto-immune disorder where the body produces disordered immunological response against itself to such an extent as to cause tissue injury.

Symptoms are painless enlargement of the thyroid gland or a feeling of fullness in the throat.

Treatment is that for myxoedema (*see* myxoedema).

---

hay fever, a condition characterized by over-secretion of nasal and eye mucous membranes caused by hypersensitivity to pollen. Prevention has been claimed with high doses of vitamin B complex plus extra calcium pantothenate (100mg) and pyridoxine (100mg) in some cases. Treatment includes vitamin C (500mg every 6 hours) which has recognized antihistamine effect. Also claimed that vitamin E (300IU) and bioflavonoids (200mg) daily may bring relief in some people.

headache, a pain or ache anywhere in the head. It is a symptom rather than an illness itself. Causes include disease of the eye, nose or throat; sinuses that are blocked or infected; head injury; air pollution or poor ventilation; medicinal drugs; alcohol; tobacco smoking; fever; infections; disturbances of the digestive tract and circulatory system; brain disorders; iron deficiency anaemia; low blood sugar; overdose of vitamin A; deficiency of nicotinamide, pyridoxine or calcium pantothenate; allergies.

Treatment depends on underlying cause so professional advice must be sought. Adequate intakes of nicotinamide, pyridoxine, calcium pantothenate and vitamin A may help relieve some headaches.

Migraine headaches, *see* migraine.

---

heart, edible, traces only of vitamins A, D and carotene and poor source of vitamin E (0.37-0.70mg per 100g). Good source of B vitamins, supplying the following (in mg per 100g): thiamine 0.21-0.48; riboflavin 0.8-1.5; nicotinic acid 10.6-14.7; pyridoxine 0.11-0.38; pantothenic acid 1.6-3.8. Good source of vitamin B_{12}, providing 13-15μg per 100g. Poor source of folic acid (4μg) and biotin (3μg). Vitamin C levels vary from 5 to 11mg per 100g.

---

heart disease, coronary heart disease (CHD) or ischaemic heart disease (IHD) are synonymous terms for diseases arising from a failure of the coronary arteries to supply sufficient blood to the heart muscle. These diseases are in most cases associated with atherosclerosis of the coronary arteries. They include myocardial infarction, angina pectoris and sudden death without infarction.

Myocardial infarction is death of part of the heart muscle due to failure of blood supply (ischaemia). Usually due to blockage of the supplying blood vessel with clot or by fat deposition on the vessel wall. *See* atherosclerosis and blood clot.

Angina pectoris, see angina.

Sudden death may occur in those who have had myocardial infarction and angina.

Heart disease can be prevented and cured by dietary and supplementary means. Regular vitamin B complex plus high potencies of vitamin E

(400-1200IU daily); vitamin C (500-1000mg daily); vitamin B$_6$ (100mg daily); lecithin (15-45g daily); replacement of saturated animal fats in the diet by PUFA and regular intakes of fish oil containing EPA and DHA may help reduce the chances of heart disease and decrease the possibility of further problems in those who have the complaints.

Mineral

Adequate intakes of certain minerals appear from epidemiological and other studies to protect against heart disease and in some cases can benefit the individual with the complaint. The minerals are:

1. calcium and magnesium, where observations suggest that those communities living in hard-water areas have fewer cases of heart disease than those living in soft-water areas. Hard water contains many minerals, but the main ones are calcium and magnesium and these are believed to exert a protective effect.

2. calcium, which in adequate quantities tends to reduce blood-cholesterol levels. Low body-calcium levels result in high blood-cholesterol levels. Calcium may act in the intestine by combining with fatty acids to form insoluble calcium soaps that are excreted. This reduces fat absorption and lowers blood fats. Both fats and cholesterol levels can be reduced with intakes of calcium between 1025 and 1200mg per day. The mineral appears to function by reducing LDL (low-density lipoprotein) cholesterol levels but allows HDL (high-density lipoprotein) cholesterol levels to be maintained. The end-result is reduction in the severity of atherosclerosis.

3. magnesium, which in adequate quantities appears to prevent cardiac spasms. Post-mortem studies on those who have died from heart disease indicate lower heart-muscle levels of magnesium than in those who have died of other causes. Magnesium is believed to dilate blood vessels in the heart; calcium causes constriction. Correct balance of both minerals ensures the heart beats smoothly. When magnesium is short the imbalance can cause constriction which in turn gives rise to cardiac spasm. Diet and supplementation should ensure adequate intakes of both minerals.

4. potassium, which helps to counteract the negative effects of sodium on the blood-pressure. Post-mortem studies indicate that in those dying suddenly from heart attacks, potassium levels in the heart muscle are also low. Low potassium concentration is associated with angina. Low magnesium and potassium levels may be localized because of heart

problems (rather than causing them) but sensible insurance against heart attacks is adequate intakes of potassium as well as the other minerals.

5. selenium, which when deficient in animals gives rise to heart problems and high blood-pressure. In human studies, those who live in areas where soil selenium and hence selenium intakes are low have the highest rates of coronary disease. Where selenium intakes are highest, rates of coronary disease are lowest. The largest trial was in China, involving more than 45,000 people, in an area where selenium is low. In this area heart disease is rife, affecting many of the population; supplementation with selenium in thousands of children reduced the rate of heart disease from 40 per 1000 to zero. The death-rate in those already afflicted was reduced from 50 per cent to 6 per cent simply by feeding small amounts of selenium (200μg per day). *See* Keshan disease.

6. chromium, which is usually low in the heart tissues of those dying from heart disease. Chromium appears to play a significant role in increasing the highly desirable HDL cholesterol levels at the expense of the less desired LDL cholesterol levels. This alone will help reduce the chances of development of heart failure.

7. manganese, which has been found in low concentration in the heart tissue of those dying from cardiac problems.

---

heavy metal poisoning, excess lead, mercury and cadmium in body can be detoxified with high doses of vitamin C (up to 3000mg daily) plus supplementary essential minerals.

---

hepatitis, inflammation of the liver. When due to viral infection can be relieved by very high doses of vitamin C (25-30 grams) for a few days preferably by intravenous injection but also orally by taking 5 grams every four hours. Medical supervision recommended.

High potency multivitamin complex needed to restore vitamins lost from the liver both during and after attack of hepatitis.

---

herpes simplex, cold sores. May respond to daily intakes of essential amino acid L-lysine (0.5-1.5g). Lysine therapy is also suitable for the treatment of genital herpes.

---

herpes zoster,   *see* shingles.

---

high blood-pressure,   may be associated with high sodium, low potassium, high cadmium intakes. *See* heart disease; salt. High cadmium intakes antagonize the uptake and metabolism of selenium in the body so the effect of this toxic mineral may be mediated through these effects or in a direct action of its own.

---

hormone replacement therapy (HRT),   treatment of symptoms of menopause with natural or synthetic female sex hormones. Similar effect on vitamins to those of contraceptive pill. *See* contraceptives, oral. Treated with similar supplements.

---

hydralazine,   blood-pressure reduction. Enhances excretion of pyridoxine.

---

hydrochloric acid,   a mineral acid, produced by the parietal cells of the stomach, that provides the acidic medium of the gastric juices needed for the early stages of food digestion. Gastric juice contains between 0.2 and 0.5 per cent hydrochloric acid. The acid is a combination of hydrogen ions (which determine acidity) and chloride ions. Hydrogen ions arise by the dissociation of carbonic acid, itself produced from carbon dioxide and water in the blood. Carbonic acid production is under the control of an enzyme carbonic anhydrase which contains zinc. Only the hydrogen ions from the dissociation of carbonic acid pass from the blood to the parietal cells of the stomach (bicarbonate ions are unable to do so), where they combine with the readily available chloride ions to form hydrochloric acid.

Excessive production of hydrochloric acid causes heartburn, gastric and duodenal ulcers.

Deficiency of hydrochloric acid production (known as hypochlorhydria) or complete lack (known as achlorhydria) can lead to malabsorption of some minerals that are usually solubilized by hydrochloric acid; chronic gastritis due to destruction of the parietal cells. The condition is associated with pernicious anaemia; gastric cancer and other cancers of the gastrointestinal tract possibly because in the absence of hydrochloric acid certain cancer-forming substances can be produced from normal food ingredients.

Supplementary forms of hydrochloric acid are:

1. dilute hydrochloric acid. Two to five ml of 10 per cent hydrochloric acid are diluted with 200-250ml of water and sipped through a straw during the course of a meal. No more than 20ml of the 10 per cent hydrochloric acid should be taken over 24 hours.

2. betaine hydrochloride, which provides 23.8mg hydrochloric acid in 100mg. Usual dose is 60-500mg dissolved in water which is drunk after meals. Also available in tablet form.

3. glutamic acid hydrochloride, which provides 19.9mg hydrochloric acid in 100mg. Usual dose is 600-1800mg which is dissolved in water and drunk after meals. Also available in tablet and capsule forms.

---

hydrocortisone,   natural corticosteroid hormone present in adrenal glands. *See* corticosteroids.

---

hydrofluorsilicic acid,   provides 13.2mg fluoride in 100mg acid. Used in controlled amounts for the fluoridation of drinking water.

---

hydroxocobalamin, B_{12a} vitamin.

---

hyperactivity,   usually occurs in children; characterized by excessive or abnormal activity. Often benefit from high doses of vitamins including nicotinamide (1-3g); pyridoxine (100-300mg); vitamin C (1g); vitamin E (up to 400IU) daily. Constant monitoring essential.

---

hypercalcaemia,   infantile. High blood level of calcium that may lead to excess calcification of bones, hardening of the arteries and possibly mental retardation. Symptoms of excessive vitamin D intake. May also occur in adults causing deposition of calcium in soft tissues.

---

hyperkeratosis, rough, bumpy skin, once known as 'toad skin'. Most obvious sign of vitamin A deficiency.

---

hypertension, high blood-pressure. *See* blood-pressure.

---

hyperthyroidism, also known as thyrotoxicosis; Grave's disease; Basedow's disease; Plummer's disease; toxic diffuse goitre; toxic modular goitre. Characterized by an excessive secretion of thyroid gland hormones which increase the metabolic rate.

All forms of hyperthyroidism give rise to the following signs and symptoms: goitre; fast heartbeat; warm, fine, moist skin; tremor; eye signs that include stare, lid lag, lid retraction, eye pain, excessive tears, irritation, sensitivity to light; nervousness; increased activity; increased sweating; heart sensitivity; palpitations; fatigue; increased appetite; weight loss; insomnia; weakness; excessive bowel movements sometimes leading to diarrhoea. In addition symptoms confined to Grave's disease include abnormal extrusion of the eyeball (exophthalmia) and an itchy, red, coarse and thick skin.

Treatment consists of:

1. iodine in high doses usually in the form of potassium iodide or sodium iodide, orally or by intravenous injection. Lasts only up to a week and functions by inhibiting incorporation of iodine into thyroid hormones.

2. antithyroid drugs that inhibit the incorporation of iodine into thyroid hormones;

3. radioactive iodine, used in female patients past their child-bearing years and in males. No evidence of increased incidence of tumours, leukaemia or cancer of the thyroid after this treatment. Therapy of choice in those above 40 years of age with Grave's disease.

4. surgery, in all age groups, to remove the whole or part of the thyroid. Sometimes hypothyroidism occurs and can be treated with thyroxine. After complete removal of the thyroid, thyroxine therapy is needed for life.

---

hypothyroidism, *see* cretinism; Hashimoto's disease; myxoedema.

I

immigrants, those from Asia are particularly prone to vitamin D deficiency, producing rickets in children and osteomalacia in adults. Reasons not known with certainty but change to Western diet including dairy products, more exposure of skin to sunshine and supplementary vitamin D recommended.

immune system, the defence mechanism that the body develops against bacterial and viral infections. Cells responsible arise in thymus gland, spleen and lymphatic system. Impaired by malnutrition and certain vitamin and mineral deficiencies, particularly vitamins A, E and C, beta-carotene and the minerals selenium, iron and zinc. The same micronutrients plus certain enzymes are believed to be essential in quenching harmful free radicals, protecting against cell and tissue degeneration, and reducing the harmful effects of irradiation and pollution. *See* disease resistance.

impotence, inability of the male to attain or sustain an erection satisfactorily for normal sexual intercourse. More common in diabetics because they appear to lack ability to convert carotenes to vitamin A which is essential for sex hormone production. Ensure adequate intakes of vitamin A as the preformed vitamin.

Mineral
Noted in patients undergoing kidney dialysis who were found to have low blood levels of zinc because the dialysing fluids lacked the mineral. Remedying this restored normal sexual function. Earlier studies on zinc

deficient populations in the Middle East and elsewhere found that lack of dietary zinc gave rise to retarded sexual development in growing children. Increasing zinc intakes allowed normal development to continue. Zinc has been shown to help in some cases of sexual dysfunction in adult males. Low testosterone (male sex hormone) levels were associated with low blood-zinc concentration resulting in low sperm counts. Increasing dietary zinc from the food and by supplementing with 30mg of the mineral daily restored sexual function to normal.

---

inborn errors of metabolism, a term introduced by Sir Archibald Garrod in 1908 to describe conditions caused by a deficiency of or an error in a single gene. This is the result of a spontaneous or induced mutation in one or both parents and so it becomes part of the genetic make-up of the foetus. These diseases are hence potentially present at the moment of conception. They are completely different from acquired congenital diseases that are due, not to genetic errors, but to defects arising in the uterus.

Several hundred inborn errors of metabolism have been described and there are probably as many more as yet undiscovered. Some of these respond to treatment with a specific vitamin, usually at levels far in excess of normal dietary intakes. The defect is usually in an enzyme that requires the specific vitamin in order to function; or defective absorption of a vitamin; or an inability to transport a vitamin or an inability to convert a vitamin to its active form.

Thiamine
1. Certain types of maple-syrup urine disease: characterized by delayed nervous system development. Due to defective enzyme that requires thiamine pyrophosphate as coenzyme. Responds to 10mg thiamine daily.
2. Lactic acidosis: characterized by persistent low blood sugar and acidosis due to accumulation of lactic acid. Deficient enzyme is pyruvate carboxylase. Responds to 10mg thiamine daily.

Nicotinamide
1. Hartnup disease: characterized by intermittent skin rash and mental disturbance, symptoms similar to pellagra. Appears partly due to impaired

intestinal absorption of tryptophane, an amino acid that is a precursor of nicotinamide. Skin and mental symptoms respond to 100mg of nicotinamide daily.

2. Hydroxykynureninuria: symptoms are mild, mental deficiency; short stature; rash on buttocks and ulceration of the mouth. Responds to 100mg of nicotinamide daily.

Pyridoxine

1. Infantile convulsions: symptoms are convulsions, excessive irritability, and acute sense of hearing immediately after birth. Responds to 10mg pyridoxine daily by mouth. Treatment must continue for many years.

2. Cystathioninuria: symptoms are mental retardation and congenital defects with an increased tendency to bleed. Pituitary gland abnormalities. Due to large amounts of amino acid cystathionine in blood and urine because body cannot metabolize it. Pyridoxal phosphate is coenzyme for the enzyme cystathioninase which is defective. Responds to high doses (more than 10mg per day) of pyridoxine.

3. Hypochromic anaemia: anaemia with high blood serum iron and increased iron stores. Due to defective enzyme delta-aminolaevulinic acid synthetase. Usually, but not always, responds to large doses of pyridoxine at levels of 20-100mg per day.

4. Homocystinuria: characterized by an excessive excretion of the amino acid homocystine in the urine. Some cases respond to very large doses of pyridoxine at levels of 200-500mg per day.

5. Xanthurenic aciduria: characterized by excessive excretion of xanthurenic acid after high tryptophane meal. Symptoms are defective mental states. Sometimes responds to large doses, up to 200mg per day, of pyridoxine.

Biotin

Propionic acidaemia: acidosis in the new-born due to accumulation of propionic acid in the blood. Caused by a defect in the enzyme propionyl — CoA carboxylase which requires biotin. Responds well to 10mg biotin daily.

Folic acid

1. Congenital defect in folate absorption: deficiency of folic acid caused

by a defect in its absorption from the food and inability to transport the vitamin. Characterized by anaemia; mental retardation; seizures; involuntary movement; impairment of voluntary movement. Anaemia responds to doses of folic acid of 40mg per day but fits may not respond.
2. Formimino-transferase enzyme deficiency: symptoms are retarded mental and physical development; blood shows increased folic acid level. Condition involves vitamin but does not respond to it.

Vitamin B_{12}

1. Malabsorption of the vitamin not due to lack of intrinsic factor. Characterized by megaloblastic anaemia that responds only to injections of vitamin B_{12}.
2. Congenital lack of intrinsic factor. Occurs early in life and is due to non-production of intrinsic factor for reasons unknown. Responds completely to injections of vitamin B_{12}.
3. Megaloblastic anaemia due to lack of specific transport protein (transcobalamin II) of vitamin B_{12} in the blood. Usually occurs in new-born. Responds to injections of 1mg vitamin B_{12} on regular and prolonged basis.
4. Lack of other specific protein (transcobalamin I) carrier of vitamin B_{12} in the blood. Characterized by low vitamin B_{12} blood levels but no other signs of deficiency.
5. Methylmalonicaciduria: acidosis in the blood of the new-born. Large amounts of methylmalonic acid in the urine. Due to inability to form the coenzyme form of vitamin B_{12} called 5'-Deoxyadenosyl cobalamin. Responds to frequent injections of high-dose (1mg) vitamin B_{12} or the coenzyme B_{12} itself.

Vitamin A

The condition is due to an inability to convert carotene to vitamin A. One case only has been described and the symptoms include night blindness, dry eyes (Bitots spots), low blood plasma vitamin A with high blood carotene level. Can be treated by administration of preformed vitamin A.

Vitamin D

1. Hereditary vitamin D-resistant rickets with hypophosphataemia: low phosphate levels in the blood but calcium levels are normal. Primary abnormality is inability to reabsorb phosphate in the kidney. Main disease

is rickets or osteomalacia and dwarfism. Treatment is very high doses of vitamin daily (2.5mg or 100000IU) but this can cause intoxication. May respond better to high oral intakes of phosphate.

2. Fanconi's Syndrome: rickets or osteomalacia with low blood phosphate resistant to normal vitamin D intakes. Due to an inability of the kidney to acidify urine resulting also in low blood potassium levels. Accumulation of the amino acid cystine in the blood and excessive excretion of amino acids in the urine. May respond to massive doses of vitamin D but possible toxic effects must be monitored.

3. Primary renal tubular acidosis: usually affects females in late childhood. Characterized by chronic acidosis, osteomalacia, calcium deposits in the kidneys, stones in the kidneys. Increased excretion of calcium and phosphate in the urine leading to low blood levels of the minerals. Treatment of the acidosis is with citrate and in some cases vitamin D is required but it is not standard therapy.

Indian childhood cirrhosis, a rapidly progressive disorder and an important cause of death in the Asian subcontinent. Characterized by excessive copper deposits in the liver and kidneys of children affected. Earlier onset than Wilson's disease but treatment is similar (*see* Wilson's disease).

---

indium, chemical symbol In with an atomic weight of 114.82. Occurrence in the earth's crust is only 0.000001 per cent.

Indium is present in all human tissue at concentrations between 0.01 and 0.07µg per g fresh tissue. Hair contains a mean level of 0.0045µg per g. Some indium is absorbed from the gastrointestinal tract of animals since it is excreted in the urine after oral feeding. When taken by mouth, indium is relatively non-toxic. Rats fed on high doses of 20 to 30mg of the mineral daily for 27 days exhibited a rough coat and some weight loss. However, when mice were fed 5µg per ml in their drinking water for life they exhibited a lower incidence of tumours than mice fed the same level of scandium, gallium, rhodium, palladium, chromium, or yttrium. The same mice (fed indium) developed high levels of copper and chromium in several organs including kidney and heart.

Indium is highly toxic when it is given by intravenous or subintravenous injection. Injuries occur to blood, heart, liver and kidneys.

---

indomethacin, anti-arthritic drug. Impairs vitamin C and thiamine utilization.

---

inositol, water-soluble member of B complex. Not a true vitamin as body can make it in limited quantities. High concentration in brain, stomach, kidney, spleen, liver and heart. Also known as bios I; myo-inositol; meso-inositol; lipotropic factor.

Present in cereals and vegetables as phytic acid, which is combination of inositol and phosphorus. Major constituent of lecithin. A colourless, crystalline substance.

Best Food Sources in mg per 100g

Food	mg per 100g
Lecithin granules	2857
Beef heart	1600
Desiccated liver	1100
Wheatgerm	690
Lecithin oil	360
Liver	340
Brown rice	330
Cereals	320
Beef steak	260
Citrus fruits	210
Nuts	180
Molasses	180
Pulses (beans)	160
Greenleaf vegetables	100
Wholemeal bread	100
Soya flour	70

Functions

As fat-solubilizing agent
Mild anti-anxiety agent
Maintains healthy hair
Controls blood cholesterol
level

Stability in Foods

Very stable to all cooking processes

Recommended Daily Intakes

Difficult to assess because of body synthesis. Probable daily intakes between 500 and 1000mg

Therapeutic Uses	Deficiency Symptoms
Reducing blood cholesterol	None that are specific
Restoring healthy hair	
With vitamin E to treat nerve	
damage	
Anti-anxiety agent	
Treating irritability	
Treating schizophrenia	

Symptoms of Excess Intake
None reported
When present as phytic acid it may immobilize some minerals but no effect on vitamins

---

insect repellant, thiamine in daily doses of 75-100mg acts in those who are prone to insect bites, probably because odour of vitamin in skin is repugnant to insects.

---

international units (IU), means of expressing vitamins in terms of biological activity. Now mainly superseded by expressing them as weight (milligrams or micrograms). Only three left that are still measured in units:

Vitamin A, one IU = 0.30 micrograms retinol
One IU beta carotene = 0.10 micrograms retinol
Vitamin D, one IU = 0.025 micrograms
Vitamin E, one IU = 1.0 milligram dl-alpha tocopheryl acetate *or* 0.91mg dl-alpha tocopherol *or* 0.74mg d-alpha tocopheryl acetate *or* 0.67mg d-alpha tocopherol *or* 1.12mg dl-alpha tocopheryl succinate *or* 0.83mg d-alpha tocopheryl succinate.

Other vitamins that were expressed once in international units are:

thiamine hydrochloride, one IU = 3 micrograms
pantothenic acid, one IU = 13.33 micrograms
vitamin C, one IU = 50 micrograms

---

intestinal surgery, post-operative nausea and distension reduced by

250mg calcium pantothenate daily. Vitamin C (1000mg per day) before and after operation will accelerate healing process.

---

intra-uterine devices,   known also as the coil or IUD. Copper has been known to be toxic to spermatozoa since the mid-eighteenth century and the metal is incorporated into intra-uterine devices. A typical copper T-shaped IUD has a copper surface of 135 square millimetres and releases about 29μg of copper daily into the uterine fluid. Localized high concentration of the mineral is believed sufficient to cause a contraceptive effect although local irritations by the device may also play a part. The end-result is inhibition of implantation of the fertilized ovum.

---

intrinsic factor,   specific protein secreted by the stomach that forms a complex with vitamin B_{12} in the diet. Complex is then absorbed in the ileum, the lower part of the small intestine. Lack of intrinsic factor gives rise to pernicious anaemia because B_{12} in diet cannot be absorbed. Factor may also be deficient in those who have had stomach or part of it removed.

Giving intrinsic factor with vitamin B_{12} may help absorb the vitamin but eventually the factor may no longer be effective as it is derived from animals. No more than 8 micrograms of oral dose of vitamin B_{12} absorbed by intrinsic factor mechanism at one time.

---

iodine,   chemical symbol I, atomic weight 126.9. An essential trace element for animals and man.

Food Content
This depends upon the soil content of iodine so food analyses are meaningless. As a general guide the following foods tend to provide our daily intakes of iodine as μg per 100g food:

Fruits, vegetables, cereals and meats	2-5
Haddock	659
Whiting	65-361
Herring	21-27
Dried kelp is the richest source at 535μg per gram	

Geographical Distribution

Worldwide soil distribution extremely variable.

Areas lacking mineral are described as 'goitre belt' since goitre is
  most prevalent disease caused by iodine lack

In the USA, it stretches across the middle of the country

In the UK it is in the Midlands and South West England hence the name
  for the disease 'Derbyshire Neck'

Prevalent also in areas of China, Africa, Continental Europe, Russia
  and South America

Food grown in these soils lacks iodine and those who rely mainly on
  locally-grown produce will not receive the mineral in their diets.

Body Content

The adult contains between 20 and 50mg iodine and most of it is
concentrated in the thyroid gland situated in the base of the neck. The
rest is in the blood as the thyroid hormones triiodothyronine (T_3) and
thyroxine (T_4).

Functions

The functions of iodine reside
solely in its presence in the
thyroid hormones
triiodothyronine and
thyroxine.

These hormones determine
the level of metabolism in the
body i.e. essentially the rate at
which we live. They are
necessary for converting food
into energy and the way we
dissipate that energy.

Deficiency

Deficiency of iodine is an
important world health
problem. At least 200 million
people suffer from diseases
traced to lack of the mineral.
Intakes less than $50\mu g$ per day
induce deficiency.

Lack of iodine gives rise to
goitre; underactive thyroid;
cretinism

Lack of thyroid hormone
(when iodine is adequate)
gives rise to myxoedema.

Deficiency Causes

Reduced dietary intakes
Excessive intakes of anti-
thryoid foods including:
brassica; cabbage; cassava;
kale; ground-nuts; soya beans;
turnips and seeds of cabbage;
mustard and rape.
Some medicinal drugs

Deficiency Symptoms

Apathy
Drowsiness
Sensitivity to cold
Lethargy
Muscle weakness
Weight gain
Coarse skin
All can be due to lack of
iodine or lack of thyroxine

Symptoms of Excess Iodine

Unlikely to happen under
normal circumstances but may
occur in medical treatment
with iodine as iodides. Treat as
medical matter requiring
professional help.

Recommended Daily Intakes

Difficult to assess in view of
varying iodine content of
foods but should be about
200µg
See separate entry

Iodine Supplements (iodine in µg per 100µg)

Ammonium iodide (87.6); calcium iodide (43.2); calcium iodobehenate
(23.5); potassium iodide (76.5); potassium iodate (59.3); sodium iodide
(84.7); iodized table salt (see separate entry); kelp (see separate entry);
sea salt (4).

iodine poisoning, symptoms of acute poisoning from ingestion of
elemental iodine are mainly due to its corrosive effects on the
gastrointestinal tract. It causes a disagreeable metallic taste; vomiting;
abdominal pain and diarrhoea. Eventually the kidneys fail to produce urine,
and swelling of the throat due to oedema or oedema of the lung follows.
The fatal dose is 2 to 3g of elemental iodine. Maximum permissible
atmospheric concentration is 0.1ppm. Large volumes of milk and starch

solutions with 1 per cent solution of potassium thiosulphate are needed in emergency treatment of swallowed iodine.

---

iodism, hypersensitivity to iodine itself or more rarely iodides after prolonged oral administration. Symptoms are: a severe cold in the head (coryza); headache; pain in the salivary glands; watery eyes; weakness; conjunctivitis; fever; laryngitis; bronchitis; skin eruptions; skin rashes; exacerbation of acne.

---

iodized table salt, the addition of sodium or potassium iodide or potassium iodate to table salt to ensure no lack of iodine in the general population. It is carried out in the USA, Switzerland, Yugoslavia, New Zealand and some countries of South America. Salt is not iodized in the UK.

In the USA iodized salt must contain 76µg iodine per g salt. Daily consumption of table salt is estimated at between 2 and 6g providing 152-456µg iodine. New Zealand suggests 84.7µg iodine per g salt. Other countries recommend lower levels in table salt that appear to be just as effective. Salt used in the processing and refining of foods is not usually iodized.

---

iron, chemical symbol Fe, from latin ferrum.

Atomic weight 55.85. Exists as ferrous iron and ferric iron. Essential trace mineral that is present in the body to the extent of 3.5 to 4.5g. Two-thirds is present as haemoglobin, the red oxygen-carrying pigment of blood. The remainder is stored in the liver, spleen, bone-marrow and muscles (where it is present as myoglobin, that acts as an oxygen reservoir within the muscle fibres). In these organs and in the blood plasma iron exists as a protein complex.

Relationship with Vitamin E

Only iron in the ferric form will destroy vitamin E. When in the ferrous form, the mineral is compatible with the vitamin. Use iron supplements only in the ferrous form (look on the pack).

Body Iron Stores

Depend upon iron absorbed from diet. Losses via all routes about 1mg daily. Menstruation increases this by about 0.8mg daily. Losses during breast-feeding about 0.4mg daily. About 24mg iron released daily from normal blood breakdown but most is conserved by the body.

Absorption from Food

Only 1 to 1.5mg absorbed daily (i.e. 10%) from 15 to 20mg in the diet. Absorption highest in childhood, reducing in later years. In food, iron is present in organic haem form and inorganic non-haem form. Haem iron is in meats and is absorbed unaided. Non-haem iron needs vitamin C for efficient absorption. Iron must be in ferrous form to be absorbed.

Iron Supplements (iron in mg per 100mg)

Iron amino acid chelate (10); ferrous aspartate (14.2); ferrous carbonate saccharated (24); ferrous citrate (23.8); ferrous fumarate (31.3); ferrous gluconate (12.5); ferrous glycine sulphate (17.8); ferrous lactate (19.4); ferrous orotate (15.2); ferrous oxalate (31.1); ferrous succinate (32.6); ferrous sulphate (20.1); ferrous tartrate (22.5); ferrocholinate (12.5).

Ferric salts are also widely used but are not recommended as they must be converted first to ferrous salts by the digestive system to be absorbed. Vitamin C appears to be essential in this respect but it can also aid the absorption of ferrous salts.

Deficiency Not Related to Anaemia

Low blood plasma levels of iron can cause generalised itching (pruritus) especially in the aged.

In children, iron deficiency can depress growth and impair mental performance.

Best Food Sources in mg per 100g	
Cockles (molluscs)	33.0
Dried brewer's yeast	20.0
Winkles (molluscs)	15.0
Wheat bran	12.9
Cooked liver	12.5
Cooked kidney	11.5
Cocoa powder	10.5
Soya flour	8.0
Parsley	8.0
Dried fruits	5.8
Sardines	4.6
Cereals	4.1
Corned beef	2.9
Wholemeal bread	2.5
Haricot beans	2.5
Beef	1.9

Functions

In haemoglobin acts as oxygen carrier in red blood cells

In myoglobin acts as oxygen reservoir in muscles

In body cells acts in oxygen transfer in cytochromes

Present in enzyme catalase which protects against peroxide poison

In developing resistance to infection

Recommended Daily Intakes

Vary with the authority — see separate entry.
Usually in the region of 10-12mg for children;
15-18mg for adults

Deficiency Symptoms

Related to the anaemia resulting from reduced haemoglobin levels:
Tiredness
Lack of stamina
Pallor
Breathlessness
Giddiness
Headaches
Insomnia
Palpitations

Ultimate test of deficiency is blood haemoglobin content. Should be within range of 12-16g per 100cc blood. A level less than 12g is considered anaemic and 10 per cent of British women have this. One per cent have haemoglobin less than 8g per 100cc at which level heart output of blood may be affected.

Therapeutic Uses

Iron-deficient anaemia
Generalized itching
Impaired mental performance
in the young

Poisoning with Iron

Accidental poisoning with
ferrous sulphate, usually in
children, can be fatal. As little
as 3g of this substance taken
as one dose has caused death
in a small child.

Symptoms of Excess Intake

Most people simply reject high
intakes of iron and excrete it
in the faeces. However the
non-absorbed iron may induce
constipation or even
diarrhoea. Excessive
deposition of iron in the
tissues can occur in
haemochromatosis, a rare
hereditary disease. It also
happens when the body
cannot rid itself of excess iron
due to certain disease
conditions. Increased body
levels resulting from consistent
high intakes in the diet or by
supplementation are very rare.

---

isoniazid,   anti-tuberculosis drug. Enhances excretion of pyridoxine.

---

isotretinoin,   isomer of retinoic acid, less toxic than tretinoin and given orally.

Itai-itai,   also known as 'ouch-ouch', a disease reported in Japan that is probably associated with high intakes of cadmium from eating rice grown on land irrigated with high cadmium-containing water. Characterized by kidney and gastro-intestinal lesions together with bone softening and severe bone pain similar to that in osteomalacia. Symptoms occurred mainly in older women, particularly those who had borne many children, and in those consuming diets low in protein, vitamin D and calcium. Cadmium may be antagonistic to dietary calcium causing severe deficiency of it.

---

itching, also known as pruritus. A generalized form is sometimes associated with old age. Blood plasma iron levels are usually low despite no iron-deficiency anaemia present. Condition apparently due to response of skin nerves to local iron deficiency. Treatment is with 60mg of elemental iron three times daily. Response is usual within a few days of therapy.

IUD, intra-uterine contraceptive device or coil. *See* contraceptives.

J

jaundice, obstructive. Yellow skin due to excessive bile pigments overflowing from liver because of bile duct blockage. Causes deficient absorption of fat soluble vitamins, particularly vitamin K, which is given by injection. Water-solubilized vitamin E required.

K

K, fat-soluble vitamin, derived from koagulation (Danish).

Occurs naturally in foods as vitamin K_1 also known as phytomenadione, phyloquinone, phytylmenadione, anti-haemorrhagic vitamin. Also produced by intestinal bacteria as vitamin K_2. Synthetic vitamin is K_3, also known as menadione and menaphthone.

K_1 was isolated from alfalfa by Dr Henrik Dam in 1935 at the University of Frieberg; K_2 was isolated from decayed fishmeal by Dr Edward Daisy of St Louis University, USA in 1939.

Best Food Sources in µg per 100g	
Cauliflower	3600
Brussels sprouts	800
Broccoli	800
Lettuce	700
Spinach	600
Pig's liver	600
Cabbage	400
Tomatoes	400
String beans	290
Beef liver	200
Meat	100
Potatoes	80
Pulses (beans)	30

Deficiency Causes

Babies:
  Poor transfer of vitamin across placenta in pregnancy
  Low levels in human milk
  Sterile intestine
Adults:
  Malabsorption of fats
  Lack of bile salts
  Coeliac disease
  Surgery on intestine
  Persistent liquid paraffin intakes
  Antibiotic therapy
  Liver disease of all kinds

Stability in Foods

Survives most domestic cooking methods. Some losses in commercial processing of foods including deep-freezing.

Function

Sole function is in control of blood clotting.

Therapeutic Uses

Haemorrhagic disease of
  new-born
Inability to absorb fats
In long-term antibiotic
  treatment
Treating toxic effects of anti-
  coagulant drops e.g.
Warfarin

Deficiency Symptoms

Usually in the deficient new-born and include:
Excessive bleeding from stomach, intestine, umbilical stump

Recommended Daily Intakes

Not established because of adequate production by intestinal bacteria in healthy person.
Probably need 500-1000µg in diet.

Symptoms of Excess Intake

None have been reported

---

kanamycin, antibiotic. Prevents absorption of vitamins K and B_{12}.

---

kelp, popular name for the seaweed Ascophylum nodosum. Also known as tangle and knotted wrack. Grows in abundance on the west-facing coasts of Europe which are exposed to the Gulf Stream, as well as in the North Temperate Zones on both the Atlantic and Pacific coasts of North America. It feeds through its fronds (leaves) and is attached to rock by holdfasts. Minerals from sea water are concentrated in the body of the plant. After collection from the sea the plant is dried at temperatures between 75 and 85°C then ground to a fine powder. It may be added in this form to foods but is usually taken in the form of compressed tablets. Sometimes the powder is extracted with water and only the aqueous extract is used — the solids content of the extract is usually about 10 per cent.

Kelp is an excellent source of many minerals but it is usually taken for its iodine content. A typical analysis of kelp is (in mg per gram): potassium 19.8; sodium 16.4; calcium 12.3; nitrogen 12.1; sulphur 4.6; magnesium 2.5; phosphorus 1.0. Trace minerals present include (in μg per gram): iodine 535; iron 220; zinc 43; manganese 38; nickel 10; copper 4; cobalt 3; bromine, chromium, lead, strontium, vanadium, all 1; molybdenum 0.1.

Another species laminaria hyperborea is particularly rich in iodine, containing from 5.8-6.8mg per gram, i.e. some ten times more potent than kelp. *See also* kelpware.

---

kelpware,   popular name for the dried thallus (filament without a root) of fucus vesiculosus, fucus serratus and fucus siliquosus. Also known as bladder-wrack, sea-wrack, bladder fucus, black-tang, cut-weed, sea-oak. Found in the Atlantic and Pacific oceans. Mineral contents are similar to those in kelp. *See* kelp.

---

keratinization,   formation of hard, dry, scaly cells in place of normal healthy cells in wet surfaces of the body, particularly around eyes, mouth and lining of reproductive tract. Symptom of vitamin A deficiency.

Keshan disease,   a congestive heart disease that is potentially fatal, affecting children and prevalent in vast areas of rural China. Clinical studies indicate that when given 1000μg selenium per week, affected children were cured of heart disease. When the selenium supplement was given to all members of a commune, incidence of the disease became zero.

---

kidney,   as a food is richest source of vitamin A, B complex and C next to liver. Also provides excellent amounts of trace minerals.

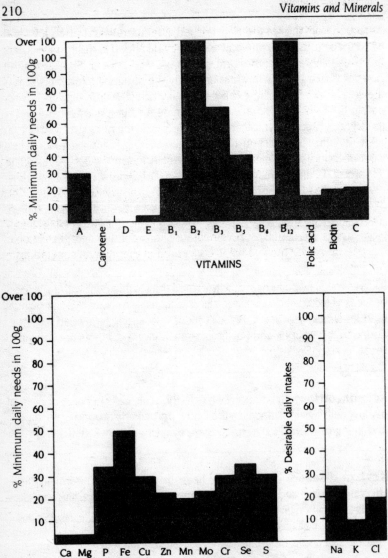

kidney stones, also known as renal stones, renal calculi or urinary calculi. Common causes of back pain, obstruction and secondary infection. Over 90 per cent are composed of calcium salts. The stones cause pain, fever, obstruction of the urinary tract, infection and blood in the urine.

Therapy and prevention involves pyridoxine (up to 100mg daily) plus magnesium (300mg daily) as amino acid chelate to dissolve calcium and prevent its precipitation.

Mineral

Evidence from clinical studies now suggests that such stones can be prevented by suppressing calcium levels with extra magnesium. Quantities required were 200-300mg elemental magnesium daily. Supplementary magnesium has been found to suppress kidney-stone formation in those prone to them; the mineral has also helped remove pre-formed stones in some cases. Vitamin B_6 supplementation may complement the action of magnesium since the vitamin is concerned in the mineral's metabolism.

L

lactoflavin(e), B_2 vitamin.

---

laetrile, water-soluble factor present in vitamin B complex. Also known as amygdalin, B_{17}, vitamin B_{17} (incorrectly); full name laevo-mandelonitrile-beta-glucuronoside. First isolated from apricot kernels in early 1950s by father and son team of Drs E. T. Krebs and E. T. Krebs Jr. White crystalline powder. Present in supplements as laetrile.

Richest sources are apricot kernels (average 5mg per kernel); peach kernels; apple pips; bitter almonds; cherry stones; plum stones; lime pips; pear pips; some grasses; some berries (figures not known).

Unstable to heat so kernels are usually eaten raw.

Functions as source of organic cyanide. Cancer cells believed to convert organic cyanide to inorganic cyanide but unable to detoxify it. Hence inorganic cyanide specifically destroys cancer cells.

Deficiency in man has not been reported.

Deficiency in animals has not been reported.

Recommended dietary intakes not set by any authority.

Toxicity is due entirely to cyanide content.

Toxic symptoms are cold sweats, headaches, nausea, lethargy, breathlessness, blue lips, low blood-pressure — all associated with excess cyanide. Injectable laetrile less toxic than oral dosing.

Controlled by DHSS and available only on prescription.

Therapy with laetrile confined to cancer but benefits very controversial. Injectable preparation preferred but regarded as only part of holistic approach.

---

lead, chemical symbol Pb from the Latin *plumbum*. Atomic weight 207.2. One of the metals known to the ancient world. Occurs in the earth's crust to the extent of 0.002 per cent, mainly as the mineral galena in which it is combined with sulphur.

Traces of lead appear to be essential for the health of some animals but never shown as a necessary trace mineral for man. Problem is one of excessive intakes rather than deficiency.

Excessive intakes may occur from food, drinking water and the air. Exhaust fumes from petrol-driven vehicles are the main source of atmospheric lead which has a maximum permissable concentration of 150µg per cubic metre. In Los Angeles air concentration was 4.5µg per cubic metre in 1969 which contributed significant extra intake. In the UK a survey of drinking water in 43 boroughs indicated that 96 per cent of the population in those boroughs consumed water with a pH less than 7.8 which was sufficiently acid to dissolve lead from piping. In soft-water areas lead piping can give rise to levels of 108µg lead per litre water. Main water supply was only 17.9µg per litre, indicating significant dissolution of lead. Food levels of lead reflect the extent of the metal in the water that irrigates the land on which the food is grown. Home-made beer and wine made in pewter vessels can also contribute significant amounts of lead by dissolution.

Total dietary intake of lead in industrialized societies is between 200 and 400µg daily. Ninety per cent of this is unabsorbed and excreted in the faeces; most of the remainder is got rid of through the kidneys. Some stays behind and a blood level above 42µg per 100ml is associated with lead poisoning.

Toxic effects are well documented in children who are more susceptible to lead poisoning than adults. Poisoning has come from accidental ingestion of lead salts; from lead toys and by sucking lead-painted articles. Acute poisoning causes intense thirst; metallic taste in the mouth; burning abdominal pain; vomiting; diarrhoea; black stools; lack of urine formation; shock; coma. Chronic poisoning is insidious, causing loss of appetite; constipation; headache; weakness; a blue or black lead-line on the gums; anaemia. Later there is vomiting; irritability; inco-ordination; neuritis leading to unsteady gait, visual disturbance, delirium; paralysis (with wrist and foot drop); kidney failure. Acute abdominal pain may result; in pregnancy the uterus violently contracts inducing abortion. Organic lead compounds like those in petrol-vehicle exhaust fumes have a specific action on nervous tissues. Mental disturbances are often a feature; and convulsions may occur.

Anaemia is often the first sign of lead intoxication but it is seldom severe and is characterized by large numbers of immature red blood cells.

---

learning disabilities,   inability to learn and concentrate in children and adolescents. Usually associated with hyperactivity. Megavitamin therapy, *see* hyperactivity.

---

lecithin, a complex mixture of choline, inositol, fatty acids and phosphorus. May be presented as liquid oil (50 per cent lecithin) in capsules or as dry granules (98 per cent lecithin). Colour varies from light yellow to dark brown depending on source, crop variation and treatment. Odourless or with a slight nut-like odour and bland taste.

High concentration in brain, liver, kidneys and bone marrow. Present in all animal and vegetable cells.

Best Food Sources in mg per 100g	
Liver	850
Meats	650
Fish	580
Eggs	350
Butter	150
Wheat	2820
Soya bean	1480
Peanuts	1113
Corn	953
Oats	650
Rice	580

Functions

Solubilizes fat
Mobilizes fat
Prevents fat build up in organs
Constituent of fatty
  membranes
Constituent of myelin sheath
  (insulator around nerves)
Provider of choline
Provider of inositol

Fatty Constituents

Vegetable lecithins provide
  polyunsaturated fats
Animal lecithins provide
  saturated fats

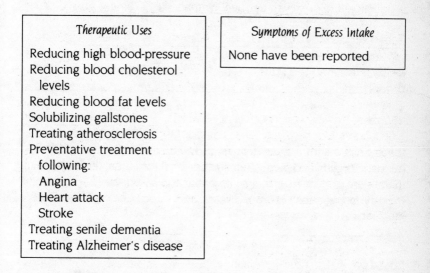

Recommended Daily Intake

Impossible to assess because of synthesis in the body.

Therapeutic Uses

Reducing high blood-pressure
Reducing blood cholesterol
  levels
Reducing blood fat levels
Solubilizing gallstones
Treating atherosclerosis
Preventative treatment
  following:
  Angina
  Heart attack
  Stroke
Treating senile dementia
Treating Alzheimer's disease

Symptoms of Excess Intake

None have been reported

---

leg cramps, *see* cramps.

---

leg ulcers, caused by a breakdown of healthy skin resulting from poor blood circulation; often a feature of deep vein thrombosis, varicose veins and diabetes. Have been treated successfully by a combination of oral zinc supplements (200mg three times daily) and directly applied zinc ointment containing zinc, silver (as silver nitrate) and allantoin (from comfrey) at the 1 per cent strength. *See also* ulcers.

---

leucocytes, white blood cells. Function as phagocytes that engulf invading micro-organisms. Efficiency depends upon mobility of the leucocytes and on their antimicrobial action. Both factors require adequate vitamin C concentration in leucocytes. Those with low resistance to infection need up to 3 grams vitamin C daily to ensure adequate levels.

Lymphocytes are white blood cells that produce antibodies to neutralize invading organisms. Vitamin C in lymphocytes essential for antibody production. Children with deficient lymphocytes exhibit normal defence response to infection with one gram of vitamin C daily.

---

lipids, general term for all fatty substances including fats, oils, phospholipids (lecithin), cholesterol, triglycerides, fatty acids. *See* under individual headings.

---

lipoic acid, known also as thioctic acid. Regarded as vitamin for bacteria, protozoa, plants and some animals. Essential for pyruvate oxidation in these species. Not regarded as essential in man but has been used as therapy in treatment of liver disease and in poisoning by non-edible mushrooms.

---

liquid paraffin, anti-constipation agent. Prevents absorption of vitamins A, D, E and K and carotenes.

---

lithium, chemical symbol Li. Atomic weight 6.9. An alkali metal. Occurrence in earth's crust is 0.005 per cent by weight as the minerals spodumene, lepidolite, petalite and triphylite.

Lithium is not considered to be an essential trace mineral in animals or man but it is usually supplied to the body in drinking water. Studies on communities differing in lithium content of their drinking water suggest that higher intakes of the mineral result in lower death-rates from heart attacks; lower number of admissions for mental disorders; lower suicide rates; lower murder rates; lower incidence of gastric and duodenal ulcers; lower incidence of gout; lower incidence of rheumatism. Low lithium levels in water were found to be 8mg per litre; high levels were 100mg per litre. Some South American Indian communities known for their quiet, peaceful ways and reduced incidence of arthritic complaints, gastroduodenal ulcers and heart disease have been found to have lithium intakes from their drinking water some 50 times more than the average Western World community.

Absorption of lithium is very efficient and is passive, requiring no specific absorption process. It is rapidly distributed throughout the body with highest concentrations occurring in the bones, the thyroid gland and the brain. Most excretion occurs through the kidneys into the urine and there are also losses in the sweat and saliva. The mineral crosses the placenta in the pregnant female and also appears in the breast milk of the nursing mother. All information on distribution throughout the body has come from studies on people given high doses of lithium. It cannot be detected easily in the body when the sole source is dietary.

Food sources of lithium are not known as levels have not been measured. Concentrations in drinking water can range from 4-150mg per litre and this represents the main source for most people.

Functions of lithium include that of a mood stabilizer. This has been utilized in psychiatry where the mineral is given as a treatment for mania and in the prevention of manic depression and depression. It could also be acting in a similar manner in those communities who have a high intake from their water supply but the evidence is based only on epidemiological studies.

How it functions is unknown. Observed effects of lithium when given in drug doses are:

1. increased turnover of the hormone noradrenaline;
2. displacement of sodium from extracellular fluids;
3. reduction of bone mineral content;
4. increased blood serum concentrations of magnesium, calcium and phosphate;
5. increased blood plasma level of parathormone (from the parathyroid glands) which controls calcium and phosphorus metabolism;
6. a reduced synthesis and release of thyroid hormones;
7. an increased release of insulin enhancing formation of muscle glycogen;
8. increase in blood plasma level of anti-diuretic hormone (vasopressin);
9. transient increase in blood plasma level of aldosterone.

Therapy with lithium in acute mania requires constant monitoring of the plasma concentration to ensure that this lies close to 0.7mg per 100ml. At this level there is no interference with sodium and potassium levels. If lithium concentration rises above 1.4mg per 100ml adverse effects will appear. Treatment must therefore be left in the hands of a medical practitioner who has access to a blood plasma monitoring service.

In the past, lithium has also been used to treat leucopenia (low white blood cell count), hyperthyroidism, Ménière's disease, tardive dyskinesia, Huntington's chorea; and in the management of migraine, cluster headache, epilepsy, premenstrual syndrome. Many of these non-psychiatric uses are anecdotal and need to be investigated further. Doses of blood serum concentrations of lithium for use in these disorders have not been standardized.

Therapeutic forms of lithium are lithium carbonate; lithium citrate; lithium chloride; lithium sulphate; lithium aspartate; lithium gluconate; lithium orotate; lithium acetate. All are classed as prescription drugs only.

Excessive intakes give rise to nausea; vomiting; diarrhoea; coarse tremor; sluggishness; defective speech at blood plasma levels greater than 1.05mg per 100ml. At higher levels, i.e. greater than 1.4mg per 100ml the mineral gives rise to manifestations of impaired consciousness; abnormal muscle tenseness; coarse tremor; twitchings; increased reflex action; epileptic fits; 'coma vigil', where the individual can react when spoken to only by moving the head or eyes.

---

liver, largest gland in the body forming one-fortieth of body weight.

Storage depot for vitamins A, D, riboflavin, pantothenic acid, biotin, folic acid, pyridoxine, vitamin B_{12} and vitamin C. Contains sufficient vitamin A, D and B_{12} to last 6 months to 2 years in well-fed person. Other vitamins must be replenished regularly every day or so.

Site for activation of all vitamins, i.e., conversion of thiamine, riboflavin, nicotinamide, pyridoxine, pantothenic acid, biotin into phosphate complexes; conversion of folic acid to folinic acid; conversion of vitamin B_{12} into its coenzyme forms; conversion of vitamin D into 25-hydroxy vitamin D; conversion of vitamin A into retinoic acid. All these transformations essential before vitamins can perform metabolic functions. *Site* for synthesis of choline and inositol and further incorporation into lecithin. *Site* for conversion of cholesterol into bile salts, dependent on vitamin C. *Site* for production of proteins needed for blood clotting, dependent upon vitamin K.

Diseases of liver can cause excessive loss of all vitamins but especially the B complex; can prevent uptake of vitamins by the liver; can reduce efficiency

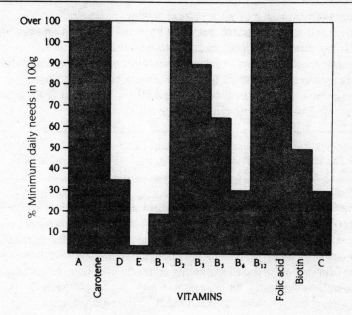

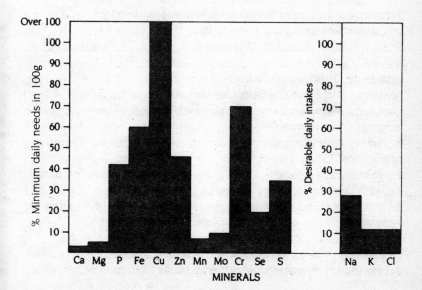

of activation of vitamins into metabolic forms.

Alcohol and some medicinal drugs can have similar effects on vitamins. *Fatty liver* due to deficiency of choline and inositol.

As *a food*, liver from all sources supplies large quantities of vitamin A and carotene with some vitamins D and E. Rich source of the B vitamins and unlike most foods of animal origin, provides some vitamin C. Excellent source of all minerals including trace elements.

LLD factor, B_{12} vitamin.

---

loss of taste, also known as hypogeusia. A symptom associated with many conditions, e.g. head colds; pregnancy; old age. Associated also with copper deficiency; zinc deficiency; and vitamin deficiencies (especially vitamins A, B_6 and B_{12}). Loss of taste perception may be associated with a deficient protein in the saliva, known as gustin, that is a zinc-containing protein. Treating gustin-deficient people with zinc supplements (25mg of the element daily) restored gustin contents of the saliva to normal and the sense of taste returned. Studies have indicated that about one third of those with hypogeusia are zinc deficient. It is worthwhile, therefore, to take extra zinc as first-line treatment in any case of taste loss.

---

losses in food processing, the term food processing includes domestic cooking techniques as well as those used in the food manufacturing industry. Losses of nutrients, particularly vitamins, may be summed up as follows:

1. Some loss of vitamins is inevitable but, except for the examples quoted below, most losses are small.

2. Manufacturing losses, when they occur, are sometimes comparable to those in domestic cooking losses.

3. When foods are further cooked at home, losses of vitamins are additional to those incurred during the manufacturing process.

4. It is easier and more convenient to recover vitamins lost during domestic cooking (e.g. by utilizing cooking water) than those lost in factory processing.

5. The importance of the losses in a particular food must be considered

in relation to the whole diet. When the food makes only a small contribution to the intake of vitamins, processing losses may not be significant. However, losses from foods that make up a significant part of the diet, like milk and cereal products for babies and cereals in some countries, can cause serious deficiencies in those relying on such diets.

6. Some processing methods confer nutritional advantages on the vitamin content of food, e.g. thiamin inhibitors in some vegetables are destroyed by cooking and nicotinic acid is liberated from its inactive bound form by the cooking of cereals.

7. Under-processing of some foods may not destroy harmful micro-organisms in those foods. Processing can improve appearance and flavour of some foods and allow preservation for all-round-the-year availability. The ideal conditions of food processing allow these advantages with only minimal destruction and loss of vitamins.

Nicotinic acid — is very stable and leaching causes the only losses. It is unaffected by heat, air, light, acidity and alkalinity, and by sulphite. One of the few vitamins to be liberated by cooking processes since in many cereals it is bound to starches and proteins in a complex called niacytin which is not digested in the gastro-intestinal tract. In wheat flour, 77 per cent of the nicotinic acid is in a bound form that is completely liberated by baking with alkaline baking powder. In Mexico maize is soaked overnight in lime water before making tortillas in order to free the vitamin.

Some loss of nicotinic acid when cooking meat but all can be recovered from the juices. Roasting beef and pork at 150°C loses less than 10 per cent of the vitamin; at temperatures of 205°C (which give an internal temperature of 98°C) losses are 30 per cent. Dry curing of meat gives rise to no losses of nicotinic acid; wet curing causes 20 per cent of it to be leached but this is recoverable.

No nicotinic acid is lost in the pasteurization and sterilization of milk or in the production of dried milk and dried egg.

Pyridoxine — is very stable to heat but pyridoxal and pyridoxamine are more sensitive. Stability in milk during sterilization or drying is reduced due to interaction with milk proteins. Losses can occur up to 20 per cent during milk sterilization; higher temperatures cause more serious losses. No destruction of pyridoxine during cooking. Three forms of the vitamin are all stable to air, acid and alkali. Canning of beans gives rise to 20 per cent loss into blanching water and 15 per cent in steam but all can be recovered by utilizing the water. Losses into thawed fluids of 20-40 per cent can occur when frozen vegetables are cooked.

Vitamin A — Both vitamin A and carotene are insoluble in water so do not suffer from losses through extraction into processing and cooking water. The main destructive agent is oxygen but in foods they tend to be protected by natural antioxidants like vitamin E.

Destruction of vitamin A and carotenes is accelerated by peroxides and free radicals formed from accompanying fats, particularly those of the polyunsaturated variety. Peroxides and free radicals in turn are formed by high temperatures and oxygen and promoted by light, traces of iron and the presence of copper.

The amounts of vitamin A left after boiling margarine in water and frying in the fat are indicated thus:

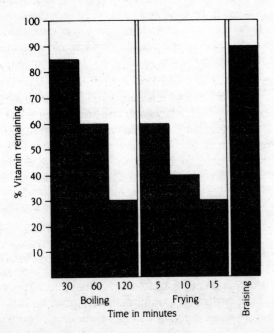

Canning green vegetables causes 15-20 per cent loss in vitamin A activity: yellow vegetables lose 30-35 per cent. Drying vegetables and fruits under mild, controlled conditions gives rise up to 20 per cent loss: traditional open-air drying methods destroy the vitamin completely.

Vitamin B$_{12}$ — unstable in the presence of alkali but stable under all other conditions of cooking. Light may destroy some but proteins in the food appear to protect the vitamin. Leaching represents main loss in food preparation.

Thiamine — apart from vitamin C, thiamine is the least stable of the vitamins. Stable only under acid conditions, destruction is catalysed by copper. Completely inactivated by sulphur dioxide, a widespread preservative added to foods, e.g. mince containing sulphur dioxide loses 90 per cent of its thiamine in 48 hours. Protein and amino acids protect thiamine in foods and starch assists by absorbing the vitamin. Cereals are added to pork to help stabilize thiamine in cooked meats.

Principal losses of thiamine are due to its water solubility: the more finely ground the food the greater the loss. Chopped and minced foods can lose from 20-70 per cent of their thiamine which can be recovered by eating the extracted liquors. Cooking meat at temperatures up to 150°C causes no destruction of the vitamin but considerable losses into the exuded juices. At temperatures of 200°C, 20 per cent of the thiamine is destroyed.

The vitamin is not lost by leaching when boiling rice in distilled water but 8-10 per cent is lost in tap water and 36 per cent is lost in well water, indicating the effects of alkalinity. Baking processes cause 15-25 per cent loss of the vitamin but adding baking powder increases it to 50 per cent.

Amongst vegetables, only potatoes contribute significant amounts of thiamine (about 15 per cent of the daily intakes) to the diet. Ready-peeled potatoes and potato chips are kept white by adding sulphite solution causing 55 per cent destruction of the vitamin present. Further frying results in 10 per cent additional loss from unpreserved variety and 20 per cent from the vegetable soaked in sulphite solution. Commercial processing causes 24 per cent losses in potatoes dipped in sulphite solution after three days' storage at 5°C: further losses on frying can be 30 per cent.

Meats, poultry and fish represent important sources of thiamine in the diet but much of the vitamin can be lost depending upon the cooking method used. These are indicated as shown in the table overleaf:

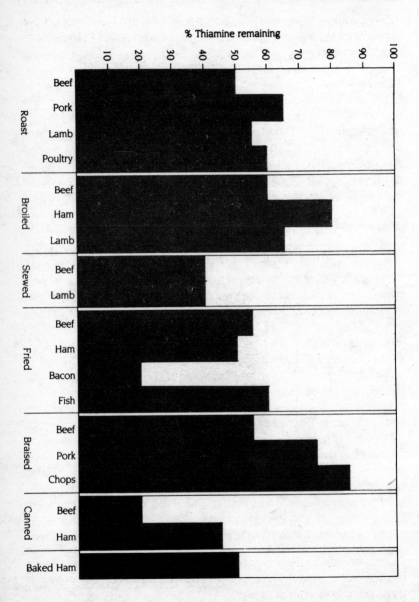

Baking of bread gives rise to losses up to 30 per cent in the finished loaf but no further breakdown occurs. Toasting of bread causes further losses up to 30 per cent.

Riboflavin — is stable to oxygen, acid and heat up to 130°C. Unstable to alkalis and light. Readily lost by leaching from chopped foods in wet processing and cooking.

Light in presence of alkali converts riboflavin to lumiflavin which in turn destroys vitamin C. In milk 5 per cent lumiflavin can cause 50 per cent loss in vitamin C content. Under any conditions, however, light remains the great destroyer of riboflavin as shown in this chart which refers to the vitamin in milk and bread after only two hours exposure:

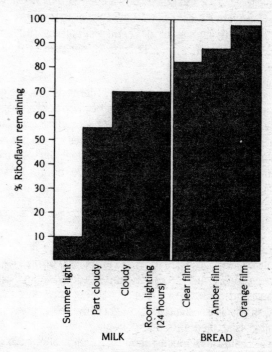

In the dark, under slightly acid conditions, riboflavin is completely stable, e.g. after 48 days in cold storage beef has the same vitamin content as that immediately after slaughter.

Milk loses riboflavin when heated. On boiling there are losses of 12-25 per cent; in pasteurization these losses are 14 per cent. Similar losses occur in meat cooking and in all cases losses are greater in the presence of light. Dry curing of meat gives rise to 40 per cent loss of riboflavin content; wet curing causes similar losses.

Folic acid — unstable only in the free form. Losses are 10 per cent on steam blanching, 20 per cent on pressure cooking and 25-50 per cent on boiling vegetables. Can be destroyed by oxidation. Losses from sterilized milk can vary from 20-100 per cent depending on time of contact with air. If vitamin C is present, there is protective effect and no folic acid is lost. If vitamin C is destroyed by subsequent reheating, folic acid is also oxidized.

It is sensitive to sunlight and destruction is catalysed by riboflavin so keep foods dark. Cumulative losses of folic acid occur in food processing and total losses can be as high as 65 per cent. Vegetables, fruits, bread and dairy products can be left with as little as 30 per cent of their folic acid content when finally eaten.

Pantothenic acid — stable under most cooking methods that are carried out in neutral conditions but destroyed by heat both on acid and alkaline side of neutrality. Wheat suffers a 60 per cent loss during manufacturing procedures involving baking powder. Meat losses are 30 per cent during cooking but most is recoverable as it is due to leaching. Six to eight per cent is lost from meats over periods up to twelve months in deep frozen state.

Biotin — nothing is known about its stability in cooking processes.

Vitamin C — most unstable of all the vitamins.

Soft fruits like strawberries, raspberries and blackcurrants lose up to 60 per cent of the vitamin when processed and stored. Vitamin C in fruit juices is very unstable and losses up to 50 per cent are common once the container is opened. Virtually all is lost after a fortnight in the refrigerator, particularly if the container is shaken after each opening.

The chart indicates how much vitamin C remains after cooking various vegetables under different conditions.

All the vitamin C leached out into the water can be recovered by utilizing the water in sauces, gravies etc.

Vitamin D — regarded as being very stable but few studies carried out. It withstands smoking of fish, pasteurization and sterilization of milk and drying of eggs. Probably loses between 25 and 35 per cent of activity during

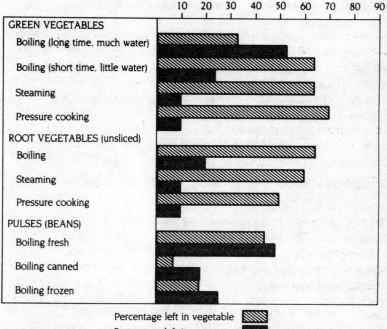

| | 10 20 30 40 50 60 70 80 90 |

GREEN VEGETABLES
  Boiling (long time, much water)
  Boiling (short time, little water)
  Steaming
  Pressure cooking
ROOT VEGETABLES (unsliced)
  Boiling
  Steaming
  Pressure cooking
PULSES (BEANS)
  Boiling fresh
  Boiling canned
  Boiling frozen

Percentage left in vegetable
Percentage left in water

the spray-drying of milk but this is allowed for in fortification.

Vitamin E — very sensitive to oxidation, particularly in the presence of heat and alkali. Serious degradation in frozen foods, e.g. potato crisps lose 48 per cent of their vitamin E after two weeks at room temperature; 70 per cent after four weeks and 77 per cent in eight weeks. Even at deep-freeze temperatures (-12°C) vitamin E losses can total 68 per cent after two weeks. French-fried potatoes at the same low temperature can lose 68 per cent and 74 per cent of the vitamin after one month and two months respectively.

Processing and refining of cereals lead to wholesale losses of vitamin E. The most serious is the decrease in the vitamin content of white flour

(92 per cent) when it is produced from wholewheat grains. Wholemeal bread provides 2.2mg per 100g compared with only 0.23mg in the white variety because the wheatgerm is removed and bleaching agents destroy vitamin E.

Cooking food in fats destroys 70-90 per cent of the vitamin E content. Greatest losses happen in the presence of rancid fats and oils and these cannot always be detected by taste. Continual use of cooking fats and oils (e.g. in chip pan) consistently destroys the vitamin in the food being fried.

Tocopherol esters are more stable than the free tocopherol. Only 10-20 per cent of the ester was destroyed under conditions that completely inactivated the free vitamin.

Boiling destroys 30 per cent of the vitamin E in sprouts, cabbages and carrots. Canning of vegetables leads to even greater losses, up to 80 per cent of the original content.

---

losses of vitamin C in cooking, depend upon cooking method:

Boiled, peeled and mashed: 30-50 per cent lost.
Boiled, unpeeled: 20-40 per cent lost.
Baked: 20-40 per cent lost.
Roast: 20-40 per cent lost.
Steamed: 20-40 per cent lost.
Chips: 25-35 per cent lost.

Losses can be minimized by keeping volume of water low. Much of the vitamin C can be recovered from the cooking water by utilizing it in sauces, gravy, etc.

---

losses of vitamin C in storage, vitamin C is lost steadily from potatoes once they leave the ground and are stored:

Main crop, freshly dug contain 30mg per 100g.
After 1-3 months' storage contain 20mg per 100g.
After 4-5 months' storage contain 15mg per 100g.
After 6-7 months' storage contain 10mg per 100g.
After 8-9 months' storage contain 8mg per 100g.

---

lumbago, pain, tenderness and stiffness in the back muscles. Has been relieved by high doses (up to 600mg) of thiamine. May also respond to 2g calcium pantothenate daily.

---

lung cancer, *see* cancer.

M

---

magnesium, chemical symbol Mg, atomic weight 24.31. Name is derived from the Greek city Magnesia where there are large deposits of magnesium carbonate. Body contains about 25g of magnesium of which half is found in the bones. The rest is distributed amongst the organs, nerves and blood.

Best Food Sources in mg per 100g	
Soya beans	310
Nuts	250
Dried brewer's yeast	230
Wholewheat flour	140
Brown rice	119
Dried peas	116
Shrimps	110
Wholemeal bread	93
Rye flour	92
Seafoods	90
Dried fruits	80
Vegetables	60
Meats	50
Bananas	42
Greenleaf vegetables	25

Functions

Cofactor in many body processes including energy production and cell replication.
Cofactor for vitamins B_1 and B_6
Stabilizes body cell structure
In growth
In repair and maintenance of body cells
Cofactor in hormones
Component of chlorophyll
Nerve impulse transmission

Deficiency Symptoms

Weakness
Tiredness
Vertigo
Convulsions
Nervousness
Muscle cramps and tremors
Tongue jerks and tremors
Involuntary eye movements
Unsteady gait
Hyperactivity in children
Irregular heartbeat
Palpitations
Low blood sugar
Painful swallowing

Deficiency Causes

Reduced dietary intake due
   to poor diet, malnutrition,
   anorexia nervosa, high fibre
   intake, loss of appetite
High dietary intake of
   phosphate calcium, vitamin
   D and saturated fats
Reduced absorption due to
   laxative abuse, infections or
   allergies (coeliac disease)
Kidney disease; diabetes;
   cancer; alcoholism; drug
   diuretics; antibiotics; heart
   drugs
Contraceptive pill
High milk intake in diet

Therapeutic Uses

Premenstrual tension
Menstrual cramps
Toxaemia of pregnancy
Morning sickness
Hypoglycaemia (low blood
   sugar)
Atherosclerosis, arteriosclerosis
Angina
Abnormal and irregular
   heartbeats
Epilepsy
Alcoholism
Kidney stones
Insomnia
Hyperactivity in children

Heart Disease

May be related to low body
magnesium levels because
death rates from coronary
heart disease are higher in
soft-water areas worldwide.
Missing mineral in soft water is
magnesium which is decreased
in the heart muscle of those
dying from heart attacks.

Effects of Excess Intakes of Magnesium

Flushing of the skin
Thirst   ⎫   These are highly unlikely in
Low blood pressure ⎬ normal individuals who take
Loss of reflexes   ⎬ too much magnesium because
Shallow breathing ⎭   intestines reject excess
                      mineral. Most likely in those
                      with kidney disease.

Can act as a purgative

Recommended Daily Intakes

Vary with authority but in the region of 400mg. See separate entry.

Magnesium Supplements (magnesium in mg per 100mg)

Magnesium amino acid chelate (18); dolomite (13); magnesium carbonate (25.2); magnesium acetate (11.2); magnesium chloride (11.8); magnesium citrate (16.2); magnesium gluconate (5.3); magnesium orotate (6.9); magnesium oxide (59.5); magnesium sulphate (9.7).

---

magnesium stearate, consists of a mixture of magnesium stearate and magnesium palmitate, prepared from magnesium and vegetable oils (or sometimes animal fats). Used in dusting powders in skin diseases and in cosmetics. Acts as mechanical barrier in barrier cream. Added to tablets as a lubricant to prevent tablets sticking during manufacture but quantity used is usually only up to 5mg per tablet.

Provides about 4.5mg magnesium in 100mg stearate so when used as lubricant adds only 0.2mg magnesium to tablet. Not used as a supplement because of its water insolubility. Inhalation of magnesium stearate by babies can cause toxic effects but no evidence that small amounts used as tablet lubricant are harmful.

Used also as a food additive. Functions as an emulsifier; an anti-caking agent; a release agent. Acceptable daily intake not limited. Permitted as a miscellaneous additive.

---

magnesium sulphate, also known as Epsom Salts. It is a common ingredient of aperient mineral waters. Rarely used as a supplement although when taken for its mild purgative effect significant amounts may be absorbed. Should not be taken by those with impaired kidney function and by children with intestinal parasitic diseases. Acts in dilute solution when swallowed by reducing the normal absorption of water from the intestine with the result that the bulky fluid contents distend the bowel and evacuation of the contents of the intestine follows in 1 or 2 hours.

Provides 9.7mg magnesium in 100mg sulphate. As a purgative dose is 5-15g sulphate in 250ml water, preferably before breakfast. For children dose is 100-250mg sulphate per kg body weight.

Used also as a food additive. Functions as a dietary supplement; as a firming agent; in brewing. Acceptable daily intake has not been determined. Permitted in boiler feed water for direct steam treatment of milk; as a miscellaneous additive.

---

manganese, chemical symbol Mn, atomic weight 54.9. An essential trace element for human beings.

Body Content and Turnover

An adult contains between 12 and 20mg.
Highest concentrations in skeleton, liver, kidneys and heart.
Daily losses in the faeces are about 4mg (via the bile)
Only 3 to 5 per cent of dietary manganese is absorbed

Therapeutic Uses

Schizophrenia
Myasthenia gravis
Anaemia (improves utilization
 of iron
Benefits claimed in the above
 conditions

Supplementation is also wise
in other conditions under
Deficiency Symptoms

Deficiency

Usually related to poor dietary intake when processed and refined foods form large part of diet. Rarely may be due to excessive copper intakes.

Best Food Sources
in mg per 100g

Cereals	4.92
Wholemeal bread	4.21
Nuts	3.54
Pulses (beans)	2.01
Fruit	1.05
Greenleaf vegetables	0.78
Liver	0.64
Root vegetables	0.58
Meats and fish	0.02
Black tea (0.5mg per cup)	

Functions

Growth
Maintains healthy nervous system
Cofactor for enzymes for energy production and health of joints
Cofactor for female sex hormones
Cofactor for nucleic acid synthesis
Production of thyroxine
Cofactor for vitamins B, C and E
Synthesis of structural proteins of body cells
Development and maintenance of healthy bones
Stimulates glycogen (animal starch) storage in liver

Deficiency Symptoms

There are no specific symptoms associated with deficiency but low blood and tissue levels reported in:
Diabetes
Heart disease
Schizophrenia
Atherosclerosis
Myasthenia gravis (muscle wasting and weakness)
Rheumatoid arthritis
Infants before weaning

Symptoms of Excess Intake

These are very rare from oral ingestion of manganese but include: lethargy; involuntary movements; lack of control of voluntary movements; changes in muscle tone; postural changes; coma.

Recommended Dietary Intakes

Suggestions are from 2.5 to 5.0mg. There are usually easily obtained from good diets. Tea can provide up to half required intake in tea-drinking countries like UK and Australia.

Manganese Supplements (in mg per 100mg)

Manganese amino acid chelate (10); manganese sulphate (24.6); manganese gluconate (11.4); manganese orotate (315.2); manganese chloride (27.7); manganese glycerophosphate (24.4); manganese hypophosphite (27.1).

---

margarine, both hard and soft are fortified with vitamins A and D to contain (in µg per 100g): vitamin A 900; vitamin D 7.94. Good source of vitamin E, providing 8.0mg per 100g. Traces only of all B vitamins but contains no vitamin C.

---

marzipan, vitamins are provided by almonds, lemon juice and eggs. Vitamin A content is 10µg per 100g, but carotene is absent. Vitamin D content of 0.13µg per 100g. Good provider of vitamin E at 9.1mg per 100g. B vitamins present are (in mg per 100g): thiamine 0.12; riboflavin 0.45; nicotinic acid 2.4; pyridoxine 0.06; pantothenic acid 0.35. Folic acid level is 45µg per 100g; biotin level is 2µg per 100g. Vitamin C content is 2mg per 100g.

Mineral
Excellent source of potassium and is also low in sodium. Rich source of calcium, magnesium and phosphorus. Good source of iron, zinc and sulphur. Mineral levels are (in mg per 100g): sodium 13; potassium 400; calcium 120; magnesium 120; phosphorus 220; iron 2.0; copper 0.08; zinc 1.5; sulphur 81; chloride 13.

---

meats, all muscle meats, whether from beef, lamb, veal or poultry (chicken and turkey). contain only traces of vitamins A. D and carotene and little vitamin E. They are completely devoid of vitamin C and provide very little folic acid and biotin. Pork is a better provider of the B vitamins but these tend to be reduced a little in the curing process to produce bacon.

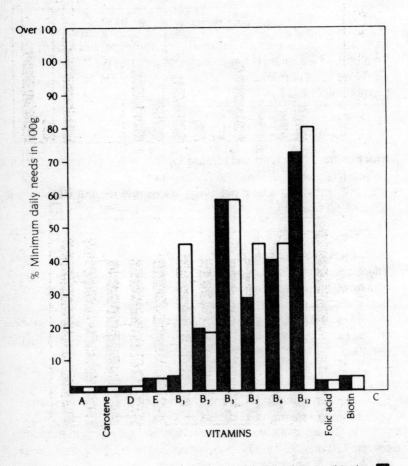

Beef. Lamb. Veal and Poultry ■
Pork and Bacon □

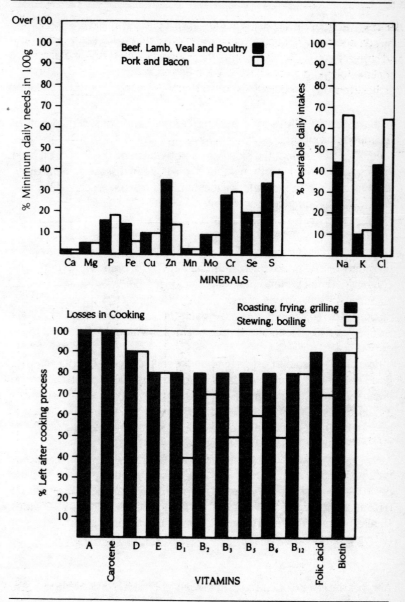

megaloblastic anaemia, characterized by appearance of large, immature red blood cells with shortened life-span. May be due to deficiency of folic acid, vitamin B_{12} or pyridoxine. Only treatment is to replace specific deficient vitamin.

---

megavitamin therapy, treating certain conditions with doses of vitamins far above the levels found even in good diets. Using vitamins as medicines but without the side-effects noted with drugs. Has been used successfully in treating arthritis, autism, colds, heart disease, hyperactivity, learning disabilities, respiratory infections, schizophrenia, senile dementia. *See* individual complaint for treatment.

---

melons, *Canteloupe,* raw, edible portion is very rich source of carotene, providing also a good amount of vitamin C. The orange-coloured flesh contains 2.0mg carotene per 100g plus 0.1mg per 100g of vitamin E. B vitamins present are (in mg per 100g): thiamine 0.05; riboflavin 0.03; nicotinic acid 0.5; pyridoxine 0.07; pantothenic acid 0.23. Folic acid level is 30μg per 100g; biotin has not been detected. Vitamin C content is 25mg per 100g.

Honeydew, raw, edible portion is moderate source of carotene but provides good amounts of vitamin C. Carotene content is 100μg per 100g for the green-coloured flesh; vitamin E level is 0.1mg per 100g. B vitamins present are (in mg per 100g): thiamine 0.05; riboflavin 0.03; nicotinic acid 0.5; pyridoxine 0.07; pantothenic acid 0.23. Folic acid level is 30μg per 100g; biotin is absent. Vitamin C content is 25mg per 100g.

Watermelon, raw, edible portion is poor source of all vitamins except pantothenic acid and C. Carotene is 20μg per 100g; vitamin E level is 0.1mg per 100g. B vitamins present are (in mg per 100g): thiamine 0.02; riboflavin 0.02; nicotinic acid 0.3; pyridoxine 0.07; pantothenic acid 1.55. Provides small amount of folic acid (3μg per 100g) but no biotin. Vitamin C content is 5mg per 100g.

Mineral
All types are low in sodium and supply very good levels of potassium. Some trace minerals present.

Canteloupe variety, levels for raw, edible portion (in mg per 100g): sodium 14; potassium 320; calcium 19; magnesium 20; phosphorus 30; iron 0.8; copper 0.04; zinc 0.1; sulphur 12; chloride 44.

Honeydew variety, levels for raw, edible portion (in mg per 100g): sodium 20; potassium 220; calcium 14; magnesium 13; phosphorus 9; iron 0.2; copper 0.04; zinc 0.1; sulphur 6; chloride 45.

Watermelon, raw, edible portion, contains the following levels (in mg per 100g): sodium 4; potassium 120; calcium 5; magnesium 11; phosphorus 8; iron 0.3; copper 0.03; zinc 0.1.

---

memory, when faulty may be symptom of thiamine deficiency. Treat with adequate doses (up to 50mg daily) of vitamin B_1. When associated with age may respond to choline. *See* senile dementia. Claims that RNA intake may help improve memory, particularly in the aged.

---

menaphthone, K_3 vitamin.

---

menaquinone, K_2 vitamin.

Meniere's disease, a disorder characterized by recurrent severe vertigo, deafness, tinnitus (noises in the ear), nausea and vomiting. Some relief gained by following regime: thiamine (10-25mg); riboflavin (10-25mg); 50:50 mixture of nicotinic acid:nicotinamide (100-250mg); all four times daily for two weeks. If relief obtained, reduce all vitamins to dose that maintains relief and continue.

Menke's syndrome, is a rare genetic disease characterized by an inability of the baby to absorb copper, resulting in progressive degeneration of the nervous system. Deterioration starts with convulsions at three months of age and death used to occur within three years. Symptoms and signs are failure to keratinize hair which looks like steel wool, hence the name 'steely-hair syndrome'; mental retardation; low body temperature; low copper levels in blood plasma and in liver; weakened skeleton; degenerative changes in the walls of the aorta. Provided diagnosis is made early in life, the condition can be controlled with intravenous copper.

---

menopause,   period in a woman's life when her secretion of female sex hormones slows down and eventually ceases. Characterized by hot flushes, headaches, giddiness, 'nerves', depression, excessive menstrual flow, increase in weight, pruritus (itching) in sexual parts.

Vitamin E (100IU with each meal) claimed to relieve hot flushes, headaches, 'nerves'. Pyridoxine (50-100mg daily) may help relieve depression. Iron (15mg) and vitamin C (200mg) daily will help replace blood losses. Calcium (1000mg) and vitamin D (6.25μg) will help prevent calcium loss from bones induced by deficiency of oestrogens.

---

menstrual cramps,   abdominal cramps that tend to occur a few days before menstruation and may continue through the first few days of the menstrual flow. Has been found to respond, along with associated leg and back cramps, to supplementary calcium, 500-1000mg in the few days preceding menstruation until it has finished.

---

menstruation,   monthly breakdown of lining of uterus leading to loss of blood in the menstrual flow.

Blood loss replaced by adequate intakes of mineral iron (24mg) with vitamin C (100mg); vitamin E (100IU); folic acid (200μg) and vitamin B_{12} (5μg). Mild depression that occurs just before menstruation often responds to pyridoxine — *see* depression. Irregular or painful menstrual periods may respond to bioflavonoids (1000mg daily).

---

mental ability,   may be increased in normal children with thiamine (1.0mg); vitamin C (100mg) and vitamin E (100IU) daily to ensure adequate intakes and so maximize potential.

---

mental disturbance, can be related to mild deficiencies of vitamins, particularly thiamine, riboflavin, nicotinamide, pyridoxine, folic acid, vitamin B_{12}. Individual may also be vitamin-dependent, requiring larger intakes than can be obtained from diet. *See* autism, depression, megavitamin therapy, schizophrenia, senile dementia.

---

mercury, Chemical symbol Hg, from the Latin *hydrargyrum*. Atomic weight 200.6. Also known as quicksilver, liquid silver. Occurs in nature as cinnabar (mercuric sulphide) with an abundance in the earth's crust of 0.5mg per kg.

Not known to have any essential role in the metabolism of any living organism. In the form of liquid or gaseous mercury it is toxic. Mercury salts and particularly organic forms of mercury are more poisonous than the element. Dental amalgams used for filling teeth cavities are so insoluble that they are usually not regarded as toxic but some doubts expressed recently on the safety of the tiny amounts eroded from fillings. Claims that cancer, heart disease, menstrual and thyroid problems relieved by removal of amalgam fillings. The most dangerous forms of mercury are the alkyl derivatives methylmercury and ethylmercury. They are usually introduced into the body from fish and grain foods.

Inorganic mercury salts, introduced by pollution into fresh and sea waters, are converted by micro-organisms into methylmercury. This is introduced into the food chain via plant-eating small fish to carnivorous large fish like tuna, swordfish and pike. When these fish are eaten by man, poisoning results. Fatal levels of contamination in such fish have been reported from Japan where industrial pollution introduced mercury salts into sea water.

Fish from inland fresh-water lakes in Sweden and North America may contain as much as 503µg mercury per 100g which is a toxic level. Canned tuna can contain from 10-80µg mercury per 100g, half as methylmercury. Deep-sea fish caught off the UK fishing grounds contain only 8µg mercury per 100g, but nearer the coasts where chemical effluents are discharged into the sea, fish may contain up to 50µg mercury per 100g. The highest tolerable weekly intake of mercury according to WHO recommendations is 300µg, of which no more than 200µg should be methylmercury.

Seeds that have been dusted with alkyl mercury compounds to prevent fungal contamination have caused poisoning in Guatamala, Iraq and

Pakistan. The poisoning was accidental since the seeds were not meant for human consumption but 459 deaths resulted from 6500 cases. Similar treated seeds fed to farm animals have given rise to mercury poisoning in humans who ate the meat from these animals.

Elemental mercury may arise from accidental breaking of thermometers, barometers; from discarded batteries, mercury vapour lamps, mercury switches; from coal burning, which can contribute 3000 metric tons per year to the atmosphere; from natural weathering of rocks and soils which contribute 230 metric tons annually; from the 'silvering' of coins; from manufacture of mercury amalgams.

Ingested mercury compounds accumulate in certain parts of the brain, eventually causing brain damage. Other affected organs include the colon and kidneys. Methylmercury causes nerve degeneration; birth defects; genetic defects; chromosome damage; excessive salivation; loss of teeth; gross muscle tremors. When applied to the skin, alkyl mercury compounds cause irritation, redness and blistering.

In babies, dusting of the skin with powders or application of ointments containing mercury causes pink disease or acrodynia. Characterized by lesions of the skin on the hands and feet; swelling of the extremities; digestive disturbances; itching of the hands and feet; pink coloration of hands, feet, cheeks and tip of nose; weakness of the muscles; arthritis.

Acute poisoning by soluble mercury compounds causes metallic taste; thirst; severe abdominal pain; vomiting; ashy discoloration of the mouth and throat; diarrhoea contaminated with blood. Later ulceration, kidney disease and colitis with severe haemorrhage may develop. Mercury vapour when inhaled causes respiratory symptoms and kidney damage.

Chronic poisoning by mercury vapour or by soluble mercury salts or by prolonged skin contact causes tremor; muscle instability; sensory disturbances; gastrointestinal symptoms; dermatitis; liver and kidney damage; anaemia; mental deterioration. A blue line on the gums may be indicative of chronic mercury poisoning.

Maximum permissible atmospheric concentrations of mercury are 50μg per cubic metre air and 10μg alkyl mercury per cubic metre of air.

Medicinal compounds of mercury include:
1. ammoniated mercury to treat impetigo and threadworm infections;
2. oleated mercury, as ammoniated mercury;
3. mercurial diuretics, used in cardiac oedema;

4. mercuric chloride, used in solution as a disinfectant for the skin;
5. mercuric cyanide, used as a disinfectant in eye solutions;
6. red mercuric iodide, used as a disinfectant in wounds; as a vaginal douche; as a skin disinfectant; to treat ringworm and lupus; to treat syphilis;
7. mercuric nitrate, used to treat syphilitic warts; eczema; psoriasis;
8. yellow mercuric oxide, used as an ointment to treat blepharitis; conjunctivitis. Prolonged use should be avoided as mercury can be absorbed through eye tissues.
9. mercuric oxycyanide, preferred over mercuric chloride as a skin disinfectant and in eye lotions;
10. mercurous chloride, once used orally as a purgative, dose 30-200mg. but now discontinued because of absorption. As an ointment or dusting powder has been used to treat itching; psoriasis and eczema; as a strong ointment (30-50 per cent) in preventing syphilis.

---

meso-inositol,   inositol.

---

metformin,   anti-diabetic drug. Prevents absorption of vitamin B_{12}.

---

methods of food processing,   *blanching* — this is required to inactivate enzymes that cause deterioration of food. It always precedes freezing and drying and is a feature of canning. Leaching occurs into the blanching water and the extent of loss depends largely on the time the vegetable is in contact with water. Temperature must be high enough to inactivate the enzymes, i.e., at least 85°C. Garden peas need one minute; sliced beans two minutes; Brussels sprouts from 3.5 to seven minutes depending on size. Temperatures vary from 93 to 99°C and oxidation may contribute to some destruction of the vitamins.

Losses during blanching are estimated to be between 13 and 60 per cent for vitamin C; 2-30 per cent for thiamine; 5-40 per cent for riboflavin. Carotene losses are less than 1 per cent but these ignore possible transformation into less active forms. Losses due to extraction into water are lessened if the water is consumed. Canning retains all leached vitamins in the liquor so this should not be discarded when the vegetable contents are eaten. Similarly with tinned meats. Microwave blanching is reported to cause less damage than steam, and a combination of microwave and hot water treatment is claimed to preserve more vitamins and produce a more palatable product. Fluidized-bed blanching which is really hot gas treatment is claimed to reduce vitamin C and carotene losses. In domestic blanching losses of vitamin C, thiamine and carotene can be prevented by rapid cooling after blanching. Cold air is best to prevent further leaching into water.

Heat sterilization — as oxygen is excluded, losses of vitamins are minimal during canning procedures. Thiamine is lost even so, particularly from meat. Best conditions to preserve vitamins are heating for a short time at high temperature rather than longer periods at lower temperatures.

Losses are less for tinned meat and fruit than for vegetables during heat sterilization because the acid conditions are protective. Minor losses only of riboflavin and nicotinic acid occur during heat sterilization of meat. Once the food has been sterilized in cans stability of the vitamins is good. Only 15 per cent of vitamin C is lost after two years' storage of vegetables in cans.

Freezing — represents one of the better methods of preserving foods since only the fresh variety is frozen when at the peak of its vitamin content. In frozen meat, most of the vitamins are well preserved but the exudate from thawing can contain appreciable amounts of the water-soluble vitamins. Vegetables must be blanched before freezing so losses are those mentioned under blanching. Similarly during the thawing process the aqueous exudate will contain vitamins so introducing frozen vegetables directly into the heating water will retain them all as long as this water is utilized in the meal. Pyridoxine, pantothenic acid and vitamin E are most affected by deep freezing.

Irradiation — causes some losses in vitamins but freeze-drying before treating with ionizing radiation reduces these losses. Most sensitive vitamins are thiamine, riboflavin, vitamin A and vitamin E. Most stable is nicotinic acid.

Freeze-drying — this low temperature dehydration is probably the best method of retaining vitamins in the preserved food. It is not, unfortunately, widespread.

Hot-air drying — causes variable losses in the different vitamins. Under the most favourable conditions some 10-15 per cent of vitamin C is lost during hot-air drying of vegetables.

Pressure cooking — the shorter time required plus the smaller volume of water used reduces vitamin losses compared with conventional boiling. Principal cause of loss is leaching rather than heat but this is limited by volume of water rather than by time of cooking. In many vegetables it has been shown that losses of thiamine in pressure cooking are 25-50 per cent, those in steaming are 50 per cent and those on boiling 75-80 per cent. Vitamin C losses are of the same order but vary amongst different vegetables.

Microwave heating — uses high-energy electromagnetic radiation, frequency 2450m Hz, wavelength 12cm, to produce very efficient cooking. Microwaves generate heat throughout the bulk of the food rather than simply applying it to the surface as in a conventional oven. Losses of vitamins may be less than or equal to those associated with conventional cooking methods but they are never more.

General principles to retain the highest vitamin content in foods cooked using domestic methods are:

1. Use fresh food rather than stored food.
2. Cook in minimum amount of water.
3. Minimum cooking at a high temperature is preferable to long cooking at a lower one.
4. Cooked foods should not be stored before eating except when deep frozen.
5. Remember that cooking of frozen foods represents the second process they have been through so the whole of the food plus cooking liquids (or thawed exudate) should be utilized. *See also* entries under eggs; fish; meats; milk; vegetables.

---

methotrexate, anti-cancer drug. Immuno-suppressant. Impairs folic acid utilization.

---

migraine, a particular type of headache caused by constriction of the blood-vessels followed by their dilation which gives rise to pulsating pain. Characterized by nausea, vomiting and visual disturbances in severe cases.

Vitamin therapy includes whole vitamin B complex (10mg potency) three times daily plus nicotinamide (100mg). calcium pantothenate (100mg). pyridoxine (50mg) all three times daily. If regime prevents attacks, reduce gradually to that intake that maintains relief.

Mineral

Extra magnesium taken at the rate of 400mg daily, preferably as the amino-acid chelate, has been claimed to prevent development of migraine headaches. A trigger factor for the development of those headaches may be high concentrations of sodium in some sufferers. One study has shown that those people could precipitate migraine attacks by sudden loads of common salt as in potato crisps, salted nuts, and high sodium foods such as pickles, sauces and preserved meats; or of sodium glutamate in highly spiced and oriental foods. Avoiding these foods led to a reduced incidence of migraines in these people.

---

milk, good source of all vitamins but seasonal variation with regard to the fat-soluble. A low sodium food that is rich in potassium and calcium

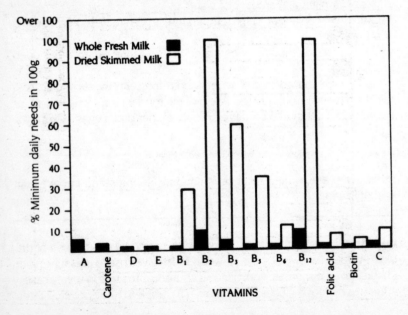

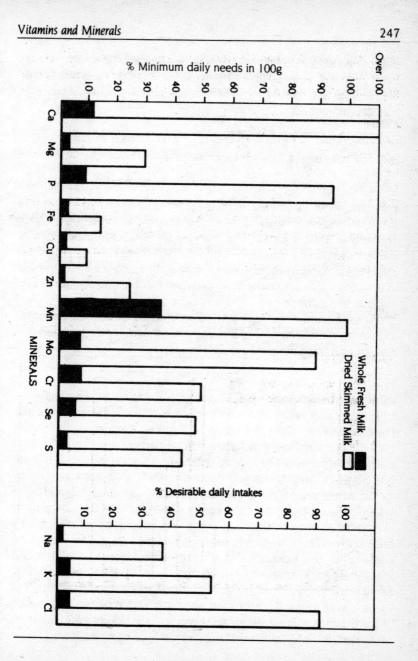

but not a good source of iron. Skimmed milk is devoid of fat-soluble vitamins but contents of water-soluble variety are similar to those of whole milk. Dried skimmed milk is very rich in all micronutrients because of concentration effect.

---

milk of magnesia,   *see* cream of magnesia.

---

mineral,   literally 'mined from the earth'. Divided into: 1. metallic elements, present in high quantities in the body and diet where daily intakes greater than 100mg, e.g. calcium, magnesium, potassium; 2. non-metallic elements, abundant in the earth, body and diet where daily intakes greater than 100mg, e.g. carbon, phosphorus, sulphur; 3. metallic elements, present in very small amounts in the body and diet, that are essential for health, e.g. chromium, copper, iron, zinc; 4. non-metallic elements, present in very small amounts in the body and diet, that are essential for health, e.g. fluorine, iodine, selenium. Any essential element not found in groups 1. and 2. is classed as a trace mineral or trace element.

---

mineral absorption,   the process whereby minerals are transferred from the food or from supplements into the intestinal cells and hence into the bloodstream. The main site of absorption of minerals is the small intestine but some are transferred in other parts of the gastro-intestinal tract. Simple minerals like sodium, potassium, chloride and iodide that are present as electrically charged atoms (known as ions) are absorbed by simple diffusion from the gut contents into the intestinal cells and there is little or no control of their absorption. Control of their level in the body comes in their excretion. Sodium, potassium, lithium and ammonium ions are monovalent, i.e. they carry only one positive charge. They cannot be chelated for this reason. Calcium, magnesium, copper, zinc, iron and manganese are all divalent, i.e. they carry two positive charges per atom. Small amounts of them may also be assimilated by simple diffusion, but in the main they must be chelated with amino acids before they can be absorbed into the intestinal cells and hence into the bloodstream. Transport of divalent minerals within the body is mainly as complexes with amino acids or with proteins but small amounts exist in the bloodstream as simple ions, e.g. calcium, which participates in the blood-clotting process. Absorption of divalent minerals therefore depends upon:

1. the quantity of protein or amino acids present in the digestive system;
2. the quality of protein or amino acids available, since the right sort of amino acids must be present;
3. competition amongst minerals for the amino acids available and the specific sites of absorption in the small intestine. For example, lead and iron compete for the same sites; cadmium and zinc compete for the same sites. Any excess of one mineral over its competitor will increase its chances of absorption.

Table 9 shows the ratios of quantities of minerals absorbed from amino-acid chelates compared with these from mineral salts and oxides.

Table 9: The ratios of quantities of minerals absorbed from amino-acid chelates compared with those from mineral salts and oxides

Mineral	Amino-acid chelates: Carbonates	Amino-acid chelates: Sulphates	Amino-acid chelates: Oxides
Copper	5.8:1	4.1:1	3.0:1
Magnesium	1.8:1	2.6:1	4.2:1
Iron	3.6:1	3.8:1	4.9:1
Zinc	3.0:1	2.3:1	3.9:1

mineral content of vegetables,   in general the mineral content of vegetables reflects that of the soil in which they are growing. Studies have indicated that even in plants growing in adjacent areas, there is wide variation in mineral content because of differing soil concentrations. Other factors may also play a part — *see* minerals in soil. Table 10 illustrates how vegetables may not always contain the concentrations of minerals expected. However it must be pointed out that most mineral concentrations in vegetables sold commercially lie somewhere in the middle of the ranges.

Table 10: Variation in mineral content of selected vegetables

Food	Figures in p.p.m. (parts per million)	Boron	Manganese	Iron	Copper	Cobalt
Snap beans	Highest content	73	60	227	69	0.26
	Lowest content	10	2	10	3	0.00
Cabbage	Highest content	42	13	94	48	0.15
	Lowest content	7	2	20	0.4	0.00
Lettuce	Highest content	37	169	516	60	0.19
	Lowest content	6	1	9	3	0.00
Tomatoes	Highest content	36	68	1938	53	0.63
	Lowest content	5	1	1	0	0.00
Spinach	Highest content	88	117	1584	32	0.25
	Lowest content	12	1	19	0.5	0.20

mineral losses in freezing are made up of leaching of minerals during

Table 11: Typical percentage losses of calcium and magnesium from frozen fruits and vegetables.

Fruits and vegetables	Calcium	Magnesium
Apricots	33	12
Asparagus	0	30
Blackberries	56	48
Black-eyed peas	7	0
Blueberries	53	0
Brussels sprouts	33	9
Cherries	22	0
Corn	57	53
Green beans	19	34
Green peas	4	31
Lima beans	33	28
Peaches	33	40
Potatoes	0	38
Spinach	0	23
Strawberries	39	31

the thawing process; losses into water during the blanching stage; losses into the water or fat during the cooking processes. Typical losses of calcium and magnesium from frozen fruits and vegetables are shown in Table 11.

mineral losses in refining, all minerals are lost to some extent during the refining of natural foods into the processed variety, but losses of trace minerals are the most significant. Some of these are shown in Table 12.

Table 12: Percentage losses of trace elements by refining of foods

	Co	Cr	Cu	Fe	Mg	Mn	Mo	Se	Zn
White flour from wholemeal	89	98	68	76	85	86	48	16	78
Polished rice from brown rice	38	75	25	—	83	27	—	—	50
White sugar from raw cane sugar	88	90	80	99	99	89	—	75	98
Refined oils from cold expressed oils	—	—	—	—	99	—	—	—	75
Butter production from milk	—	—	—	—	94	—	—	—	50

Gross minerals too are lost (see Table 13). In the UK and some other countries calcium and iron must be replaced at levels of between 94 and 156mg calcium and not less than 1.65mg iron per 100g flour in white flour, but there is no legislation regarding all other minerals.

Table 13: Percentage losses of gross minerals by refining of wheat and sugar

	Ca	Cl	K	Na	P	S
White flour from wholemeal	60	0	77	78	71	32
White sugar from raw cane sugar	96	99	98	99	99	99

mineral relationships, the minerals in the body are all in balance with one another so that excess or otherwise of one or more will affect the levels of others. Their relationships are summed up in the mineral wheel shown in Figure 1.

On this wheel an arrow pointing to a particular mineral means that a deficiency of that mineral may be caused by an excess of the mineral from whence the arrow comes. For example, a high calcium intake may reduce the amount of zinc; high cadmium intakes will cause copper levels to drop. When the line between two minerals contains two opposing arrows, each mineral may influence the other. A low potassium intake will allow sodium to accumulate and conversely an excess of sodium in the diet will lower potassium levels in the body.

The wheel allows other relationships to be worked out. Calcium and/or phosphorus deficiency may allow an excess of manganese to develop. This high level can cause depression of potassium which allows sodium to accumulate. There is no direct line between calcium and sodium and potassium but calcium levels can indirectly affect those of the other two

Figure 1: Mineral relationships

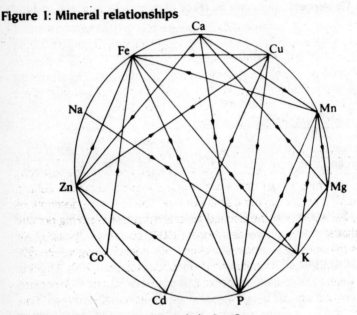

Ca - Calcium, Cd - Cadmium, Co - Cobalt, Cu - Copper.
Fe - Iron, K - Potassium, Mg - Magnesium, Mn - Manganese.
Na - Sodium, P - Phosphorus, Zn - Zinc

elements. Hence calcium deficiency may have an effect upon blood-pressure. In another example calcium and/or phosphorus in excess will depress zinc levels leading to a skin disease called parakeratosis. This complaint can therefore be caused by excessive intakes of calcium and phosphorus as well as a reduced dietary intake of zinc.

mineral waters, have now been officially defined under EEC regulations. 'Natural mineral water' means water which originates in an underground water table or deposit and is extracted for human consumption from the ground through a spring, well, or other exit. 'Natural mineral water fortified with gas from the spring' means an effervescent mineral water whose carbon dioxide content includes carbon dioxide from the same water table or deposit as the water. 'Naturally carbonated mineral water' means an effervescent natural mineral water whose carbon dioxide content is the same after decanting (if it is decanted) and bottling as it was at source. It includes a natural mineral water to which carbon dioxide from the same water table or deposit as the water has been added if the amount added does not exceed the amount previously released during decanting or bottling. The only treatments allowed for natural mineral water are filtration or decanting; total or partial removal of carbon dioxide by physical methods; the addition of carbon dioxide only to mineral waters that are naturally effervescent. Hence chlorination, fluoridation and softening of natural mineral waters are not allowed.

Natural mineral waters vary widely in their content of minerals. A low mineral content water must not contain more than 500mg of mineral salts per litre. A very low mineral content water must not contain more than 50mg of mineral salts per litre. A water rich in mineral salts must contain more than 1500mg of mineral salts per litre. The following descriptions can only be used where the claimed mineral has a content in mg per litre above that stated: contains bicarbonate (600); contains sulphate (200); contains chloride (200); contains calcium (150); contains magnesium (50); contains fluoride (1.0); contains iron (1.0); contains sodium (200). An acidic mineral water must contain more than 250mg free carbon dioxide per litre. A mineral water suitable for a low-sodium diet must contain less than 20mg per litre.

The upper limits on trace mineral contents (both essential and toxic) of natural mineral waters are (in μg per litre): arsenic (50); cadmium (5.0); cyanides (50); chromium (50); mercury (1.0); nickel (50); antimony (10); selenium (10); lead (10). No limits are suggested for nitrates and nitrites but in view of the undesirability of high intakes of these, they should be absent or present only in low concentration in natural mineral waters.

Mineral waters when sold in bottles or drunk at source as at spas have been popular for centuries as a remedy for various complaints, particularly those of the rheumatic kind. With modern knowledge that such diseases may be associated with mineral imbalance there would appear to be some logic in increasing mineral intakes for their diuretic, laxative and replacement effects. Many people prefer mineral waters because the water has not been softened, chlorinated, fluoridated and has had the minimum of pipe feeding before they drink it.

---

minerals in soil,   man derives his food from plants or from animals that have eaten plants or from fish that have eaten plants. All plants whether growing on land or in water must derive their minerals from the soil or the sea. These sources are the ultimate source of all minerals. The richness of a soil as well as depending on the macro-elements nitrogen, phosphorus and potassium must also have present other less abundant but just as essential trace minerals. Deficiency of macro-elements does exist. Some lands are low in phosphate, hence the importance of the natural phosphate-rich fertilizer guano. Potassium is lacking in some areas and deficiency is made up by treating the land with potassium, often obtained from rich inland lakes like the Dead Sea. Nitrogen is usually supplied in the form of nitrates. Zinc deficiency is not unknown and it reflects in the health of the farm animals who live off plants grown on the soil. Supplementation of animal feeds with zinc is more usual than treating the soil.

Mineral deficiencies in the soil can produce disease in localized areas. Lack of iodine in the soil causes goitre. Magnesium deficiency of the soil in certain areas of France has been associated with a particular type of cancer. Some regions in Poland had a high incidence of leukaemia. The causative agents were found to be toxins produced by the soil micro-organism Aspergillus flavus. This fungus flourishes in soil that is deficient in iron, copper and magnesium and has excessive concentrations of silicon and potassium. When this imbalance was corrected by correct fertilization of the soil (extra trace elements plus dolomite to supply calcium and magnesium) the fungus was controlled and the incidence of leukaemia dropped. Low levels of manganese and chromium in the soil appear from epidemiological studies to increase the chances of heart disease and atherosclerosis in those living in the area. In South Africa, molybdenum, copper and iron deficiencies in the soil have led to oesophageal cancer.

Mineral excesses of a toxic element in the soil can also produce disease.

In Japan, faulty treatment of waste water from a mine led to pollution of a river with cadmium. The mineral was deposited in the soil from which the plants absorbed it. When the rice was eaten, the local population accumulated cadmium in the body and, combined with a low calcium and vitamin D intake, a concentration was reached that resulted in a bone disease that caused excruciating pain. *See* Itai-itai disease. Adjustment of the diet to give the correct balance of the essential minerals cured the complaint. In the Netherlands, some areas of high silicon content in the soil had a high incidence of all types of cancer that was reduced by treating the soil with calcium. This inhibited the uptake of silicon by plants. Excessively high soil concentrations of zinc and chromium have been associated with gastrointestinal cancer in some parts of the world. In India a raised water table made the topsoil in one area more alkaline. This increased the uptake of molybdenum and fluoride by sorghum plants (the staple diet). These uptakes led to copper deficiency. The result was that the population eating these plants were copper deficient but had excessive intakes of molybdenum and fluoride. The result was a crippling bone disease called genu valgum which was only remedied by balancing the intake of the essential minerals.

Uptake from the soil can be affected by:

1. high levels of humic acid which can bind minerals, making them unavailable;
2. the presence of other minerals, e.g., low levels of potassium or high levels of phosphate will render iron insoluble;
3. pH. This is a measure of acidity or alkalinity of the soil. From pH 0-6 is acid, from pH 8-14 is alkaline; pH 7 is neutral. At neutral pH most minerals are fully available to the plant. In highly acid soils only potassium, iron, manganese, copper and zinc can be absorbed. In highly alkaline soils phosphorus, potassium, sulphur and boron are freely available for absorption. *See also* Mulder's chart.

---

molybdenum, chemical symbol Mo, atomic weight 95.9. Essential in soil and plants for processes 'fixing' or utilizing nitrogen from the air. Essential trace element for animals and man.

Functions

Prevention of dental caries
Iron metabolism
Uric acid excretion
  (nitrogen excretory product)
Maintains normal sexual
  function in male

Body Content

Adult content is 9mg with
most in the liver. Fifty per cent
of dietary mineral is absorbed.
Excretion is mainly in the
urine.

Recommended Daily Intake

Suggested only by the US
Food and Nutrition Board at
500µg.

Best Food Sources
in µg per 100g

Buckwheat	485
Beans — canned	350
Wheatgerm	200
Liver	200
Soyabeans	182
Wholegrains	120
Cereals	90
Organ meats	75
Eggs	50
Cocoa	50
Vegetables	26
Fruits	16
Alcoholic beverages	10

Deficiency Symptoms

Irritability
Irregular heartbeat
Lack of uric acid production
Coma

Deficiency

Associated solely with reduced
dietary intakes caused by:
  Eating foods from
    molybdenum deficient
    soils
  High intakes of refined and
  processed foods

Deficiency May Result in

Dental caries
Sexual impotence in men
Cancer of the gullet

Therapeutic Uses	*Effects of Excess Intake*
May be of benefit in those conditions resulting in deficiency but no clinical trials carried out yet. Has been used to remove excess copper from body.	Gout (at intakes of 10-15mg daily) Increased excretion of copper causing deficiency. In animals this can give rise to loss of hair colour.

monosodium glutamate, also known as MSG; sodium hydrogen L-glutamate. A food additive that functions as a flavour enhancer. Acceptable daily intake up to 120mg per kg body weight — not to be given to infants under 12 weeks old. Provides 12.3mg sodium per 100mg. Permitted miscellaneous additive. Prohibited in foods specially made for babies and young children. *See also* Chinese restaurant syndrome.

morning sickness, *see* nausea.

mouth ulcers, also known as canker sores; aphthous ulcers; aphthous stomatitis. Acute painful ulcers on the moveable oral mucosal lining, occurring singly or in groups. Reports of successful prevention of mouth ulcers by taking oral zinc supplement equivalent to 20-25mg element daily. Existing ulcers may respond to directly applied zinc creams, preferably with the mineral as zinc gluconate or mouthwashes containing zinc. *See also* ulcers.

mucous membranes, wet surfaces of the body including nose, eyes, mouth, respiratory system, digestive tract, anus and genital tracts.

Vitamin A protects all mucous membranes and maintains their health. Deficiency of vitamin leads to drying out of membranes resulting in ulceration and liability to infection — *see* keratinization.

Inflammation can result from deficiency of nicotinic acid and riboflavin. Polluted atmosphere can destroy membrane — best protected with vitamins

A and E. Tobacco smoking irritates mucous membranes of respiratory tract — best protected with beta-carotene.

Mulder's chart,   in soil a complicated mixture of minerals is presented to a plant. The uptake of a particular mineral is under the influence of other minerals which can either stimulate or antagonize the absorption of that mineral. Zinc absorption by a plant is dependent upon phosphorus, iron and calcium. High phosphorus levels antagonize the uptake of zinc, copper and potassium; they also stimulate the uptake of magnesium. Inter-relationships are shown in Figure 2.

Figure 2: Plant uptake of minerals

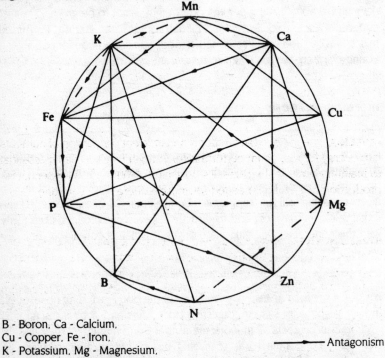

B - Boron, Ca - Calcium,
Cu - Copper, Fe - Iron,
K - Potassium, Mg - Magnesium,
Mn - Manganese, N - Nitrogen,
P - Phosphorus, Zn - Zinc.

———► Antagonism

– – ► Stimulation

muscle cramps, prolonged painful contractions of a muscle. May appear as spasms where the muscles cannot perform a specific task but allows the use of them for other movement. Known as occupational cramp, an example of which is 'writer's cramp'. Can be caused by an imbalance of certain minerals; also as a result of stress, bad posture or fatigue. May respond to extra calcium in the diet, usually between 640 and 800mg of the element daily. This therapy has been found to relieve 'growing pains' in children; night cramps; aching legs; muscle cramps of pregnancy. Night cramps may also respond to extra potassium in the diet. *See* fatigue.

---

muscle pain, may be related to biotin deficiency. Treat with 2 to 5mg daily by mouth.

---

muscle spasms, also known as restless legs. Often occurs during sleep and relieved by walking or moving affected leg. Treated with vitamin E (100IU with each meal *or* 400IU in one dose daily).

---

muscles, need good blood supply and efficient conversion of nutrients into energy for maximum performance. Vitamin E (400IU daily) essential to maintain healthy blood-vessels. Vitamin C (500mg daily) essential for production of carnitine, needed for muscle energy. *See* carnitine.

---

muscular dystrophy, muscle disease characterized by progressive weakness and degeneration of muscle fibres but without evidence of nerve degeneration. Symptom of vitamin E deficiency in many animal species and can be cured by vitamin treatment. No evidence of relationship between vitamin E and human muscular dystrophy but occasionally cases have responded to high doses of vitamin E, preferably with the trace mineral selenium.

Benefit in rare cases claimed with ubiquinone, a natural vitamin-like substance, produced in the body under the influence of vitamin E.

---

muscular tics, also known as tremors and twitches. Repeated and largely involuntary movements of muscles varying in complexity. May become prominent under conditions of emotional stress. Caused by an impulse conductance abnormality at the junction of nerve and muscle, possibly due to a mineral imbalance. Most likely deficiencies are in potassium and magnesium. Supplementation with these minerals can often relieve persistent tics, tremors and twitches. May also be caused by excess toxic minerals like lead, in which case the condition is relieved by removal of the toxic mineral with agents calcium, zinc and vitamin C.

myelin, fatty sheath that covers nerves and spinal cord and acts as insulator. Composed of cholesterol, PUFA and phosphatidyl choline complexed with lipid called sphingosine. Myelin loss due to degeneration is factor in multiple sclerosis. Vitamin B_{12} and PUFA essential for healthy myelin sheath.

myocardial infarction, *see* heart disease.

myo-inositol, inositol.

myxoedema, also known as hypothyroidism. The condition is caused by thyroid hormone deficiency in the adult. Symptoms and signs may be subtle and insidious at onset. The facial expression is dull; there is puffiness and swelling around the eyes; eyelids droop; hair is sparse, coarse and dry; skin is coarse, scaly, dry and thick; memory is poor; there is intellectual impairment with gradual change in personality; sometimes this leads to frank psychosis commonly called 'myxoedema madness'. Often carotene is deposited in the palms and soles causing yellow coloration. The tongue may be enlarged. Heartbeat rate is slow and the heart is often enlarged. Tingling in the hands and feet is often present. Reflexes are quick to contract but slow to relax. There may be excessive bleeding at menstrual periods. Constipation, low body temperature and anaemia are often present. Vitamin B_{12} absorption is adversely affected because of decreased intrinsic factor synthesis.

   Treatment is replacement therapy with a variety of thyroid hormone preparations including synthetic thyroxine; synthetic triiodothyronine; combinations of both; desiccated animal thyroid. Average maintenance dose of 150-200μg L-thyroxine daily is the preferred treatment. At least 60 per cent of this is absorbed. In infants and young children maintenance dose is 2.5μg per kg body weight per day. Triiodothyronine tends to be used to initiate therapy because it has a rapid action and turnover, but this detracts from its use in long-term therapy where thyroxine is preferred.

   Iodides cannot be used since the thyroid does not have the ability to convert them to the thyroid hormones. *See also* cretinism.

N

natural vitamins, those that are:

1. derived from natural sources (e.g. d-alpha tocopherol);
2. produced by fermentation (e.g. vitamin B_{12});
3. presented in a natural environment (e.g. vitamin E in wheatgerm oil or soyabean oil);
4. presented in a food (e.g. vitamin B complex in yeast).

Advantages are:

1. biologically more active (e.g. d-alpha tocopherol);
2. better absorbed (e.g. fat-soluble vitamins need fats or oils present as well);
3. better utilized in presence of other factors (e.g. vitamin C and bioflavonoids occur in foods together and function in body together);
4. retained by body longer (e.g. natural vitamin E).

---

nausea, feeling of discomfort in region of stomach with aversion to food and tendency to vomit. Side-effect of many medicinal drugs.

Morning sickness — nausea of the early stages of pregnancy. Has been treated with pyridoxine (but seek medical advice).

Travel sickness — nausea associated with various forms of travel. Has been treated with pyridoxine (25mg) and ginger (160mg) before trip and if necessary during it. Half dose effective for children.

neomycin,   antibiotic. Prevents absorption of vitamin D.

---

nervous system,   health depends upon adequate vitamin B complex and vitamin E. Thiamine at intakes between 50 and 600mg daily has relieved sciatica, trigeminal neuralgia, facial paralysis, optic neuritis and peripheral neuritis. Psychosis and mental deterioration have responded to vitamin B_{12}, preferably by injection.

Choline is of benefit in some cases of Alzheimer's disease and senile dementia. A combination of vitamin E and inositol has helped in some nerve diseases associated with muscle degeneration. Huntington's chorea treated with high potencies of whole vitamin B complex has relieved mental deterioration of the disease. Mild depression will often respond to vitamin B_6 therapy alone.

Nicotinic acid in high doses (1-3g daily) has been used successfully in schizophrenia. Paraesthesia relieved by 50mg pyridoxine daily.

Deficiencies of thiamine, riboflavin, nicotinamide, pyridoxine and vitamin B_{12} all cause damage to nervous system. Preferable therefore to treat any mild mental or nervous condition with high potency of whole vitamin B complex.

---

neuritis,   general term for degeneration and inflammation of one or more nerves. Symptom rather than disease.

Optic, inflammation of the eye nerve.

Peripheral, affecting simultaneously several nerves, usually those of the limbs. Caused by thiamine deficiency, diabetes, alcohol, heavy metal poisoning. Also known as polyneuritis.

Treatment — *see* nervous system.

---

niacin,   water-soluble vitamin, member of the vitamin B complex. Synonymous with nicotinic acid. Presented also as niacinamide, synonymous with nicotinamide. Generally accepted as vitamin B_3. Also known as vitamin PP (pellagra-preventing) or PP factor. Nicotinic acid known since 1867 but demonstrated as a vitamin only in 1937 by Dr Conrad Elvehjem.

Best Food Sources in mg per 100g	
Yeast extract	67.0
Dried brewer's yeast	37.9
Wheat bran	32.6
Nuts	21.3
Pig's liver	19.4
Chicken	11.6
Soya flour	10.6
Meat	10.5
Fatty fish	10.4
Wholegrains	8.1
Cheese	6.2
Dried fruits	5.6
Wholemeal bread	5.6
Brown rice	4.7
Wheatgerm	4.2
Eggs	3.7

Functions

Acts as coenzymes NAD (nicotinamide adenine dinucleotide) and NADP (nicotinamide adenine dinucleotide phosphate) in cell respiration

Produces energy from sugars, fats and protein

Maintains healthy skin, nerves, brain, tongue, digestive system

Significant amounts produced in the body from the amino-acid L-tryptophane — 60mg L-tryptophane makes 1mg niacin

Stability in Foods

Usually stable but see Losses in Food Processing entry.

Therapeutic Uses

Childhood schizophrenia
Alcohol addiction
Tobacco addiction
Arthritis
Reducing blood cholesterol
  (niacin only)

Symptoms of Excess Intake

Niacinamide (more than 3g):
  Depression
  Liver malfunction

Niacin:
  Flushing of face
  Sensation of heat
  Pounding headache
  Dry skin
  Abdominal cramps
  Diarrhoea
  Nausea

Deficiency Symptoms	Deficiency Results in

Summed up as 3 D's
  Dermatitis
  Diarrhoea
  Dementia
	Pellagra characterized by:
	  Rashes
	  Dry scaly skin
	  Wrinkles
	  Coarse structure of skin

Deficiency Causes

Alcohol
Anti-leukaemia drugs

(continuing *Deficiency Results in*:)

Loss of appetite
Nausea and vomiting
Inflamed mouth
Inflamed digestive tract

Insomnia
Irritability
Stress
Depression

Avoid

High doses during pregnancy (both types of vitamin) and when suffering from gastric and duodenal ulcers (niacin).

Recommended Daily Intakes

Should be at least 19mg but see separate entry.

niacinamide, active form of nicotinic acid. Known also as nicotinamide.

nickel, chemical symbol Ni. Atomic weight 58.7. Occurs in nature as chalcopyrite, penthandite, garnierite, nicollite, nillerite; abundance in earth's crust 180mg per kg. It is an essential trace mineral for rats, chicks and swine, but functions not known.

Deficiency in animals impairs iron absorption leading to low iron levels in the tissues and organs and to iron-deficiency anaemia.

Not known to be essential for man but traces of the mineral are found in all human tissues.

Functions in animals include an antagonistic action to the hormone adrenalin; intensifying the action of insulin; increasing blood fats; stabilizing RNA and DNA in the tissues.

High blood levels are found in those who have suffered a heart attack; those with serious burns; those who have suffered a stroke; women with toxaemia of pregnancy; women with cancer of the uterus; those with lung cancer.

Low blood levels are found in those with cirrhosis of the liver; those with chronic kidney failure.

Food sources are provided by contamination, e.g. from the alloys used to line cooking utensils; from machines used to process and refine food, from pasteurization equipment; from margarine, where it is used as a catalyst in its production; from cigarette smoke. In tobacco some nickel combines with carbon monoxide to form the toxic nickel carbonyl, a known carcinogen (cancer-producing substance) for rats.

Toxic effects of excess oral nickel intakes in man are unknown. Nickel carbonyl from tobacco smoke may be a factor in causing lung cancer in man. Acute toxic effects of nickel carbonyl are frontal headache; vertigo; nausea; vomiting; chest pain; cough. Nickel when in contact with the skin of sensitive people can cause dermatitis.

Excessive oral intakes in young chicks cause pigmentation changes in the skin; swelling in the legs; dermatitis; fat-depleted liver; oxygen-depleted liver. The mineral accumulated in liver, bone and aorta.

---

nicotinamide,   active metabolic form of nicotinic acid. Known also as niacinamide, vitamin B_3.

---

nicotinic acid,   niacin, vitamin B_3.

---

night blindness,   inability to see in the dark due solely to vitamin A deficiency.

---

niobium, also known as Columbium, it has the chemical symbol Nb with an atomic weight of 92.9. Its abundance in the earth's crust is similar to that of nickel. The mineral is named after Niobe, the daughter of Tantalus.

The levels of niobium in human tissue are comparable to those of copper and exceeded among the trace elements only by iron, zinc and rubidium. The mineral is also widely distributed in nearly all vegetable and animal foods, with concentrations within the range 0.5 to $3.0\mu g$ per g fresh weight. Hence a typical diet will give an intake of at least $600\mu g$ per day of which one half is absorbed and subsequently excreted in the urine.

Human tissue levels of niobium are as follows (in μg per g fresh weight): blood 0.004; kidney 0.01; liver 0.004; lung 0.02; lymph nodes 0.06; muscle 0.03; testis 0.009. Bone contained less than $0.07\mu g$ per g of ash. UK diets provide between 16 and $24\mu g$ per day. If niobium is fed to mice and rats at a level of $5\mu g$ per ml drinking water for their lifetime, signs of toxicity appear. In mice the extra niobium increased the incidence of liver fatty degeneration, decreased median lifespan and longevity and suppressed growth. In rats, the mineral supplement elevated copper, manganese and especially zinc levels in a number of organs especially in the heart and liver where marked changes occurred. Hence there is some relationship between niobium and other minerals, and metabolic actions can be affected. After injection of niobium into rats, the mineral preferentially accumulated in testis, ovary, kidney, lung, liver and spleen. It is likely that niobium may have a role in metabolism but this awaits further study.

---

nitrates, *see* nitrosamines.

---

nitrites, *see* nitrosamines.

---

nitritocobalamin, B_{12c} vitamin.

---

nitrofurantoin, urinary anti-infective. Impairs folic acid utilization.

---

nitrosamines, toxic substances associated with certain types of cancer. Readily formed in the digestive tract from amines and nitrites, both present in food, drugs, cosmetics and the environment. Nitrites used extensively as food preservatives and readily formed from nitrates. Nitrosamines more likely to be produced in stomach in absence of acid.

Vitamin C prevents formation of nitrosamines and neutralizes preformed variety, so vitamin should be taken at every meal.

---

nucleic acids, comprise both ribonucleic acids (RNA) and deoxyribonucleic acids (DNA). Essential components of all living cells, they are necessary for cell growth and hereditary information. Reduced synthesis leads to consequences of ageing including poor memory. Have been used to slow down ageing process, usually given by injection.

Vitamins needed for healthy RNA and DNA production in human beings include vitamin A, vitamin E, pyridoxine, folic acid, vitamin B_{12} and choline. Present in dried yeast to extent of 12 per cent of weight.

---

nuts, include almonds, Barcelona, Brazil, chestnuts, hazel, walnuts and pecan.

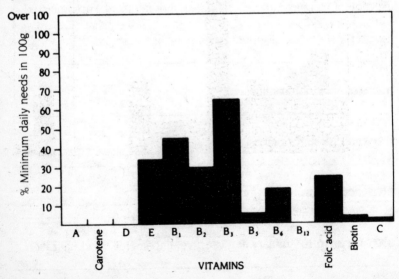

Kernels of all nuts are completely devoid of carotene and in the ripe state contain traces only of vitamin C. Provide good quantities of vitamin E but only two types present, alpha-tocopherol and gamma-tocopherol. Brazil nuts, chestnuts, peanuts and walnut kernels contain mainly gamma-tocopherol. Individual figures for all kernels are total tocopherols. All kernels supply good quantities of the B vitamins. *See* individual nuts.

In the raw state, nuts are a sodium-free food that supply useful amounts of all other minerals, particularly manganese.

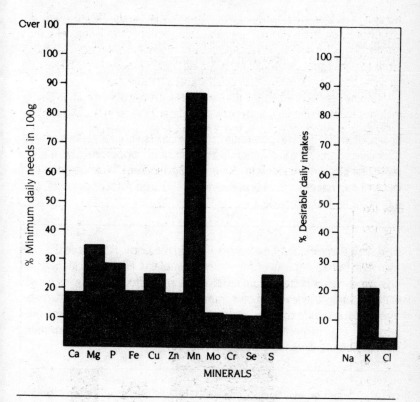

O

---

oatmeal, when raw is rich source of B vitamins providing (in mg per 100g): thiamine 0.50; riboflavin 0.10; nicotinic acid 3.8; pyridoxine 0.12; folic acid 0.060; pantothenic acid 1.0; biotin 0.020; vitamin E 0.9. Devoid of vitamins A, D, C and carotene.

Mineral
Low sodium food rich in potassium, magnesium, sulphur and phosphorus. Excellent source of trace minerals iron, zinc and copper. As raw, it gives the following mineral levels (in mg per 100g): sodium 33; potassium 370; calcium 55; magnesium 110; phosphorus 380; iron 4.1; copper 0.23; zinc 3.0; sulphur 160; chloride 73.

---

oedema, retention of excessive water in the body. Not a disease in its own right but a symptom of some other complaint. Has been claimed that high potencies of certain vitamins have a diuretic effect in removing excess water: vitamin C at levels of one gram or more; vitamin E at levels greater than 500IU; pyridoxine at levels of 200mg. May be effective for mild oedema, e.g. in premenstrual syndrome, but most oedema requires stronger acting drugs (medicinal or herbal).

---

offal, organ meats. Supply vitamin C in addition to all other vitamins, unlike other meat products. Liver and kidney are particularly rich in vitamin A, nicotinic acid, pantothenic acid and vitamin B_{12}. *See* under individual foods.

---

oil of evening primrose, seed oil containing substantial amounts of gammalinolenic acid (GLA) a member of an essential fatty acid family. Usually produced in body from linoleic acid but claims that in some conditions synthesis blocked or not sufficient. Reports that GLA beneficial in multiple sclerosis; in premenstrual syndrome; in skin disorders; in alcoholism; in hyperactivity in children; in arthritis and other inflammatory conditions; in disorders of the immune system. GLA functions as percursor of hormones known as prostaglandins. Usual intakes are 3 to 6 capsules per day (500mg oil containing 40mg GLA per capsule).

---

okra, African plant known also as gumbo. Provides 90µg carotene per 100g in raw state. B vitamins present are (in mg per 100g): thiamine 0.10; riboflavin 0.10; nicotinic acid 1.3; pyridoxine 0.08; pantothenic acid 0.26. Good source of folic acid at 100µg per 100g. Good source of vitamin C at 25mg per 100g.

Mineral
Practically devoid of sodium, it supplies good levels of potassium, calcium, magnesium and phosphorus. Useful quantities of trace minerals iron and copper. In raw state it supplies the following minerals (in mg per 100g): sodium 7; potassium 190; calcium 70; magnesium 60; phosphorus 60; iron 1.0; copper 0.19; sulphur 30; chloride 41.

---

onions, contain no carotene and traces only of vitamin E. Poor source of B vitamins made poorer by boiling. Levels are (in mg per 100g), for raw and boiled respectively: thiamine 0.03, 0.02; riboflavin 0.05, 0.04; nicotinic acid 0.4, 0.2; pyridoxine 0.10, 0.06; pantothenic acid 0.14, 0.10. Folic acid levels (in µg per 100g) are 16, 8; and biotin levels are 0.9, 0.6 for raw and boiled onions respectively. Vitamin C content reduced from 10mg to 6mg per 100g on boiling. Frying virtually destroys the B vitamins and vitamin C; only 0.4mg nicotinic acid per 100g survives.

Mineral
Low sodium food providing good levels of potassium and sulphur. Spring variety is a good source of calcium, iron and copper. Mineral levels for

raw and boiled respectively (in mg per 100g) are: sodium 10, 7; potassium 140, 78; calcium 31, 24; magnesium 8,5; phosphorus 30, 16; iron 0.3, 0.3; copper 0.08, 0.07; zinc 0.1, 0.1; sulphur 51, 24; chloride 20, 5.

As fried (in mg per 100g): sodium 20; potassium 270; calcium 61; magnesium 15; phosphorus 59; iron 0.6; copper 0.16; zinc 0.1; sulphur 88; chloride 38.

Raw, spring variety contains (in mg per 100g): sodium 13, potassium 230; calcium 140; magnesium 11; phosphorus 24; iron 1.2; copper 0.13; sulphur 50; chloride 36.

---

organ meats,   *see* offal.

---

orotates,   synthetic complex of minerals with orotic acid. Some evidence that orotates are absorbed more efficiently than mineral salts from the intestine and they may act as carriers of certain minerals across cell membranes. Orotic acid has been named vitamin B_{13} in the past but as ample quantities are produced within the body as an intermediate in nucleic acid metabolism it is no longer regarded as a vitamin. Mineral orotates have been claimed to be beneficial in many clinical conditions. They are useful in replacing mineral deficiencies but some of the benefits in other conditions may be related to the orotic acid moiety.

---

orotic acid,   known also as whey factor, animal galactose factor, vitamin B_{13}. No longer regarded as a vitamin.

Richest food sources are liquid whey and root vegetables but traces usually present in all foods containing the vitamin B complex.

Stable to food processing methods.

Functions as intermediate in metabolism of RNA and DNA in human beings and is produced in adequate quantities under normal circumstances.

Essential growth factor for micro-organisms.

Deficiency in man has not been reported.

Deficiency in animals has not been reported.

Recommended dietary intakes not set because need in diet not established.

Toxicity is low. Up to 4 grams orotic acid daily by mouth has caused no harm over many days treatment.

Therapy with orotic acid claimed in multiple sclerosis (given by injection); in chronic hepatitis (given as calcium orotate over many months); in gout (4 grams daily of orotic acid for six days).

orthomolecular medicine, *see* megavitamin therapy.

osteomalacia, a disease characterized by softening of the bones and low body levels of calcium due specifically to vitamin D deficiency in the adult. *See* vitamin D.

osteoporosis, honeycombing of the bones due to loss of calcium that is not replaced. Associated mainly with post-menopausal period of life; long-term corticosteroid treatment. Symptoms are bone pain and ease of fracture. Treated with high intakes of calcium (1000mg daily) plus fluoride plus adequate vitamin D to ensure absorption (400IU) *or* hormone replacement therapy in post-menopausal state.

Mineral
The bones most commonly affected are the spinal vertebrae, the femur (thigh bone) and the radius (shorter arm bone). The condition is associated with the menopausal and post-menopausal female; prolonged use of oral corticosteroid drugs; excessive excretion of calcium on some medicinal drug treatments; overproduction of adrenal cortex steroid hormones; multiple myeloma; gastrectomy; prolonged immobilization. Dietary causes include insufficient intake of calcium over long periods; non-replacement of lost calcium in poorly-fed women with multiple births over many years; non-replacement of calcium lost in breast-feeding; increased effect of fluoride on copper deficiency, inducing osteoporosis of the legs; increased overnight loss of calcium after the menopause; increased urinary loss of calcium on high-protein diets. Symptoms may be absent until bone fracture occurs. Sometimes there is aching pain in the bones, particularly the back. X-ray analysis and biochemical measurements of the blood and urine are essential for correct diagnosis and to differentiate the condition from osteomalacia.

During the menopause and post-menopausal periods, medical treatment of osteoporosis is confined to hormone replacement therapy (HRT) with female sex hormones. This therapy is still being assessed for possible long-term, serious side-effects. Dietary treatment involves supplementation with calcium; with calcium and vitamin D to help absorb the calcium; sometimes with added fluoride to stimulate calcium resorption into the bones. Typical supplementary regimes are: 1000-1500mg calcium daily, preferably with 400IU vitamin D; 1000-1500mg calcium daily with 400IU vitamin D plus 45mg per day sodium fluoride. In view of the toxicity of sodium fluoride, this regime should be taken only under medical supervision. Regular exercise is also an important factor in preventing and in treating osteoporosis. Adequate intake of calcium during life before the menopause also contributes to prevention of the disease once the menopause starts.

A *decreased mineral density* in the lumbar vertebrae of female athletes who have a reduced number of menstrual periods has been observed. Similar findings were noted in young women whose periods had stopped for reasons other than pregnancy. In all cases, calcium intake was suggested to be increased, from 800-1500mg per day.

---

otosclerosis, *see* deafness.

---

oxygen, occasionally causes eye problems (retrolental fibroplasia) in premature babies in oxygen tents. Prevented by administration of vitamin E, usually by injection.

P

PABA, para-aminobenzoic acid.

Paget's disease, also called osteitis deformans. A chronic degenerative disease of the bones occurring in the elderly and most frequently affecting the skull, backbone, pelvis and long bones. In the early stages of the disease calcium is lost from the bones. Characterized by deep, dull, aching bone pain that can cause headache, deafness, blindness when the skull is affected; bowing of the legs when these limbs are affected. Usual medical treatment is prolonged course of the hormone calcitonin but this may be complemented by extra calcium. Supplementary treatment consists of 500-1000mg calcium three times daily between meals, preferably in a form that does not supply phosphorus. Bone pain was relieved by this treatment which is believed to stimulate the body's own production of calcitonin.

pangamic acid, from 'pan' everywhere and 'gami' family. Water-soluble factor present in vitamin B complex. Also known as B_{15}; vitamin B_{15} (incorrectly); D-gluconic acid 6-(bis(1-methybethyl) amino acetate. First isolated from apricot kernels in 1951 by father and son team of Drs E. T. Krebs and E. T. Krebs Jr. Present in supplements as calcium pangamate; sodium pangamate. May also be dimethylglycine.

Richest food sources (in µg per 100g) are: rice bran (200); maize (150); dried brewer's yeast (128); oatflakes (106); wheatgerm (70); apricot kernels (65); wheat bran (31); pig's liver (22); barley (12); wholemeal flour (8).

Unstable to food processing. Lost and destroyed during cooking methods.

Doubt of correct structure of pangamic acid — now generally accepted as D-gluconic acid 6-(bis(1-methybethyl) amino acetate.

Functions as stimulator of carriage of oxygen to blood from lungs and from blood to muscles and vital organs; as lipotropic agent to keep fat in solution; as detoxifying agent on poisons and free radicals; as stimulator of anti-stress hormone production.

Deficiency in man has not been reported. Symptoms are not specific but may be related to above functions.

Deficiency in animals has not been reported.

Recommended dietary intakes not set by any authority.

Toxicity is low. Safe in doses up to 300mg daily but occasional transient flushing of skin. Calcium pangamate better tolerated than sodium pangamate.

Therapy with pangamic acid claimed to be beneficial in heart disease; in atherosclerosis; in bronchial asthma; in diabetes (USSR studies).

---

pantothenic acid, from 'panthos' meaning everywhere. Water-soluble vitamin, member of the vitamin B complex.

Usually presented in oral supplements as calcium pantothenate; in cosmetics and toiletries as dexpanthenol and pantothenol.

Generally accepted as vitamin B_5. Also known as chick antidermatitis factor. Anti-stress vitamin.

Isolated from rice husks by Dr R. J. Williams of the University of Texas in 1939. Occurs naturally as D-pantothenic acid.

Functions	Therapeutic Uses

As coenzyme A in:
  Production of energy
  Production of anti-stress
    hormones
  Controlling fat metabolism
  Formation of antibodies
  Maintaining healthy nerves
  Detoxifying drugs
	Rheumatoid arthritis
	Paralytic ileus
	Allergic skin reactions
	Reduction of mucous secretion
	  in respiratory allergies
	Stress situations

Best Food Sources in mg per 100g	
Dried brewer's yeast	9.5
Pig's liver	6.5
Yeast extract	3.8
Pig's kidney	3.0
Nuts	2.7
Wheat bran	2.4
Wheatgerm	2.2
Soya flour	1.8
Eggs	1.8
Poultry	1.2
Meats	1.1
Wholegrains	0.9
Pulses (beans)	0.8
Wholemeal bread	0.6
Vegetables	0.3

Stability in Foods

Easily destroyed, even at deep-freeze temperatures.

See Losses in Food Processing.

Deficiency Causes

Stress
Antibiotics

Deficiency Symptoms

Aching, burning, throbbing feet

Loss of appetite
Indigestion
Abdominal pain

Respiratory infections

Fatigue

Insomnia
Depression
Psychosis
Headaches

Recommended Daily Intakes

Should be at least 10mg but see separate entry.

Difficult to assess because of production by intestinal bacteria.

Symptoms of Excess Intake

None have been reported.

para-aminobenzoic acid, member of the vitamin B complex but not a true vitamin for man. Known also as PABA, vitamin Bx, bacterial vitamin H, anti-grey hair factor. Growth factor for bacteria that is blocked by sulphonamide drugs, first reported by D. D. Woods at Oxford in 1942. PABA is present as part of the structure of folic acid but no evidence that humans can make folic acid from it. Likely that intestinal bacteria can but body unable to utilize the folic acid produced.

Richest food sources are: liver, eggs, molasses, brewer's yeast, wheatgerm. Few figures are available but baker's yeast contains 6mg per kg; brewer's yeast up to 100mg per kg.

Stability in food processing unknown.

Functions in man not known.

Deficiency in man gives no specific symptoms.

Functions in animals in synthesis of body protein and in red blood cell production, possibly after conversion to folic acid. Helps utilization of pantothenic acid. May act as skin cancer preventative.

Deficiency in animals causes anaemia, premature greying of hair.

Recommended dietary intakes not set by any authority. In medicines the maximum dose is restricted to 30mg potency in the UK but there are no specified legal limits on its amount in a food as long as that amount is regarded as safe.

Toxicity is low but high intakes can cause nausea, vomiting, itching, skin rash and liver damage. *Contra-indicated* when on sulphonamide treatment.

Therapy with oral PABA in vitiligo. As lotion or cream is effective as sunscreen agent to prevent sunburn. May also prevent skin cancer. Has been used in digestive disorders, nervousness, depression.

---

para-amino salicylic acid,   anti-tuberculosis drug. Impairs absorption of vitamins A, D, E and K and of B_{12}.

---

paraesthesia,   tingling or pricking feeling or sometimes numbness in the skin. Symptom of multiple sclerosis, nerve disease, blood-vessel disease. Relieved by pyridoxine (50mg daily) but very high doses (2000mg) may cause it.

---

paralytic ileus, *see* surgery.

---

parathyroid hormone, also known as parathormone. A polypeptide hormone containing 84 amino acids, synthesized in the parathyroid glands (adjacent to or embedded in the thyroid gland), that controls the distribution of calcium and phosphate in the body. Secretion of the hormone is stimulated by a decrease in blood calcium. A high concentration of the hormone causes transfer of calcium from the bone reservoirs to the blood; a deficiency lowers blood calcium levels, causing tetany. Hormone also functions by promoting formation of the active form of vitamin D within the kidney. This is probably how the hormone mediates in its action of increasing the absorption of calcium from the intestine. The hormone also decreases the kidney reabsorption of phosphate, allowing the mineral to be excreted.

Parkinson's disease, a chronic disease of the central nervous system characterized by slowness and poorness of purposeful movement, rigid muscles and tremor. Also known as Parkinsonism, shaking palsy.

Drug *levodopa*, used to bring symptomatic relief, is neutralized by pyridoxine therefore supplements of vitamin should *not* be taken whilst on drug. Side-effects of levodopa may be lessened by taking vitamin C (500 to 1000mg daily).

---

peanut butter, supplies good quantities of vitamin E and the B vitamins. Vitamin E content is 7.6mg per 100g. B vitamins present are (in mg per 100g): thiamine 0.17; riboflavin 0.10; nicotinic acid 19.9; pyridoxine 0.50; pantothenic acid 2.1. Folic acid level is 53µg per 100g. Traces only of vitamin C. Similar vitamin contents in both smooth and crunchy peanut butter.

Mineral
Excellent source of potassium, magnesium, phosphorus and chloride; also the trace minerals iron, copper and zinc. High in sodium because of added salt. It supplies the following minerals (in mg per 100g): sodium 350;

potassium 700; calcium 37; magnesium 180; phosphorus 330; iron 2.1; copper 0.70; zinc 3.0; chloride 500.

---

peanuts,   kernels supply good quantities of vitamin E and B vitamins. Some B vitamins reduced when peanuts are roasted and salted. Vitamin E contents of fresh kernels and those that have been roasted and salted are identical at 16.9mg per 100g. B vitamins present (in mg per 100g), for fresh kernels and those that have been roasted and salted respectively, are: thiamine 0.90, 0.23; riboflavin 0.10, 0.10; nicotinic acid 21.3, 21.3; pyridoxine 0.50, 0.40; pantothenic acid 2.7, 2.1. Folic acid level in fresh kernels is 100μg per 100g, but is not detectable in the roasted and salted variety. Traces only of vitamin C in fresh and roasted peanuts.

Mineral
Excellent source of potassium, calcium, magnesium, phosphorus and sulphur; also the trace minerals iron, copper and zinc. Fresh nuts are low in sodium, but roasting and salting them increases sodium content significantly. Figures given are for fresh and roasted and salted respectively (in mg per 100g): sodium 6, 440; chloride 7, 660. Identical quantities for the following: potassium 680; calcium 61; magnesium 180; phosphorus 370; iron 2.0; copper 0.27; zinc 3.0; sulphur 380.

---

pears,   edible portion of eating variety has poor content of all vitamins either in raw state or as canned variety. Loss of B vitamins and vitamin C during canning. Carotene content is 10μg per 100g; traces only of vitamin E in both eating and canned pears. B vitamins present are (in mg per 100g), for eating and canned pears respectively: thiamine 0.03, 0.01; riboflavin 0.03, 0.01; nicotinic acid 0.3, 0.2; pyridoxine 0.02, 0.01; pantothenic acid 0.07, 0.02. Folic acid content is 11μg per 100g for fresh, edible portion of fruit and 5μg per 100g for canned fruit. Biotin is 1μg per 100g and a trace respectively. Vitamin C is reduced from 3mg to 1mg per 100g when fruit is canned.

Cooking variety have similar concentrations of vitamins to eating pears with only slight losses on stewing, with and without sugar. Carotene levels for raw, cooking pears, stewed without sugar and stewed with sugar respectively, are (in μg per 100g) 10, 9 and 8. Traces only of vitamin E. B vitamins present are (in mg per 100g), for raw, cooking pears, stewed without sugar and stewed with sugar respectively: thiamine 0.03, 0.03, 0.02; riboflavin 0.03, 0.03, 0.02; nicotinic acid 0.2, 0.2, 0.2; pyridoxine 0.02, 0.02, 0.02; pantothenic acid 0.07, 0.05, 0.05. Folic acid levels are respectively 11, 5 and 5μg per 100g; biotin levels are stable at 0.1μg per 100g respectively for the three states of cooking pears.

Mineral
Virtually free of sodium with useful potassium levels. Small amounts of all the other minerals.

Eating variety — raw, edible portion contains levels of the following (in mg per 100g): sodium 2; potassium 130; calcium 8; magnesium 7; phosphorus 10; iron 0.2; copper 0.15; zinc 0.1; sulphur 5; chloride only trace.

Cooking variety, stewed without sugar and with sugar respectively (in mg per 100g): sodium 3, 2; potassium 85, 78; calcium 6, 5; magnesium 3, 3; phosphorus 13, 12; iron 0.2, 0.2; copper 0.09, 0.09; zinc 0.1, 0.1; sulphur 3, 2; chloride 2, 2.

Canned, provides (in mg per 100g): sodium 1; potassium 90; calcium 5; magnesium 6; phosphorus 5; iron 0.3; copper 0.04; sulphur 1; chloride 3.

---

pellagra, specific disease associated with deficiency of nicotinic acid and characterized by skin, mucous membrane, central nervous system and gastrointestinal symptoms. Symptoms may appear alone or in combination. Treatment is 300 to 1000mg nicotinamide daily in divided doses.

Similar disease in dogs known as canine black tongue.

---

penicillamine, anti-arthritic drug. Enhances excretion of pyridoxine.

---

pentamidine isethionate, anti-protozoal drug. Impairs folic acid utilization.

---

pernicious anaemia, particular type of anaemia characterized by non-specific symptoms, loss of appetite, constipation alternating with diarrhoea, and vague abdominal pains. More specific is 'burning of the tongue' or glossitis. Considerable weight loss. Later there is nervous involvement with tingling in the extremities, irritability, depression, delirium, and paranoia. Loss of sensation in lower extremities.

Only treatment is vitamin B_{12} by injection which continues throughout life.

PGA, folic acid.

phagocytes, white blood cells that engulf and destroy invading micro-organisms. *See* leucocytes.

pheneturide, anti-convulsant drug. Reduces conversion of vitamin D to 25-hydroxy vitamin D.

phenformin, anti-diabetic drug. Prevents absorption of vitamin B_{12}.

phenylbutazone, anti-arthritic drug. Impairs folic acid utilization.

phenytoin, anti-convulsant drug. Reduces body levels of folic acid and 25-hydroxy vitamin D.

phlebitis, presence of a thrombosis in a vein that causes painful, tender and swollen lump, usually in the leg. Daily intake of 200IU vitamin E believed to prevent condition. Treatment needs daily intake of at least 600IU vitamin E.

phosphorus, chemical symbol P. Atomic weight 30.9. Present in the body (combined with oxygen) as phosphates and is a constituent of all plant and animal cells. With daily intakes between 1.5 and 2.0g from a wide variety of food, deficiency is highly unlikely. A greater problem may be excessive intakes of phosphates from soft drinks, processed foods and junk foods.

Best Food Sources in mg per 100g	
Yeast extract	1900
Dried brewer's yeast	1753
Dried skimmed milk	950
Wheatgerm	930
Soya flour	600
Hard cheeses	520
Canned fish	520
Nuts	370
Cereals	290
Evaporated milk	250
Wholemeal bread	240
Eggs	218
Meats and poultry	200
Fish (fresh)	170
Yogurt	140
All high protein foods	

Body Distribution

Person weighing 70kg contains between 550 and 770g phosphorus of which 90 per cent is in the bones and teeth as calcium phosphate (hydroxyapatite).

Muscles (9 per cent) and nerves (1 per cent) account for rest of body phosphorus.

Absorption

Depends upon vitamin D for absorption from the food and into bone from the blood.

Relationship with Calcium

Contrary to previous beliefs that phosphate content of the diet had a crucial influence on calcium absorption, it is now accepted that dietary relationship between the two is not important. However, for babies the calcium: phosphorus ratio of 2:1 in human milk is considered more desirable than that of 1.2:1 in cow's milk. Dried milks are now adjusted to the more favoured ratio of 2:1 and the levels of both minerals reduced to those of human breast milk.

Functions

Phosphorus functions only as phosphates in the body in the following ways:

Structural components of bones and teeth

In the production of energy.

In the 'burning' of sugar for energy

As a cofactor for many enzymes

As activators for the vitamin B complex

To aid absorption of dietary constituents

To maintain the blood at slightly alkaline conditions (pH 7.39-7.41)

As components of Ribonucleic acids (RNA) and Deoxyribonucleic acids (DNA), the basic constituents of life processes.

Deficiency Symptoms

Debility
Loss of appetite
Weakness
Bone pain
Joint stiffness
General malaise
Osteomalacia

Irritability
Numbness
'Pins and Needles'
Speech disorders
Tremor
Mental confusion

Therapeutic Uses

Low phosphate levels induced by disease must be treated by medical practitioner who can monitor response. Simple supplementation to ensure adequate dietary intakes can be carried out using supplementary forms listed below.

Excessive Intakes

Can cause diarrhoea
Can cause calcification in organs and soft tissues
Can prevent absorption of iron, calcium, magnesium and zinc

Deficiency	Deficiency Effects
Considered highly unlikely in view of widespread distribution in foods but many medical conditions can induce low blood phosphate levels.	Shortened red blood cell life (leading to anaemia) Subnormal white blood cells leading to reduced resistance to infection

Phosphorus Supplements (phosphorus in mg per 100mg)

Bonemeal (18.5); sodium phosphate (8.7); effervescent sodium phosphate (21.8); potassium phosphate (17.8); calcium phosphate (18.7); calcium glycerophosphate (14.7); magnesium glycerophosphate (15.9); sodium glycerophosphate (9.8).

phylloquinone, K_1 vitamin.

phytic acid, also known as inositol hexaphosphate. Provides 28.2mg phosphorus per 100mg. Has long been known to be a constituent of cereals, vegetables and most plant materials. It can combine with metals of nutritional importance to form phytates that are stable in the normal digestive system and so cannot be absorbed. Those most affected are calcium, iron and zinc. There is some evidence that animals, including man, who have high phytic acid intakes can induce an enzyme called phytase which hydrolyses the phytic acid-metal complexes liberating the mineral. The phytic acid content of a normal, balanced diet is unlikely to affect the essential minerals to a significant extent. Problems may arise in those eating high-cereal, high-vegetable content diets where these foods are the sole source of minerals. Examples were seen in young children on a poor diet in Ireland in the 1940s. Phytic acid is concentrated in the aleurone layer of the wheat grain and is present in high concentration in high-extraction flours and in the bran. Phytic acid contents are (in mg per 100g): bran 4225; wholemeal flour 805; white flour 200. These Irish children lived on wholemeal flour products with little dairy produce for three years. The reduced absorption of calcium as a result caused high rates in the incidence of rickets. Reducing the extraction rate of flour to 85 per cent, combined with more milk and dairy products in their diets, caused the rate in incidence of rickets to drop. Similar problems have been encountered with Asian immigrants in the UK. Although low vitamin D level in the body was the main cause of the increased incidence of rickets and osteomalacia, high intakes of phytic acid in chapatis and low intake of calcium from dairy sources were also factors.

In the preparation of bread, much of the phytic acid content of the flour is destroyed. The traditional long-proving technique of breadmaking causes 50 per cent of the phytic acid of wholemeal bread to be destroyed. Techniques that use shorter proving times, like those utilizing vitamin C, give rise to losses of phytic acid totalling one third of that in the original wholemeal flour. Most destruction is due to the enzyme phytase present in wheat and in yeast. Once this is inactivated by the baking process, further destruction is initiated by the high oven temperature.

Problems with phytic acid are more likely to arise with high intakes of raw bran, cereals and vegetables. The main source is high extraction flours but oats, high-bran breakfast foods, soya and other beans also contribute meaningful quantities of phytic acid. When the phytate:zinc ratio in these diets exceeds 15:1, the availability of zinc decreases drastically. The zinc in wholemeal bread is 3.0mg per 100g but is less readily available than

Table 14: Zinc, phytic acid and dietary fibre contents of cereal foods

Cereal food	Zinc mg/100g	Phytic acid mg/100g	Phytic acid: Zinc ratio	Dietary fibre g/100g
Wholemeal flour	2.4	850	35	9.6
White flour	1.5	200	13	7.5
Wholemeal bread	1.8	610	33	8.5
Brown bread	1.8	440	25	5.1
White bread	0.6	90	15	2.7
Bran-based cereals	3.6	2200	60	26.7
Cornflakes	0.3	60	21	11.0
Wheat-based cereals	2.8	820	29	12.3
Oatmeal	3.4	940	27	7.0

that in white bread which is only 0.9mg per 100g. This is less important in the UK where three-quarters of the zinc in the diet comes from animal, fish and dairy-based foods than in those countries where cereals and vegetables supply the greater part of dietary zinc.

Table 14 indicates the zinc, phytic acid and dietary fibre contents of cereal foods. Ratios of greater than 15 reduce zinc bioavailability.

Meat extenders and replacers derived from soya beans can also provide phytic acid which can bind zinc. This is illustrated in Table 15. Ratios of greater than 15 decrease zinc bioavailability.

Table 15: Phytic acid produced from meat extenders and replacers

Product on a dry weight basis	Zinc (mg/100g)	Phytic acid (g/100g)	Molar ratio Phytic acid:zinc
Meat extender	4.3	1.6	37
Mince additive	3.5	1.4	39
TVP (Textured Vegetable Protein) beef	4.2	1.3	31
TVP pork	4.1	1.8	43
TVP mince	5.0	1.8	36
TVP unflavoured	4.4	1.9	43
Beef	17.0 (av.)	0	—
Pork	6.6 (av.)	0	—

phytomenadione, K_1 vitamin.

phytonadione, K_1 vitamin.

picolinates, combinations of minerals with picolinic acid. Recent research suggests they may be more bioabsorbable than mineral salts. For example, poor absorption of zinc may result from metabolic faults or dietary deficiencies that prevent the body from making picolinic acid from the essential amino acid tryptophan. Picolinic acid was shown to be effective in raising zinc levels in the blood of rats deprived of tryptophan. Tryptophan deficiency in experimental rats was found to cause hair loss and tremors in addition to zinc deficiency.

Chromium picolinate has been claimed to be better absorbed than conventional chromium salts. In addition, at a daily intake of 1.6mg it lowered blood cholesterol levels in people with high cholesterol; reduced high blood sugar levels in non-insulin dependent diabetics and increased muscle gains in weight-lifters. These are very preliminary observations and research is continuing.

Plummer's disease,   *see* hyperthyroidism.

---

pollution,   atmospheric produced by carbon monoxide and lead from exhaust fumes, ozone, nitrogen dioxide, sulphur dioxide and dust.

Vitamin C protects against carbon monoxide and lead. Vitamin E protects against ozone and other oxidizers. Also protects vitamin A against destruction by ozone and nitrogen dioxide. Polluted atmosphere prevents ultra-violet light reaching skin so vitamin D is not synthesized and dietary intake must be increased.

---

polymixin,   antibiotic. Prevents formation of vitamin K by intestinal bacteria.

---

polyunsaturated fatty acids,   originally called vitamin F applied to linoleic, linolenic and arachidonic acids. Now unofficially applied to linoleic acid alone since this is the precursor of the other two in the body. Known also as PUFA, essential fatty acids, EFA. Essentiality first demonstrated by G. O. Burr and M. M. Burr in 1929 who found those acids needed by rats for health and survival. Main sources of linoleic acid are vegetable and seed oils. Recently PUFA from fish body oils called EPA (eicosapentaenoic acid) and DHA (docosahexaenoic acid) found to be essential.

Richest food sources of linoleic acid (in grams per 100g) are: oil of evening primrose (72.70); safflower oil (71.63); soyabean oil (49.66); maize (corn) oil (47.75); wheatgerm oil (41.54); peanut oil (27.70); olive oil (10.51). Oil of evening primrose contains in addition to linoleic acid, gammalinolenic acid (average 8 per cent).

Functions are constituents of cell membranes and myelin sheath of nerves; precursors of hormones called prostaglandins; constituents of cholesteryl esters; constituents of triglycerides (body fats).

Deficiency in animals and man causes mild skin complaints including scaly dermatitis. May cause infantile eczema.

Recommended dietary intake — none laid down by any authority but many recommended that most of fat intakes (25-35 per cent of total calorie intake) should be as PUFA oils.

Therapy has proved beneficial in mild skin complaints; in atopic eczema; in infantile eczema; in premenstrual tension; in multiple sclerosis; in thrombosis prevention; in reducing high blood cholesterol levels. EPA and DHA appear beneficial in increasing blood clotting time (i.e., thinning the blood); in angina pectoris; in reducing high blood fat concentrations; in preventing thrombosis formation.

---

potassium, chemical symbol K, from the Latin *kalium*. Atomic weight 39.1. Alkali metal that is found mainly as sylvite (potassium chloride) and in the aluminosilicates orthoclase and microcline and as carnallite. Occurrence in earth's crust is 2.59 per cent.

The body potassium content of a person weighing 65kg is about 140g. Of this, only 3.1g is present in the extracellular fluid. The remaining 137g occurs inside body cells and of this, four-fifths is present in skeletal muscles. The quantity in the skeleton is negligible.

Dietary intakes of potassium are between 1960 and 5870mg daily with a usual intake of 2.54g equivalent to 4.85g potassium chloride.

Food sources of potassium are widespread but very variable in content. The best sources are (in mg per 100g): dried fruits 710-1880; soya flour 1660-2030; molasses 1470; wheat bran 1160; raw salad vegetables 140-1080; chipped potatoes 1020; nuts 350-940; breakfast cereals and mueslis 100-600; savoury biscuits 140-500; fresh fruit 65-430; boiled vegetables 50-400; fish 230-360; meat and poultry 33-350; fruit juices 110-260; wholemeal flour 360; wholemeal bread 220; white bread 100; eggs 140; cheese 100-190; brown rice 190; polished rice 110. Beverages are particularly rich sources, e.g. instant coffee 4000; Indian tea 2160;

roasted coffee 2020; cocoa powder 1500; drinking chocolate 410.

Absorption of potassium from the diet is passive requiring no specific mechanism. Absorption takes place throughout the small intestine and is dependent on the potassium concentration within the intestinal contents. Absorption takes place as long as this concentration is greater than that of the blood. Secretion of potassium probably takes place in the large bowel. Rapid movement of intestine contents through the small and large intestine is unfavourable to absorption. Under these conditions, such as persistent diarrhoea, low body potassium can develop.

Excretion of potassium reflects its dietary intake. Out of a daily intake of 2.35g, 2.15g is excreted in the urine with 0.39g in the faeces. The negative balance of 0.19g is due to normal cellular breakdown which releases potassium eventually into the urine. Such breakdown of cellular proteins increases in diabetes, underfeeding and after injury. Potassium can also be displaced from the cells by hydrogen ions. Any condition giving rise to acidosis is thus liable to cause cellular depletion of potassium.

Diuretic drugs, particularly the thiazide variety, act by increasing the output of sodium and water from the kidneys but at the same time potassium excretion is increased. Supplementation with this is therefore usual. In severe kidney failure, potassium is not excreted in the urine and excessive levels build up in the blood and tissue. The consequences are discussed below.

Faecal excretion is low in a healthy person, probably not exceeding 200mg daily. The digestive juices contain significant amounts but these are usually re-absorbed in the lower gut. Diarrhoea can cause large losses in the faeces in amounts up to 3.52g in 24 hours. This is particularly serious in infants suffering from diarrhoea induced by protein-energy malnutrition who may lose as much as 10-30 per cent of total body potassium. Heart failure may result. Similar losses may appear in infants or adults with chronic diarrhoea brought on by other causes (e.g. infection) and it is important in these cases that potassium as well as water losses are replaced by supplementation.

Sweat losses of potassium are usually negligible since sweat contains only about 352mg per litre. Excessive perspiration can lead to more significant losses but these do not approach those of sodium in importance.

Functions of potassium are:

1. in maintaining a normal balance of water within body cells as the major positively-charged ion within these cells;

2. as an essential activator in a number of enzymes particularly those concerned with energy production;
3. to help stabilize the internal structure of body cells;
4. in assisting specialized cell particles to synthesize proteins;
5. in nerve impulse transmission in conjunction with sodium;
6. to increase the excitability of heart and skeletal muscle to make them more receptive to nerve impulses;
7. in preserving the acid-alkali balance of the body in conjunction with bicarbonate, phosphate and protein as well as with sodium, calcium and magnesium;
8. in stimulating the normal movements of the intestinal tract.

Causes of potassium deficiency are:

1. drug therapy with: (a) thiazide and other diuretics including frusemide, chlorthalidone, ethacrynic acid, mercurials and carbonic anhydrase inhibitors; (b) long-term use of corticosteroids and ACTH; (c) overuse of laxatives; (d) excessive intake of liquorice and the drug carbenoxolone from liquorice; (e) high-dose sodium penicillin and carbenicillin; (f) intravenous infusions of glucose and salt solutions not containing potassium; (g) ion-exchange resins used to reduce blood cholesterol; (h) low sodium diets.
2. surgical operations — ileostomy, colostomy; extensive bowel resection; gastric drainage. Other deficiency causes are extensive burns; extensive injury; diabetes mellitus; Cushing's syndrome; excessive excretion of aldosterone; diabetes insipidus; periodic familial paralysis; chronic diarrhoea; persistent vomiting; influenza; megaloblastic anaemia; ulcerative colitis; kidney disease; severe heart disease; chronic respiratory failure; prolonged fasting; therapeutic starvation; bizarre diets, especially in the elderly; anorexia nervosa; alcoholism; clay eating; cystic fibrosis; alkalosis.

Symptoms of deficiency include vomiting; abdominal distension; paralytic ileus; acute muscular weakness; paralysis; paraesthesia ('pins and needles'); loss of appetite; low blood-pressure; polydipsia (intense thirst); drowsiness and confusion leading to respiratory failure; coma; an inability to concentrate urine; increased toxicity of digitalis.

Treatment of low potassium levels is with:

1. oral or intravenous potassium chloride solutions;
2. increased dietary intake of potassium-rich foods;
3. drugs such as triamterene or spironolactone taken with potassium-losing diuretics.

Potassium phosphate may be given by injection as an alternative to potassium chloride in the presence of acidosis.

Excess of potassium causes effects first on the muscles of the skeleton and of the heart, giving rise to muscular weakness and mental apathy. Intravenous potassium in excess may stop the heart. High oral doses can cause ulceration of the small bowel, particularly if the tablets are of the enteric-coated type (i.e. treated to prevent dissolution in the stomach to ensure they dissolve in the small intestine) which produce a localized high concentration of potassium. Lower doses of salts may cause nausea, vomiting, diarrhoea and abdominal cramps.

Causes of potassium excess include kidney failure; insufficient production of adrenal gland hormones; shock after injury in which condition potassium leaks out of the damaged cells into the blood. Treatment is withdrawal of potassium salts and of foods; in serious cases medical expertise is necessary.

Supplementary form of potassium is usually potassium chloride which provides 52.4mg potassium in 100mg chloride but potassium acetate, bicarbonate, citrate, gluconate, sulphate, acid tartrate, tartrate and phosphates have also been used. Amino acid or protein complexes are also available which are claimed to be better absorbed than potassium salts. These complexes also replace protein losses which may accompany excessive potassium excretion.

Food additives that contain potassium are: potassium acetate; potassium alginate; potassium benzoate; potassium bromate; potassium carbonate; potassium chloride; tripotassium citrate; tetrapotassium diphosphate; potassium ferrocyanide; potassium gluconate; potassium bicarbonate; potassium dihydrogen citrate; potassium hydrogen glutamate; potassium dihydrogen orthophosphate; dipotassium hydrogen orthophosphate; potassium hydroxide; potassium lactate; potassium malate; potassium metabisulphite; potassium nitrate; potassium nitrite; tripotassium orthophosphate; potassium pectate; potassium persulphate; potassium polyphosphates; potassium propionate; potassium salts of fatty acids; potassium sodium tartrate; potassium sorbate; potassium sulphate; dipotassium tartrate; monopotassium tartrate; pentapotassium triphosphate.

potassium sorbate, a food additive used as a preservative, E202. Acceptable daily intake up to 0.25mg per kg body weight. Provides 26.1mg potassium per 100mg. Permitted in certain foods; in certain wines, quantity restricted.

---

potatoes, all potatoes, old and new, cooked in every way, contain only traces of carotene and vitamin E per 100g. Poor source of B vitamins but regarded as an important provider of vitamin C in the Western diet.

As they are an important item in the Western diet because of the amount eaten, potatoes in all forms are regarded as supplying significant quantities of potassium, phosphorus, sulphur and chloride plus the trace minerals iron, copper, zinc, chromium and selenium.

For amounts of nutrients present see Vegetables.

Substantial losses of vitamin C occur from potatoes when they are stored and during all cooking methods. Keep water volume low to minimise losses in boiling; much can be recovered by utilizing cooking water.

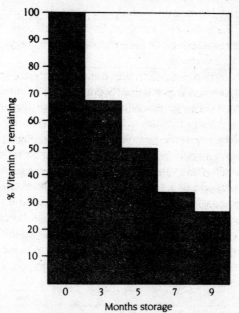

Stored potatoes — % vitamin C remaining (30mg per 100g freshly dug)

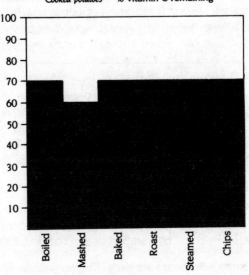

Cooked potatoes — % vitamin C remaining

PP factor, nicotinic acid.

precursors, substances that occur in food that are not vitamins in their own right but can give rise to vitamins in the body or during cooking processes.

Examples are: Carotenes, some of which are converted to vitamin A in the intestine and liver; L-tryptophane, an essential amino acid of food proteins, converted to nicotinic acid in the liver under the influence of thiamine, riboflavin, pyridoxine and biotin; Niacytin, a bound form of nicotinic acid that occurs in maize and other cereals, unavailable to the body unless cooked under alkaline conditions which liberates nicotinic acid; 7-dehydrocholesterol in the skin is converted to vitamin D by the action of sunlight or particular wavelengths of ultra-violet light. Vitamin D itself is inactive but is a precursor of 25-hydroxy D and 1,25-dihydroxy D which are its active forms in the body.

pregnancy, all authorities recognize that all vitamins and some minerals must be increased in dietary intake but no agreement on extent of increase. Blood levels of vitamin A, nicotinamide, pyridoxine, vitamin B_{12} and ascorbic acid markedly decreased in pregnant women suggesting all should be supplemented. Some evidence that low vitamin levels may lead to some birth defects in offspring. Daily supplementation with good all-round multivitamin preparation recommended throughout pregnancy since availability from diet highly unlikely. Folic acid is a special case.

High levels of any vitamin should not be taken during pregnancy, apart perhaps from folic acid. Vitamin A supplements should not be more than 7500IU (250μg) daily; vitamin B_6 (pyridoxine) supplementary intakes should not rise to more than 25mg daily. Amounts required may be above those on general sale and so should be obtained from a medical practitioner.

---

prickly heat, known also as milaria, characterized by small pimples on skin surface that irritate, cause scratching and eventual bleeding of the affected area. Induced by retained sweat. Treated and prevented by daily dose of 1000mg vitamin C for adult weighing 150lbs, proportionally less for children depending on weight.

---

primidone, anti-convulsant drug. Reduces conversion of vitamin D to 25-hydroxy vitamin D.

---

processed meats, such as canned meat, pastes, sausages, beefburgers and pies all supply significantly less vitamins than the meat from which they were made. Reduced levels are due to processing losses and dilution of the meat with fat and flour.

---

prostaglandins, hormones produced within the body that control many metabolic processes. All prostaglandins are made from certain polyunsaturated fatty acids which in turn are derived from the dietary polyunsaturated fatty acids, linoleic acid and alpha linoleic acid. Each acid is the starting material for a separate series of prostaglandins.

Prostaglandins can make blood thick, so increasing chances of thrombosis, or thin, preventing thrombosis. Production of 'thinning' prostaglandins are stimulated by vitamin E. PUFA from fish body oils, called EPA and DHA, also thin the blood, reducing its ability to form thrombosis because they are precursors of 'thinning' prostaglandins.

prostate gland,   the male accessory gland that rests just below the bladder and completely surrounds the bladder's narrow neck called the urethra. When it is enlarged, the prostate pinches off the urethra, restricting the flow of urine. When the prostate is inflamed prostatitis is the result, requiring anti-bacterial treatment. Enlarged prostate, from whatever reason, is usually treated by surgery. Maintaining a healthy prostate appears to require adequate zinc intakes. Both the healthy prostate and the semen usually contain high concentrations of zinc. Those with prostate problems almost invariably had low zinc levels in the gland and in their semen. Supplementation with an average of 25mg elemental zinc daily relieved the symptoms in some men with enlarged prostates. More importantly, adequate intakes of the mineral throughout life may cut down the chances of developing an enlarged prostate. Low saturated-fat diets combined with high-fibre intakes may also contribute.

prostate problems,   usually due to inflammation or enlargement. Supplement needs include PUFA (safflower oil, oil of evening primrose) 3g daily plus mineral zinc (25mg daily).

protein,   nutrient that is supplied in the diet, digested to amino acids and absorbed in the gastrointestinal tract then rebuilt by the body into its own proteins required for growth and repairing of body cells, tissues, muscles and organs.

Synthesis by body requires vitamin A: high protein intakes require concomitant vitamin A intake. Also pyridoxine. *Blood clotting proteins* require vitamin K for synthesis. *Nucleoproteins* are complexes of protein and nucleic acids and need vitamin B_{12} for synthesis. *See* nucleic acids.

psoriasis, common chronic and recurrent skin disease characterized by dry, silvery, scaling eruptions and plaques of various sizes due to overproduction of epithelial cells. Has been treated with oral and topical (applied to skin) vitamin A, retinoic acid and synthetic vitamin A derivatives.

---

psoriatic arthritis, - a particular form of arthritis that is associated with the skin complaint psoriasis. Occurs in a minority of those with psoriasis but is very painful and disabling. May occur in spine, toes and fingers as a spondylitis; in back joints as sacroiliitis. Studies in Denmark indicate that some cases respond to the mineral zinc, taken as zinc sulphate (220mg, three times daily). Stiff joints became mobile; grip strengthened; swelling was reduced; pain and morning stiffness disappeared. Benefit may be due to the activity of zinc in the body's own immune system that attacks the inflammatory response in arthritis. The skin complaint psoriasis may also respond.

---

pteroyglutamic acid, folic acid.

---

pteroyl monoglutamic acid, folic acid.

PUFA, *see* polyunsaturated fatty acids.

---

pulses, include beans, lentils and peas.

All pulses are good sources of carotene, vitamin E and the vitamin B complex. They contribute good levels of vitamin C also but as all water-soluble vitamins are lost into the cooking water, this should be utilized in some way to recover the vitamins. Lentils however are lower in carotene and vitamin C contents.

All are virtually free of sodium (unless it is added during cooking) but supply important quantities of potassium and the trace minerals to the diet. The charts indicate the contribution of pulses to the daily intakes of vitamins and minerals.

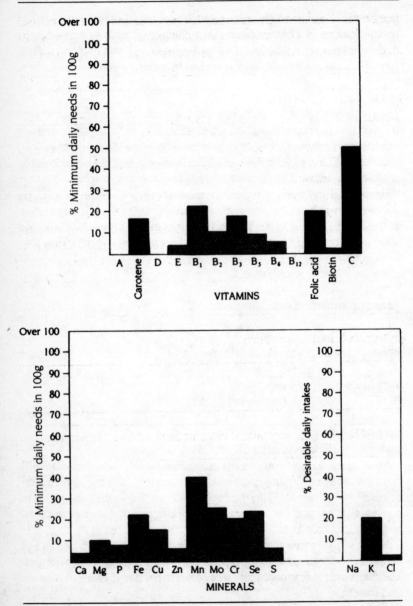

purpura, haemorrhages under the skin that occur without definite cause or due to slight injury. Has been treated with oral vitamin E, 400-600IU daily, until purpura disappears. *See also* bruises.

---

pyridoxal, B_6 vitamin.

---

pyridoxal-5-phosphate, the active form of vitamin B_6 (pyridoxine). Pyridoxine is metabolized in the body by the enzyme pyridoxal-5-phosphatase into pyridoxal-5-phosphate.

Pyridoxal-5-phospate is the form of the nutrient which is actually assimilated by the cells.

Clinical studies have identified subjects lacking in pyridoxal-5-phosphase, and consequently exhibiting signs and symptoms of vitamin B_6 deficiency, yet with normal pyridoxine levels. Pyridoxal-5-phosphate can be of clinical use when pyridoxine has failed.

The optimum daily intake is 50mg.

---

pyridoxamine, B_6 vitamin.

---

pyridoxine, B_6 vitamin.

---

pyrimethamine, antimalarial drug. Impairs folic acid utilization.

Q

---

quercetin, a B type flavone that appears to have anti-inflammatory properties in induced arthritic conditions of experimental animals and to control allergies. In this, quercetin is effective in preventing tissue release of histamine in response to allergens. It is histamine that is the primary culprit in allergy attacks triggered by pollens, animal hairs, moulds, house dust etc. in susceptible people. Histamine is believed to be responsible for the classic symptoms of allergies, e.g. swollen, runny nose, excessive mucus discharge, sneezing, itchy eyes, etc. Histamine is stored in the mast cells and basophils of the blood and tissues. Quercetin has a strong affinity for mast cells and basophils, and strengthens cell membranes, so preventing the release of histamine. It is thus useful against allergies induced by histamine. Typical therapeutic doses are 1000-3000mg daily.

R

recommended daily intakes, known in USA as recommended daily allowances (RDA). Daily minimum requirements of vitamins needed to prevent symptoms of deficiency disease but not necessarily sufficient to maintain optimum health. Safety factors added to average minimum requirements to deal with three variables:

1. to take account of individual variations in requirements — safety factor covers 95 per cent of population.
2. to take account of possible increases caused by minor stresses of life but extra needs during infections, injuries and other illnesses are ignored.
3. to take account of different availability of vitamins in various foods.

Figures vary amongst countries reflecting variation in how they are arrived at. Also number of vitamins with recommended intakes differ amongst several authorities. For figures *see* Table 16.

Mineral
See Table 17.
   Belgium also suggests the following RDAs for nutrients not in the tables: biotin 150µg; vitamin K 100µg; essential fatty acids 3.0g; chromium 125µg; chlorine 3500mg; copper 2.5mg; fluorine 2.5mg; manganese 3.5mg; molybdenum 300µg; phosphorus 1000mg; potassium 4000mg; sodium 2500mg; selenium 125µg.

regional enteritis, *see* Crohn's disease.

Table 16: Recommended dietary intakes of vitamins for adults

Vitamin	Unit	Sex	Ar	Au	Be	Bu	Can	Car	Ch	Cz	De	FDR	Fi	Fr	GDR	Hu	In	It	Ja	Ko	Me
VITAMIN A	µg	Female	750	750	1000	220	800	750	1000	900	800	900	750	800	800	750	750	750	540	600	750
		Male	–	–	–	200	1000	–	–	1000	1000	1000	–	1000	–	–	–	–	600	–	–
THIAMINE	mg	Female	0.9	1.1	1.5	1.1	1.0	0.9	1.4	1.6	1.1	1.4	0.8	1.3	0.9	1.0	1.0	1.0	0.8	1.0	0.8
		Male	1.2	–	–	1.5	1.5	1.2	1.5	2.0	1.2	1.6	1.6	1.5	1.0	1.2	1.2	1.2	0.9	1.1	1.0
RIBOFLAVIN	mg	Female	1.4	1.4	1.7	1.5	1.5	1.1	1.4	1.4	1.2	1.6	1.3	1.5	1.5	1.5	1.1	1.2	1.1	1.2	1.2
		Male	1.8	–	–	1.8	1.7	1.6	1.5	2.0	1.6	2.0	1.4	1.8	1.6	–	1.4	1.6	1.3	1.6	1.4
NIACIN	mg	Female	14	13	18	18	15	14	16	18	15	16	17	15	18	15	13	16	13	13	13
		Male	20	18	–	22	20	19	15	22	18	19	19	18	20	18	16	18	15	18	15.8
PYRIDOXINE	mg	Female	–	1.5	2.0	–	2.0	1.5	–	1.8	2.0	1.6	–	2.0	–	–	2.0	–	–	–	–
		Male	–	–	–	–	1.5	2.0	–	2.4	–	1.8	–	2.2	–	–	–	–	–	–	–
PANTOTHENIC ACID	mg		–	5.0	5.0	–	–	–	–	–	–	8.0	–	–	–	–	–	–	–	–	–
VITAMIN B$_{12}$	µg		2.0	2.0	3.0	–	3.0	2.0	–	–	3.0	5.0	–	3.0	–	–	1.0	2.0	–	–	2.0
VITAMIN C	mg	Female	30	30	60	65	30	30	60	50	45	75	30	80	70	30	40	45	50	50	30
		Male	–	–	–	100	–	–	–	80	–	–	–	–	–	–	–	–	–	55	–
BIOFLAVONOIDS	mg	Female	–	–	–	–	–	–	–	–	–	–	–	–	–	–	–	–	–	–	–
		Male	–	–	–	–	–	–	–	–	–	–	–	–	–	–	–	–	–	–	–
VITAMIN E	mg	Female	–	–	10	–	8	12	–	10	12	12	–	15	–	–	–	–	–	–	–
		Male	–	–	–	–	6	15	–	12	15	–	–	–	–	–	–	–	–	–	–
VITAMIN D	µg		2.5	10.0	7.5	–	2.5	2.5	10.0	–	2.5	2.5	2.5	10.0	2.5	2.5	5.0	2.5	2.5	10.0	2.5
FOLIC ACID	µg		200	200	400	–	200	200	–	200	100	–	–	400	–	–	100	–	–	–	200

Key: Ar: Argentina; Au: Australia; Be: Belgium; Bu: Bulgaria; Can: Canada; Car: Caribbean; Ch: China; Cz: Czechoslovakia; De: Denmark; FDR: West Germany; Fi: Finland; Fr: France; GDR: East Germany; Hu: Hungary; In: India; It: Italy; Ja: Japan; Ko: Korea; Me: Mexico; Ne: Netherlands; No: Norway; NZ: New Zealand; Ph: Philippines; Pol: Poland; Por: Portugal; Ro: Rumania; Si: Singapore; Sp: Spain; Sw: Sweden; Ta: Taiwan; Th: Thailand; Tu: Turkey; UK: United Kingdom; USA: United States of America; USSR: Russia; WP: West Pacific. WHO/FAO: World Health Organization/Food and Agriculture Organization.

		Me	Ne	No	NZ	PK	Pol	Por	Ro	Si	Sp	Sw	Ta	Th	Tu	UK	USA	USSR	WP	WHO/FAO
VITAMIN A	Female μg	1000	850	750	750	550	1500	1500	1500	750	750	900	750	750	750	750	800	1500	750	750
	Male					650											1000			
THIAMINE	Female mg	1.0	0.8	1.0	1.0	0.9	1.5	1.2	1.8	0.80	0.9	1.0	1.1	0.6	0.9	0.9	1.0	1.5	0.9	0.9
	Male	1.4	1.0	1.4	1.2	1.2	2.0	1.5	2.1	0.96	1.2	1.4	1.3	0.9	1.2	1.2	1.4	1.8	1.1	1.2
RIBOFLAVIN	Female mg	1.2	1.2	1.5	1.7	0.9	1.8	1.4	2.0	1.20	1.3	1.5	1.3	0.8	1.2	1.3	1.2	2.0	1.6	1.3
	Male	1.7	1.4	1.7		1.2	2.3	1.8	2.4	1.44	1.8	1.7	1.4	1.2	1.8	1.7	1.6	2.4		1.8
NIACIN	Female mg	16.0	15	15	13	13	15	14	15	13.0	16	14	15	11	12	15	13	18	14.2	15
	Male	22.5	19	18	18	16	20	18	18	15.8	20	18	20	16	17	18	18	20	18.0	20
PYRIDOXINE	Female mg	–	–	–	2.0	–	2.0	–	1.7	–	–	–	1.8	–	–	–	2.0	1.8	–	–
	Male												2.0					2.1		
PANTOTHENIC ACID	mg	–	–	–	–	–	–	–	–	–	–	–	–	–	–	–	4.7	10	–	–
VITAMIN B₁₂	μg	–	–	–	3.0	–	5.0	–	–	2.0	2.0	–	3.0	–	2.0	–	3.0	–	2.0	2.0
VITAMIN C	Female mg	50	50	30	60	70	70	75	75	30	30	55	60	30	50	30	60	64	30	30
	Male					75	75		85			60						75		
BIOFLAVONOIDS	Female mg	–	–	–	–	–	25	–	16	–	–	–	10	–	–	–	–	17	–	–
	Male				13.5		30		18				12					20		
VITAMIN E	Female mg	–	–	–	13.5	–	25	–	10	–	–	–	10	–	–	–	8	–	–	–
	Male						30						12				10			
VITAMIN D	Female μg	–	2.5	2.5	10	–	–	–	2.5	2.5	2.5	2.5	2.5	10.0	–	2.5	5.0	–	2.5	2.5
	Male																7.0			
FOLIC ACID	μg	–	–	–	200	–	400	–	–	200	–	–	400	–	200	300	400	–	200	200

Table 17: Recommended dietary intakes of minerals for adults

		Ar	Au	Be	Bu	Can	Car	Ch	Cr	De	FDR	Fi	Fr	GDR	Hu	In	It	Ia	Ko	Ma
CALCIUM	Female mg	600	700	1000	750-1400	700	500	600	800	800	700	600	800	800	500	450	600	600	600	450
	Male	700	800	–	650-1100	800	–	–	–	–	800	700	–	–	–	–	–	–	–	–
IODINE	Female µg	–	120	150	–	100	–	–	–	225	–	–	120	–	–	–	–	–	–	–
	Male	–	150	–	–	150	–	–	–	–	–	–	–	–	–	–	–	–	–	–
IRON	Female mg	14-28	15	10	20	14	6.19	15	14	18	18	12	18	15	18	32	18	12	18	28
	Male	5-9	12	–	13	10	6	12	12	10	12	8	10	10	12	24	10	10	10	9
MAGNESIUM	Female mg	–	–	350	–	250	250	–	350	300	220	–	350	–	–	–	300	–	–	–
	Male	–	–	–	–	300	300	–	400	350	260	–	–	–	–	–	350	–	–	–
ZINC	Female mg	–	16	15	–	9	–	–	8	15	–	–	–	–	–	–	15	–	–	–
	Male	–	–	–	–	12	–	–	–	–	–	–	–	–	–	–	–	–	–	–

		Me	Nr	No	NZ	Ph	Pol	Por	Ro	Si	Sp	Sw	Ta	Th	Tu	UK	USA	USSR	WP	WHO/FAO
CALCIUM	Female mg	500	800	800	600	500	800	800	900	450	400	800	600	400	500	500	800	800	400	400
	Male	–	–	–	–	–	–	–	–	–	500	–	–	500	–	–	–	–	–	500
IODINE	Female µg	–	–	–	200	–	100	–	–	–	–	–	110	–	–	140	150	–	–	–
	Male	–	–	–	–	–	125	–	–	–	–	–	145	–	–	–	–	–	–	–
IRON	Female mg	18	12	18	15	18	12	15	20	19	28	18	15	16	23	12	18	15	14	28
	Male	10	10	10	12	10	–	13	12	6	14	10	10	6	7	10	10	–	5	14
MAGNESIUM	Female mg	–	–	–	300	–	350	–	–	–	–	–	–	–	–	–	300	400	–	–
	Male	–	–	–	350	–	400	–	–	–	–	–	–	–	–	–	350	600	–	–
ZINC	Female mg	–	–	–	–	–	–	–	–	–	–	–	–	–	–	–	15	–	–	–
	Male	–	–	–	–	–	–	–	–	–	–	–	–	–	–	–	–	–	–	–

retinal, vitamin A aldehyde, retinaldehyde, active form of vitamin A in sight process.

retinene, old name for retinal.

retinoic acid, vitamin A acid, active form of vitamin A in growth. Used on skin in treating skin complaints including skin cancer.

retinoid, term to describe vitamin A and its derivatives both natural and synthetic.

retinol, vitamin A.

retrolental fibroplasia, eye problem in premature babies. *See* oxygen and vitamin E.

rheumatism, general term indicating diseases of muscle, tendon, joint, bone or nerve resulting in discomfort and disability. Often used to include rheumatoid arthritis, osteoarthritis, spondylitis, bursitis, fibrositis, myositis, lumbago, sciatica and gout. Vitamin therapy as for rheumatoid arthritis. *See* gout.

rheumatoid arthritis, *see* arthritis.

riboflavin(e), B_2 vitamin.

ribonucleic acid (RNA), *see* nucleic acids.

rickets,   disease in children characterized by lack of mineralization of bones and due to deficiency of vitamin D.

Symptoms are restlessness, poor ability to sleep and constant head movement. Infants do not sit, crawl or walk early and closing of the soft joints in head bones is delayed. Weight-bearing eventually bends the bones causing bow legs, knock-knees in the legs and pigeon breast.

Therapy is doses up to 20000IU daily with calcium and phosphorus.

---

rosehip syrup,   in undiluted form is a very rich source of vitamin C. Traces of vitamin E present. Traces only of thiamine, riboflavin, nicotinic acid, pyridoxine, pantothenic acid, folic acid and biotin. Vitamin C content is 295mg per 100ml.

---

rubidium,   alkali metal with the chemical symbol Rb and atomic weight 85.47. It is widely distributed in very small quantities throughout the earth's crust. Its close relationship with potassium means that both have similar actions on (i) contraction of the heart muscle (ii) neutralizing the toxic action of lithium (iii) in the motility of spermatozoa (iv) the fermentation capacity of yeast (v) the utilization of energy producing intermediates in mitochondria (vi) the transmission of nerve impulses and (vii) the response of muscles to stimulation.

In animals, rubidium can replace potassium to a certain extent in kidneys and muscles when potassium is lacking but this temporary response inevitably disappears, leading to death. There is no evidence that rubidium is an essential element for either animals or man. However, it may have its own role in some neurophysiological mechanism based on the finding that (i) its level is lower in the conductive tissue of the heart than in the heart muscle itself (ii) the rubidium content of brain differs markedly in various regions of the brain and these levels decrease with age (iii) the mineral can enhance the turnover of brain neurotransmitters (iv) it diffuses rapidly through the membranes of the artificial kidney (v) it causes increased EEG activity in monkeys, although this has not been demonstrated in human beings.

Rubidium is rapidly and efficiently absorbed, assimilated and excreted by the digestive tracts of animals in a manner similar to that of potassium, suggesting identical and shared transport systems. All soft tissues of the human body have rubidium concentrations that are high compared to those of other trace elements. The body content of rubidium is about 360mg. No particular organ or tissue is a rich source of rubidium and levels throughout the body are steady between 4 and 6μg per g fresh tissue. The mineral is generally retained in body tissues: e.g. after intravenous administration of the labelled material, between 39 and 134 days were needed to excrete half the dose in the urine. These figures are comparable to those for potassium.

Foods vary tremendously in their content of rubidium and blood levels reflect the amounts taken in the diet. Dietetically treated patients suffering from phenylketonuria or maple syrup-urine disease had depressed levels of rubidium in the blood compared to those on normal diets. Whether these were the result of the diets or the disease was not apparent. Most foods contain 1.5–5.0μg/g rubidium and a normal daily intake is 4.2mg in Finland. In the UK it is between 3 and 6mg per day; in the USA 1.28–4.98mg per day and in Italian diets at about 2.5mg per day. Meat and dairy products provide the highest amounts, but Brazil nuts are rich in the mineral. All foods examined contained some rubidium.

Rubidium-82 is used in the imaging of the heart muscle for diagnostic purposes. The same radioactive element can be used to assess blood flow through the heart.

---

rutin,   bioflavonoid, particularly rich in buckwheat. Used to treat bleeding gums and strengthen capillary walls at daily intakes of 60 to 600mg. Preferably taken with vitamin C (up to 500mg daily) at same time.

S

---

salt, strictly speaking a salt is a combination of a metallic element or ammonia with an acid group. Examples are sodium sulphate, potassium chloride, magnesium acetate, calcium phosphate, ammonium chloride, potassium iodide, zinc carbonate, sodium bicarbonate, sodium citrate, potassium tartrate. In these cases, the part of the salt of most interest to the body is the metallic or ammonia bit but chloride, iodide and phosphate can also be utilized because they contain chlorine, iodine and phosphorus respectively.

In common parlance though, salt has come to mean sodium chloride or common salt since this is the most widespread in our diet. When dissolved in water, sodium chloride splits into positively-charged sodium ions (cations) that are electrically neutralized by negatively-charged chloride ions (anions). Hence salt is neutral because there are equal numbers of sodium and chloride ions. All other water-soluble salts split when in solution into positively-charged metal or ammonia ions and negatively-charged acid group ions.

Each 100mg sodium chloride contains 39.3mg sodium and 60.7mg chloride. Salt is the main source of both sodium and chloride in the diet. Other sodium salts present in the diet include sodium bicarbonate, sodium nitrite, monosodium glutamate, sodium benzoate, sodium alginate and sodium sulphite. Like sodium chloride, these too are in the main added to foods. All foods contain an inherent amount of sodium in them but there are wide variations in the quantity. See the individual foods for their sodium content.

Salt requirements are relatively low. It is doubtful if salt need be added to any food for its nutritional value. There is evidence that early man managed and some primitive communities today manage to survive on a diet to which no salt was or is added. Intakes of natural sodium expressed as sodium chloride are as little as between 30 and 600mg salt per day and these primitive communities have adapted to such small quantities. As civilization progressed man discovered that salt evaporated from sea water or mined from the ground could be used to preserve food. This assumed importance for storing food out of season so salt became highly valued. Roman soldiers were paid partly in salt, hence the word 'salary' for remuneration. As methods for isolating salt improved and as its transport became easier the mineral was cheaper and available to all. Its consumption increased, not because it was needed but because of its flavour-enhancing qualities. Today the population in the West consumes between 8 and 14g salt daily. They could equally well manage on 3.5-7.0g salt daily. High salt consumption leading to high blood levels can be harmful in several conditions (*see under* sodium) but the most important is on blood-pressure which is a factor in the development of heart attacks, strokes and kidney failure.

Dietary salt and high blood-pressure appear to be related on the basis of animal experiments and epidemiological studies. In animals with inherent forms of high blood-pressure and in rats bred in stock colonies an increased salt intake raises the blood-pressure. This rise can be partly offset by increased potassium intake. Once high blood-pressure is established in these species, lowering the salt intake will not always result in decreased blood-pressure.

In human epidemiological studies it was concluded that sodium intake and blood-pressure are not always related within any particular community. There is, however, a direct relation between potassium excretion, the sodium/potassium ratio in the urine and blood-pressure. The higher the blood level of potassium the lower the blood-pressure. In Africa, tribesmen who move from rural areas to the cities develop higher blood-pressure that is in part related to an increased salt intake. In one study, where Africans were deliberately given an extra 16g salt in their daily diets, their blood-pressure rose. One reason for this effect of salt is that people who have some inherent abnormality in their kidneys cannot excrete the excess sodium.

Prevention of high blood-pressure by reducing salt intake has been proved to be effective in animal experiments. No parallel work is available on human beings but babies fed on a low salt diet for the first year of life had lower blood-pressure levels than those fed normal salt intakes.

Treatment of high blood-pressure by reducing salt intake is effective in some individuals. Very low salt-containing diets were found to reduce high blood-pressure before the introduction of diuretics and other drug treatments. Simply halving salt intake to 3.5g (one level teaspoonful) daily can reduce blood-pressure by the same amount as that by one tablet of blood-pressure-lowering drugs. These drugs are more effective if salt intake is reduced at the same time. The higher the blood-pressure the more effective are the drugs on a salt-restricted diet. Those people with only mildly raised blood-pressure can sometimes reduce their blood-pressure to normal values and maintain it by simple salt restriction.

The positive effect of salt restriction and sodium restriction from other sources is enhanced if the intake of potassium is increased at the same time. It is likely too that adequate intakes of calcium and magnesium are also important in reducing high blood-pressure to normal values or in maintaining these values.

Salt retention is also associated with other conditions:
1.   Premenstrual oedema. Many women gain weight and experience a bloated feeling a few days before their periods. Symptoms include swelling of the abdomen, ankles and fingers and they are due to retention of water. This oedema can be prevented or reduced by cutting down on the salt intake and at the same time increasing potassium intake by eating more fresh fruit and vegetables and by drinking fresh fruit and vegetable juices.
2.   Crash dieting. Fasting or severe calorie-restricted diets that are favoured for rapid weight loss are effective in the short term, but resumption of normal meals after several days can result in sodium retention and hence oedema.
3.   Heart failure. When the arteries of the body, including those of the heart, become constricted, the heart works harder to pump out blood and its muscle may become damaged. The kidneys respond by retaining sodium in an attempt to assist the heart but the result is retention of water in many parts of the body including that around the heart. A vicious circle results because the heart works harder when oedema is present, and the usual consequence is heart failure. Diuretic drugs help remove this excess water but their action is improved if salt (i.e. sodium) intake is restricted at the same time.
4.   Liver disease. The kidneys may respond to liver damage as they do to heart muscle damage by retaining sodium and hence water. Salt and sodium restriction in the diet can complement conventional medical

treatment but the possibility of abnormally low body levels of sodium must be considered.

5. Kidney disease. In some kidney complaints the organ has lost the ability to rid the body of excess salt and high blood-pressure results. Some salt and sodium restriction is therefore necessary but the extent of this is the province of the medical practitioner since in severe kidney disease sodium reduction may exacerbate the condition. In nephrotic syndrome where massive amounts of protein are lost in the urine there is often retention of water and sodium. This is one kidney disease where dietary salt restriction can safely be undertaken in conjunction with diuretic and other drug treatments. Sometimes in rare cases the kidney is unable to retain sodium and excessive quantities are lost in the urine. Here sodium restriction is undesirable and extra salt may have to be eaten; this should only be done under professional advice.

Restricted salt regime is a diet where dietary sodium is reduced to about one-third of normal by eliminating salt added at table; reducing that added during cooking processes to a minimum; selecting foods with low sodium levels. Foods which are rich sources of sodium should be avoided. On this regime the intake of sodium is 2.3g equivalent to 5.9g salt. General guidelines are:

1. no table salt allowed;
2. salt added during cooking and baking powder must be reduced to a minimum;
3. ham, bacon, sausages, tinned meats, tinned fish, shellfish, cheese, sauces, biscuits, scones and shop cakes must not be eaten;
4. bread of any type is restricted to five thin slices per day; butter intake must not exceed 30g (one ounce);
5. meat and fish in small helpings are allowed;
6. sodium-containing vegetables like beetroot, celery, carrots, radish, turnip and watercress are allowed in small quantities as long as no extra salt is added to them. Potatoes cooked in their skins without added salt are allowed;
7. one egg per day is allowed, as is a total of 250ml (half-pint) of milk;
8. intake of fruits and nuts (unsalted) is unlimited;
9. there is no restriction on sugar, honey, jams, rice and sago;
10. salads without added salt are allowed but dressings are not permitted unless they are of the low sodium type.

Low sodium diets are more difficult to organize at home without expert dietary instructions and supervision. One important aspect is that salt-free bread and butter are essential. This is easier when both are home-made but they are available in some shops, as are salt-free polyunsaturated margarines. The sodium intake on the following daily regime is no more than 1.2g equivalent to 3.1g salt.

Daily allowance of milk is 250ml (half-pint), preferably of the low sodium variety; that of low-sodium butter or margarine is 30g (one ounce). *Breakfast*: fruit or fruit juice; low salt cereal; milk from allowance and sugar; one egg (unsalted); low sodium bread or toast; butter from allowance; jam or marmalade; coffee or tea with milk from allowance. *Lunch*: fruit or fruit juice; 90g (3 ounces) unsalted meat, poultry or fresh white fish, either grilled or fried in vegetable oil; potato or rice or pasta; permitted vegetable; salad with low-sodium dressing; low-sodium bread and butter from allowance; fruit sweetened with honey or sugar; tea or coffee with milk from allowance. *Evening meal*: fruit or fruit-juice; 60g (2 ounces) meat or fish or one egg; permitted vegetable and salad with low-sodium dressing; low-sodium bread with butter or margarine from allowance; tea or coffee with milk from allowance. *Bedtime*: remainder of milk allowance.

The following must be avoided: all cured, tinned and pickled meats and fish; canned vegetables and soups; cheeses; bottled sauces; pickled vegetables; sausages; any foods with the ingredients bicarbonate of soda, baking powder, sodium benzoate, monosodium glutamate or any sodium salt listed under sodium-food additives. Potassium chloride may be substituted to flavour some foods but the taste will be found to be different from that when sodium chloride is used.

---

scandium, chemical symbol Sc with an atomic weight of 44.96. Although widely dispersed in water, it has an abundance of only 6μg per g in the earth's crust. Also known as ekaboron.

Scandium is an essential mineral for the mould Aspergillus niger and the fungus Cercospora granati. In the human being, the scandium concentration in patients with uraemic heart failure (due to diseased kidneys) was higher (0.02–0.9ng per g tissue) than in nonuraemic controls (0.003–0.1ng per g). Levels are lower in those with higher blood pressure than in those with normal blood pressure. There is more scandium in the conductive tissue of heart than in the adjacent heart tissue. Cancer patients contain less scandium in their hair than do the general population. Lung tissue shows great variation with levels between 0.49 and 3.0ng per g tissue.

The requirement of micro-organisms for scandium and the redistribution of tissue scandium in disease suggest that the trace element might have some physiological action in higher forms of life. If there is a requirement it must be very low because of the relating low amounts in the food. These are only 0.005–0.1µg per g dry weight of fruits, vegetables and grains. Nuts provide only 2 to 20ng per g. Italian diets provide 170ng per day and urinary excretion was less than 10ng per day, indicating that the body retains some.

Schilling test,   specific for detecting vitamin B_{12} deficiency induced by non-absorption of vitamin from diet. Small amount of radioactive vitamin B_{12} given by mouth followed some time later by high dose intravenously to flush out absorbed vitamin. Radioactivity in urine measured over 24 hours. Test repeated with radioactive vitamin plus intrinsic factor. Differences in two amounts excreted in urine allows diagnosis to be made.

---

schizophrenia,   a group of mental disorders in people who exhibit: 1. disturbance of logical associations; 2. limited range of emotional response; 3. autism; 4. mixed feelings to an incapacitating degree. Has been treated with folic acid and pyridoxine or folic acid alone at high potencies. Others respond to nicotinamide plus vitamin C. Occasionally vitamin B_{12} injections may help. *See* megavitamin therapy.

---

scurvy,   disease specific to vitamin C deficiency. Symptoms are lassitude, weakness, irritability, vague muscle and joint pains, loss of weight, bleeding gums, gingivitis, loosening of the teeth. Minute haemorrhages under the skin followed by large haemorrhage in thigh muscles. Therapy with vitamin C at oral doses of 200-2000mg daily.

---

sea salt,   mainly sodium chloride but contains significant quantities of other salts. A typical composition (in g per 100g) is: sodium chloride 77.82;

magnesium chloride 9.44; magnesium sulphate 6.57; calcium sulphate 3.44; potassium chloride 2.11; magnesium bromide 0.22; calcium carbonate trace.

---

sea food.   *Crustacea* include crab, lobster, prawns, crayfish, scampi and shrimps that provide meaningful quantities only of vitamin E among the fat-soluble vitamins. All contain moderate amounts of the vitamin B complex but are relatively rich in B_{12}.

Molluscs include cockles, mussels, oysters, scallops, whelks and winkles. Their vitamin content is similar to that of crustacea. Some oysters provide vitamin C but most seafoods contain virtually none.

All seafoods are important providers of the essential trace minerals as well as the gross minerals.

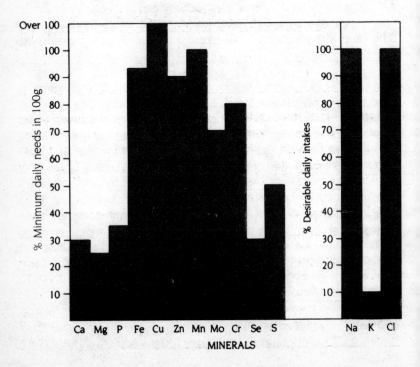

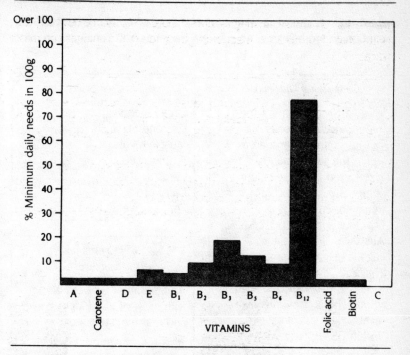

seabonal supplementation, extra vitamin A required during winter because of low environmental temperatures. Extra vitamin D required during winter because sunshine is shorter-lasting and weaker and body is more covered. Extra vitamin C required during winter because of prevalence of respiratory infections and intake of fresh fruit and vegetables in diet is decreased. Extra vitamin B complex should be taken during winter to help overcome stress of low environmental temperatures.

---

seborrhoeic dermatitis, chronic, reddish, scaling inflammation of skin often occurring with acne, rosacea and psoriasis. In infants, responds to biotin therapy, 5mg daily until cured. In adults, sometimes responds to pyridoxine therapy with ointment of 10mg pyridoxine per gram base in addition to biotin given orally.

selenium,   chemical symbol Se, atomic weight 79.0. Name derived from the moon goddess Selene. An essential trace mineral in animals and man.

Geographical Distribution

Irregular distribution of the mineral occurs in soils of various countries and areas within the same country. This is reflected in the selenium contents of the food grown in those areas.

Low levels in Europe; USA; Australia; New Zealand.

High levels in Formosa; Japan; Thailand; Philippines; Puerto Rico; Venezuela; Costa Rica. Within UK, Norfolk has high levels.

Within USA, Wyoming and Dakota have high levels.

Epidemiological studies indicate that those who live in areas of low selenium soils have more cancer and heart complaints than those living in high selenium soils.

Best Food Sources

Organ meats	40
Fish and Shellfish	32
Muscle meats	18
Wholegrains	12
Cereals	12
Dairy products	5
Fruit and vegetables	2

Body Content and Absorption

Adult content is about 20mg with most of it in kidneys, liver and in the male, testes.

Absorption is more efficient from organic selenium (as found in growing yeast) than from the inorganic variety.

Deficiency

Can be induced by living on diets high in refined and processed foods
Also by living off foods grown on selenium deficient soil
Has been seen in babies fed on dried milk rather than breast milk
No specific symptoms of deficiency but conditions induced include
  Keshan Disease and White Muscle Disease

Functions

Preservation of normal liver function
Maintaining resistance to disease
Protects against toxic minerals
Promotes male sexual reproductive capacity in production of prostaglandins (hormones)
Maintains healthy eyes and sight
Maintains healthy hair and skin
Act as anti-inflammatory agent
Maintains healthy heart
Protects against toxic substances produced in body
May protect against cancer
Works together with vitamin E in production of ubiquinone (see entry)
Protects the body as an anti-oxidant

Recommended Daily Intake

Suggested only by the US Food and Nutrition Board as no more than 200µg from food. Supplementary selenium should not exceed this.

Therapeutic Uses

Arthritis
High blood-pressure
Angina
Keshan disease (see entry)
Hair, nail and skin problems
Detoxification of arsenic, cadmium and mercury
Cataracts
In animals it has been successful in treating:
  Nutritional muscular dystrophy (white muscle disease)
  Liver disease
  Infertility in males
  Cancer

Selenium Supplements (selenium content)

Selenium-rich yeast (up to 1000µg per gram); sodium selenite (45.7µg per 100µg).

Total selenium supplementation should not exceed 200µg daily.

Symptoms of Excess Intake

Dental caries in children
Hair loss
Skin depigmentation
Abnormal nails
Lassitude
Garlicky odour on breath (in absence of garlic)

Relationship to Vitamin E

Selenium can spare vitamin E (it can partly replace it)
Selenium is 50 to 100 times more active an antioxidant than the vitamin
Protective enzyme glutathione peroxidase requires both selenium and vitamin E
Combined selenium and vitamin E gives better relief from angina than either one alone
Both trace mineral and vitamin needed for efficient resistance to infection
Cancers (experimented) in animals were inhibited by both selenium and vitamin E preferably also with vitamin C
Skin cancers induced by excessive ultra-violet light were inhibited by selenium plus vitamins E and C
Best ratio is 100IU vitamin E: 25µg selenium
The beneficial effect of combined selenium and vitamin E is greater than the additive effect of each alone, i.e. they are synergistic

---

selenium sulphide, used only as a shampoo in the treatment of dandruff and seborrhoeic dermatitis of the scalp. It is highly toxic if taken internally. If swallowed, the stomach should be emptied by aspiration and lavage and a purgative such as sodium sulphate (30g in 250ml water) given as a solution. Vitamin C, 10mg per kg body weight, given by mouth assists the removal of selenium sulphide through the kidneys.

Hair levels of selenium are increased after the application of shampoos containing selenium sulphide.

---

selenium yeast, provides up to $1000\mu g$ selenium per gram of yeast. Produced by adding inorganic selenium salts to growing yeast which incorporates the trace mineral into its protein. This involves replacement of the sulphur in the sulphur-containing amino acids by selenium. The main protein constituent is selenomethionine. Selenium in yeast protein is better absorbed, better utilized and less toxic than inorganic selenium salts.

---

senile dementia, due to a degenerative process with a large loss of cells from certain brain areas. Condition is more common in women and appears usually in seventh or eighth decade of life, i.e., later than Alzheimer's Disease. For treatment *see* Alzheimer's Disease.

---

shingles, acute infection of the central nervous system caused by a virus and characterized by skin blisters and pain in the nerve endings of the skin. Also known as herpes zoster.

Has been treated with vitamin C by injection at a dose of 3 grams every 12 hours plus one gram orally every two hours. Pain was relieved and blisters dried up within 72 hours. Some people respond to injections of vitamin B_{12}, $500\mu g$ daily, and are clear by third day. High oral doses of whole vitamin B complex recommended in all cases to help clear up nerve lesions. Continue after blisters have dried up. May also respond to high daily intakes (up to 3g daily) of amino acid L-lysine in addition to vitamin supplementation.

---

silicon, chemical symbol Si. Atomic weight 28.1. Found in nature as silica (silicon oxide) in quartz, sand, sandstone; as silicates in feldspar, kaolinate, anorthite. The second most abundant element on earth (next to oxygen), constituting about 27.6g per 100g in the earth's crust.

Silicon and silicon salts are so insoluble that only trace amounts are found in body tissues. It has been shown to be an essential trace element for the growing rat and chick; deficiency in these species leads to abnormalities in the bones. In addition, it is an essential component of cartilage where it is important for the strength and elasticity of the gristle. Silicon helps keep arterial walls elastic, an important feature of blood-pressure control. All connective tissue of the body contains silicon. All studies have been carried out on animals but similar functions probably apply to human beings also.

Toxic effects of silicon are confined to the inhalation of silica as dust from coal, glass manufacture, ceramics production and sand-blasting of rocks. The resulting disease is silicosis where particles of silica are deposited in the lungs, setting up irritation and eventually loss of elasticity.

Silicon compounds used in tabletting include silicon dioxide.

---

silicon dioxide,   also known as silica, colloidal silica. Provides 46.8mg silicon in 100mg.

---

silver,   chemical symbol Ag, from the Latin *argentum*. It is a heavy metal with atomic weight 107.87. Found native or associated with copper, gold and lead and constitutes 0.00001 per cent of the earth's crust. There is no evidence that silver is essential for any living organism nor is it ranked among the more toxic trace elements. It occurs naturally in very low concentrations in soils, plants and animal tissues but can gain access to foods from silver-plated vessels, silver-lead solders and silver foil used in decorating cakes and confectionery.

Foods contain very little silver and measurements indicate contents of less than a few nanograms (one thousandth of one microgram) in fruits and vegetables and fruit juices to 10ng per gram of bananas. Cow's milk is a rich source with levels of 27 to 54μg per litre. Western diets usually provide between 10 and 45μg per day but intakes of less than 1μg daily have been reported in some diets.

Low intakes are reflected in low tissue levels which vary between 0.001μg silver per g tissue (lymph nodes) to 0.0025μg per g heart muscle and 0.006μg per g in liver. Hair is richer with levels between 0.13 and 0.60μg per g. Even higher levels (7.3μg) have been found in non-ferrous smelter workers. Chronic and acute renal failure are conditions where liver silver is markedly elevated.

When given intramuscularly or by intravenous injection, administered silver is readily excreted, mainly (93 per cent) via the faeces. Oral silver is 99 per cent excreted in the faeces. Bile accounts for some excretion but the very poor bioavailability of silver is reflected in the negligible amounts detected in human urine.

Within the body, silver interacts metabolically with copper and selenium. Silver accentuates signs of copper deficiency and the latter mineral can reverse the silver toxicity symptoms of depressed growth, low haemoglobin and lowered elasticity of the aorta. The mechanisms of this relationship are not known. What is apparent is that excessive silver promotes degeneration of the liver in vitamin E-deficient rats and chicks.

Silver can also alleviate selenium toxicity. Although not proved completely, it appears that (i) silver is easily reduced, inducing peroxidation and hence increasing the requirements for selenium and/or vitamin E and (ii) silver complexes with selenium to prevent the formation or function of the enzyme glutathione peroxidase.

Silver has been used for purification of drinking water. Although regarded as non-toxic, on prolonged administration, silver salts can lead to greyish-blue discoloration of the skin known as argyria. Silver salts can be irritating to the skin and mucous membranes e.g. in the treatment of mouth ulcers with silver nitrate where it is used as a cauterizing agent.

---

skin cancer, *see* cancer.

---

skin colour, dark pigmentation of skin reduces effect of ultra-violet light in producing vitamin D in the skin. Hence a long exposure to sunlight is necessary to produce sufficient vitamin D or ensure sufficient by eating D-rich foods or by supplementation.

---

skin depigmentation,   *see* vitiligo.

---

skin diseases,   sometimes related to mild deficiency of vitamins and some will respond to oral intakes of vitamins plus direct application to skin. Vitamins particularly important to healthy skin are A, riboflavin, nicotinic acid, pyridoxine, biotin, C and E. Adequate polyunsaturated fatty acids are also important. *See* acne, dermatitis, eczema, seborrhoeic dermatitis, psoriasis.

---

slimming,   regimes that reduce daily calorie intake to 1000 calories or less will usually cause concomitant decrease in vitamin and mineral in diet to levels below recommended daily intake. Multivitamin and multimineral supplement essential on daily basis whilst slimming.

---

smell,   sense may be reduced by vitamin A deficiency; restored by intramuscular injection of high potencies of the vitamin. Zinc deficiency may also cause loss of sense of smell.

---

smoking,   *see* acetaldehyde and lung cancer.

---

sodium,   chemical symbol Na, from the Latin *natrium*. Atomic weight 23.0. An alkali metal that occurs naturally as sodium chloride, sodium bromide, sodium silicates and sodium carbonates. Abundance in earth's crust is 2.8 per cent.

Adult body content (65kg weight) of sodium in a healthy individual is about 92g, equivalent to 234g sodium chloride. More than half the sodium is in the fluids that bathe the cells (extracellular); 34.5g is present in the bones; less than 11.5g is retained within the cells (intracellular). Bone sodium is not generally available as an immediate reserve since it is enmeshed in the crystals of the insoluble bone minerals. If sodium is injected into the body as common salt, it quickly equilibrates with both intracellular and extracellular sodium, but exchange with bone sodium is almost negligible.

The total exchangeable sodium in the body is therefore about 64.4g and it is this sodium that changes rapidly, depending upon its intake from the diet and the excretion of the mineral.

Daily intakes of sodium from the food are from 1.61-6.90g which corresponds to 4.10-17.55g common salt. The food as eaten contributes only 4.6g sodium daily (corresponding to 11.7g common salt), the remainder being added as table salt.

In babies, the ideal sodium content of food is that of human breast milk (180mg per litre). Unmodified cow's milk contains 770mg per litre so it should not be fed to babies in the first three months of life. Animal experiments indicate that too much salt in a baby's diet can cause high blood-pressure and even death. UK and USA health authorities recommend that salt should not be added during the processing and preparation of infant foods.

Foods as they occur in nature do not generally have high amounts of sodium but the mineral is added in large amounts as sodium chloride (common salt) during cooking, refining, processing and preservation of foods or as sodium bicarbonate in baking powder or as monosodium glutamate. Bakers, for example, add salt to bread at a level of about 1 per cent; butter, bacon, processed meats, tinned foods in general are all salted in preparation. An ordinary diet without salt supplementation in this way will provide ample sodium for body needs; added salt at the table is simply an acquired taste.

Rich sources of sodium are (in mg per 100g): yeast extract 4640; bacon 1900; smoked fish 1000-1800; salami 1800; sauces 1100-1400; cornflakes 1200; canned or boiled ham 1200; savoury biscuits 610-1200; processed cheese and cheese spread 1360; Danish Blue cheese 1420; Camembert cheese 1410; Stilton cheese 1150; corned beef 910; Edam cheese 980; salted butter 870; margarine 800; sausage 780; Cheddar and other hard cheeses 610; cottage cheese 450; bread 560; fresh and tinned shellfish 210-550; tinned vegetables 230-330.

Moderate sources of sodium are (in mg per 100g): sweet biscuits 200-500; self-raising flour 350; cream cheese 300; root vegetables 60-140; eggs 140; fresh fish 100; raw meats 60-90; yogurt 64-76; pulses 30-60; cornflour 52; oatmeal 33; single cream 42; dried fruits 30.

Poor sources of sodium are (in mg per 100g): fresh fruit 1-30; unsalted nuts 1-20; green vegetables 2-13; fruit juices 1-4; rice 6; flour 2-4; sago 3; lard

2. For other levels see individual foods.

Foods of animal and fish origin usually contain more sodium than wholegrains, fruits, vegetables, unsalted nuts and fruits. Poultry supply only moderate amounts.

Absorption of sodium as common salt or in any soluble form from the intestines is passive so excessive intakes are as easily absorbed as moderate ones. There is no control of absorption as with most other minerals so the gastrointestinal tract plays little part in controlling body levels.

Excretion of sodium is mainly via the kidneys and the resulting urine usually contains from 920-2300mg sodium per litre. Increased intake of the mineral leads to increased excretion and normal healthy kidneys have no difficulty in excreting the excess as long as there is sufficient water excreted. There is a limit to the amount by which the kidneys can concentrate urine (specific gravity of about 1.035 is the maximum), so high intakes of sodium, usually as salt, must be accompanied by large volumes of water. Excessive salt intakes usually induce thirst which when slaked compensates for the increased requirements of water. The highest excretion of sodium occurs about midday, with the lowest at night.

Control of urinary excretion of sodium is under the influence of hormones. These act upon the kidney tubules by stimulating or slowing the reabsorption of sodium within the kidney. One hormone is aldosterone which is elaborated in the adrenal cortex. When the body sodium is depleted, e.g. by excessive sweating or by starvation, aldosterone is secreted and this stimulates the kidney to reabsorb and hence conserve the sodium in the urine. In Addison's disease, aldosterone is no longer produced because the adrenal cortex is destroyed and sodium is excreted in large, uncontrolled amounts. The result is muscular weakness and low blood-pressure. Treatment is to give sufficient sodium in the form of salt to replace the losses and to supply the hormone by injection. Diseased kidneys as in renal failure are unable to conserve sodium and the individual becomes markedly depleted.

Excessive amounts of aldosterone and other adrenal cortex hormones will cause increased retention of sodium. This also happens in congestive heart disease and in certain types of kidney disease. The usual result is high blood-pressure.

Faecal excretion of sodium is very small, usually only about 115mg daily. All the digestive juices contain large amounts of sodium but most of this is reabsorbed in the large intestine. In diarrhoea, reabsorption is inefficient and significant daily losses of sodium up to 2070mg are possible in the faeces. These must be replaced in chronic diarrhoea to prevent body depletion.

Excretion through the skin is usually negligible, but when sweating is excessive losses can be significant. Sweat contains from 460-1840mg sodium per litre but in those who are acclimatized to heat this is maintained at 960mg per litre. In tropical climates or whilst indulging in heavy manual work excretion of sweat can reach up to 14 litres so sodium loss then becomes serious and more significant than urinary loss. Without supplementary salt in these conditions, sodium depletion soon follows. Miner's cramp is one such condition.

Sodium balance in a healthy individual should be zero. For example, with a good intake of 3105mg and no salt added at table, excretion should be 2990mg in the urine plus 115mg in the faeces; sweat excretion is negligible if the individual is sedentary. Under conditions of hard exercise or manual work sweating can induce a negative balance, i.e. more sodium is excreted than eaten. Excessive intakes and certain diseases can cause positive balance where the extra sodium in the diet is not excreted. Negative balance is usually treated by increased oral intake of sodium; positive balance by diuretic drugs.

Deficiency of sodium is highly unlikely on any diet but it can be associated with dehydration as in heat exhaustion brought on by high temperatures, hard exercise, manual work; in babies it can be caused by diarrhoea. The extracellular fluid volume is reduced, as is the blood volume. The blood thickens, veins collapse, blood-pressure is reduced and the pulse becomes rapid. These changes cause dryness of the mouth even though thirst may be absent. There is usually mental apathy, loss of appetite and sometimes vomiting. Muscle cramps are usually present. Dehydration is also indicated by sunken features — particularly the eyes, which recede — and a loose, non-elastic skin.

Deficiency of sodium may occur without water depletion; the condition is called water intoxication. It occurs after heavy sweating when the thirst is quenched with water to which no sodium has been added; in the treatment of sodium deficiency if too much water is given by mouth or intravenously; in the treatment of dehydration if only water is given. Symptoms include loss of appetite; weakness; mental apathy; muscular twitchings; convulsions; coma induced by excessive retention of water by the brain. Treatment is to ensure that salt is added to replacement fluids in the above conditions.

Causes of low blood sodium levels may also be due to kidney failure; hormonal imbalance, e.g. excess production of anti-diuretic hormone or vasopressin; lung cancers; lung infections; meningitis; myxoedema; lack of adrenal and pituitary hormones; oedema as in heart failure, liver cirrhosis, nephrotic syndrome, nephritis, toxaemia of pregnancy; high blood glucose levels; porphyria. Treatment of low blood sodium in these conditions is salt replacement, hormones and successful correction of the underlying disease.

Excess of sodium in the body accumulates primarily in the extracellular fluids. As the concentration rises the body responds by passing more water into the extracellular fluids to dilute out the sodium so oedema results. Consequences of high salt intake that is not excreted are therefore high blood-pressure; enlarged heart; abnormal ECG tracings; enlarged kidneys, leading to nephritis. Epidemiological evidence shows that high blood-pressure in some countries is associated with habitual high salt intakes. Elevation of blood serum sodium concentration is indicative of a deficit in body water relative to sodium.

Causes of high blood sodium levels include diabetes insipidus where vasopressin is deficient; kidney failure; high blood calcium; low blood potassium; excessive sweating without access to water (e.g. infants, bedridden or comatose patients); excessive diarrhoea, especially in children; grossly excessive intakes of sodium with limited access to water. Treatment is water replacement usually accompanied by drug diuretic treatment; restriction of sodium in the diet; occasionally kidney dialysis.

Functions of sodium are:

1. in maintaining a normal balance of water between body cells and the surrounding fluids. Potassium also contributes to this.
2. in nerve impulse transmission where the flow of sodium into the nerve cell and the opposite flow of potassium out of the cell sets up an electrical impulse that travels down the nerve to the muscle;
3. in all muscle contraction including that of the heart where the correct balance of sodium and potassium is essential for a smooth response;
4. in preserving the acid-alkali balance of the body in close relationship with bicarbonate, phosphate and protein and the minerals potassium, calcium and magnesium;

5. as a constituent of ATPase, the enzyme responsible for splitting adenosine triphosphate in the production of energy;
6. the active transport of the nutrients amino acids and glucose into body cells.

Supplementary form of sodium is sodium chloride which provides 39.3mg sodium in 100mg chloride.

Recommended daily intake has not been suggested by any authority since insufficiency in the diet is highly unlikely.

Food additives of sodium, apart from those found in natural foods, include sodium acetate; sodium alginate; sodium aluminium phosphate, acidic and basic; sodium ascorbate; sodium benzoate; sodium biphenyl-2-yl oxide; sodium bicarbonate; sodium carbonate; sodium caseinate; sodium chloride; sodium hydrogen citrate; trisodium citrate; tetrasodium diphosphate; trisodium diphosphate; sodium ferrocyanide; sodium gluconate; sodium heptonate; sodium dihydrogen citrate; sodium hydrogen diacetate; disodium dihydrogen diphosphate; disodium dihydrogen ethylenediamine — NNN'N'-tetra-acetate; sodium hydrogen glutamate (monosodium glutamate); sodium hydrogen malate; sodium dihydrogen orthophosphate; disodium hydrogen orthophosphate; sodium hydrogen sulphite; sodium hydroxide; sodium lactate; sodium malate; sodium metabisulphite; sodium nitrate; sodium nitrite; trisodium orthophosphate; sodium pectate; sodium polyphosphates; sodium propionate; sodium 5'-ribonucleotide; soaps or sodium salts of fatty acids; sodium sesquicarbonate; sodium sorbate; sodium stearoyl-2-lactate; sodium sulphate; sodium sulphite; disodium tartrates; monosodium tartrates; pentasodium triphosphate; sodium potassium tartrate; sodium hydrogen malate.

Drugs containing sodium include sodium alginate, sodium bicarbonate — antacids; sodium acetate and sodium lactate — metabolic acidosis; sodium phosphate, sodium sulphate and sodium tartrate — purgatives; sodium ascorbate — vitamin; sodium calcium edetate — treatment of heavy metal poisoning; sodium carboxymethylcellulose — bulking and swelling agent; sodium citrate — cough mixtures; sodium cromoglycate — asthma; sodium fusidate — corticosteroid; sodium hyaluronate — eye preparation; sodium lauryl sulphate — laxative; sodium lauryl sulphoacetate — laxative; sodium nitroprusside — angina treatment; sodium oleate — haemorrhoid treatment; sodium perborate — gingivitis; sodium picosulphate — laxative; sodium pyrrolidone carboxylate — skin cleanser; sodium ricinoleate —

gingivitis; sodium saccharin-sweetener; sodium salicylate — asthma; sodium valproate — epilepsy.

sodium pump, the mechanism whereby potassium levels inside body cells and sodium levels outside them are kept constant. Cells' membranes are permeable to both minerals when in solution; the concentration gradients are such that potassium tends to flow out of cells and sodium flows in. To maintain the balance of high levels of potassium inside and sodium outside the cells energy is required which is provided by splitting of high-energy phosphate bonds of adenosine triphosphate. The minerals are transported on the backs of glucose and some unknown carrier. Certain factors can affect the efficiency of the sodium pump causing it to slow down. One is ouabain, a plant drug that acts like digitalis; the other is phlorizin, the toxic principle of apple, pear, plum and cherry trees (but not their fruits). Vasopressin, the sodium-excreting hormone from the adrenals, slows down the sodium pump. This increases the blood-pressure and it has been shown recently that the sodium pump is slower in those people with high blood-pressure.

soups, all soups as eaten provide some B vitamins but little else apart from lentil and tomato soups which provide also vitamin A, carotene and vitamin D. All figures refer to canned, condensed as eaten and dried as eaten, soups. B vitamins present are (in mg per 100g) in the ranges quoted: thiamine 0.01-0.07; riboflavin 0.01-0.05; nicotinic acid 0.1-0.8; pyridoxine 0.01-0.07. Folic acid detected only in soups based on tomatoes and mushrooms and at levels of 2-12μg per 100g. Thiamine level of dried oxtail soup as eaten is 0.8mg per 100g which is mainly derived from the flavouring agent.

Lentil soup provides also 40μg vitamin A per 100g; 430μg carotene per 100g and 0.28μg vitamin D per 100g, due mainly to ham ingredient plus traces of vitamin C.

Tomato soup provides also 210μg carotene per 100g and traces of vitamin C.

Mineral
All provide high sodium levels (except specific low sodium varieties) but

are good sources of potassium, calcium, magnesium, phosphorus, chloride and the trace elements depending upon type.

All figures refer to mineral levels of canned, condensed as eaten and dried as eaten in the following ranges (in mg per 100g): sodium 350-6120; potassium 16-920; calcium 3-140; magnesium 3-48; phosphorus 10-260; iron 0.2-4.3; copper 0.02-0.33; zinc 0.1-2.4; chloride 290-9030.

---

soya flour, excellent source of B vitamins that is even better when defatted. Devoid of sodium but rich in potassium, calcium, magnesium, phosphorus and iron.

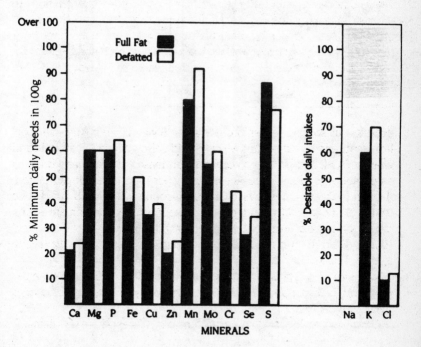

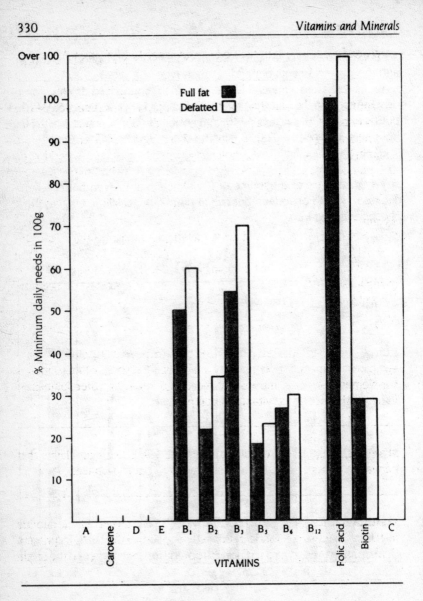

spirits, all alcoholic spirits are completely devoid of all vitamins.

spironolactone,   diuretic. Reduces availability of vitamin A.

---

spirulina,   blue-green alga, used as a staple food by the Aztecs of Mexico and now being developed as a high-protein food supplement rich in vitamins and minerals. The vitamins present are (in mg per 100g): carotene 250; vitamin E 19.0; thiamine 5.5; riboflavin 4.0; nicotinic acid 11.8; pyridoxine 0.3; pantothenic acid 1.1; inositol 35.0; folic acid 0.05; biotin 0.04; vitamin B_{12} 0.2.

Mineral
Range of mineral contents of dried material (in mg per 100g) is: calcium 104.5-131.5; magnesium 141.0-191.5; phosphorus 761.7-894.2; iron 47.5-58.0; sodium 27.5-41.2; potassium 1331-1540; chloride 400-440; manganese 1.8-2.5; zinc 2.7-3.9. There are also traces of bismuth, chromium, cobalt and selenium.

---

sprue,   tropical disease characterized by sore mouth, fatty diarrhoea and symptoms of malnutrition. Inability to absorb fat-soluble vitamins means supplementation of all must be by injection or orally as water-solubilized variety. Also needs for vitamin B complex.

---

stamina,   dependent on blood vitamin E levels. Russian claims that pangamic acid synergizes effect of vitamin E. *See* endurance.

---

stannous fluoride,   tin fluoride, provides 75.8μg tin and 24.2μg fluoride in 100μg. Used as a fluoride gel directly applied to the teeth to prevent dental caries. Added also to fluoride toothpastes but may stain the teeth.

---

sterility,   *see* fertility.

---

steroids, *see* corticosteroids.

---

stilboestrol, synthetic oestrogen. Reduces body levels of pyridoxine.

---

stomatitis, inflammatory condition of the mouth which may occur as a primary disease or as a symptom of some other disease, e.g. sprue. May respond to daily intake of 300mg nicotinamide orally. *See also* glossitis, gingivitis.

---

stress, increases body's requirements of vitamin B complex and particularly pantothenic acid because of its role in producing anti-stress hormones. Also vitamin C for the same reason. During stressful periods increase vitamin B complex and C intakes to ten-fold minimum daily requirements at least.

Oxidative stress — increase also vitamin E intake to at least 400IU daily. *See* vitamin E.

Physical stress — *see* athletes.

---

stretch marks, also known as striae. Apply vitamin E cream as soon as possible and supplement diet with 400IU daily in divided doses.

---

stroke, cerebrovascular disease due to atherosclerosis of brain blood-vessels and high blood-pressure.

Prevention or post-stroke treatment should include high intakes of vitamin E (400-600IU), vitamin C (500-1000mg), safflower oil or evening primrose oil, 3g all daily, lecithin (5-15g daily), fish oils containing EPA and DHA (3g daily) and a switch from saturated dietary fats to polyunsaturated oils.

---

strontium, named from its discovery in the ore from the lead mines of Strontian in Scotland. Chemical symbol Sr. Atomic weight 87.6. An alkaline earth metal.

No evidence that it is essential for animal and human life. It behaves as calcium and accompanies it in foods rich in calcium, e.g. milk, grains, fresh vegetables. Dietary strontium, like calcium, is concentrated in the bones. The quantity of strontium in biological material is usually about one-thousandth that of calcium.

Cow's milk is richer in both strontium and calcium than human milk. Bottle-fed babies tend to receive intakes of strontium some four times greater than those breast-fed. Some of it is retained. Breast-fed babies excrete more than they receive because their urinary volume is increased. In all babies, the ratio strontium to calcium is higher in the urine and faeces than in the bones. These results suggest that in infants at least the body discriminates against strontium in favour of calcium.

In general, the strontium level of plant foods is higher than those of animal products except when these contain bones. The mineral tends to be concentrated in the bran rather than the endosperm of grains and in the peel of root vegetables. The vital source of strontium is Brazil nuts. Milk and milk products contribute a major percentage of the strontium in a mixed diet. Amounts between 11 and 32 per cent of the total daily strontium intakes come from these food sources. UK diets provide from 0.7 to 1.1mg strontium daily; those in India contain from 3.1 to 4.7mg per day, and in the USA 1.2-2.9, 2.1-2.4, and 0.79-2.43mg have been found to be the usual daily intake in three different institutions. Drinking water can contribute a substantial portion of strontium intake. In Israel, for example, the drinking water can provide from 1.0 to 1.6mg of the mineral per litre so that a usual water intake of 1500 to 2500ml in the diet will provide between 1.5 and 4.0mg strontium daily. These levels of stronium in water are unusual, however, since most drinking water contains less than 1mg of the mineral per litre.

In general the metabolism and distribution of strontium mimics that of calcium with the major sites of retention being the skeleton, teeth and aorta. An adult contains 323mg of the mineral of which 99 per cent is present in the bones. These levels increase with age in bones, lungs and aorta. Strontium occurs in the enamel and dentin of teeth in concentrations similar to those in bones. It is deposited primarily before eruption and during tooth calcification. Levels in bone are 110mg per g; those in dental enamel are 120mg per g.

Although the metabolism of strontium is similar to that of calcium it is not identical. Absorption from the gastrointestinal tract, transfer across the placenta, excretion through the kidney and transfer into milk are all more efficient with calcium than strontium. Parallels between the two minerals are as follows:

(i)   Calcium and strontium are better absorbed by young than old animals.
(ii) The stresses of pregnancy and lactation increase the absorption of both minerals.
(iii) The duodenum is the greatest site of absorption of both minerals but the ileum represents the most effective site.
(iv) Vitamin D, lactose and the amino acids lysine and arginine enhance the absorption of both calcium and strontium.
(v)   Fibres like alginates (from seaweed) and cellulose (from plants) can depress the absorption of both minerals.
(vi) Parathyroid hormone accelerates the resorption of bone strontium and bone calcium.
(vii) When magnesium is deficient, both calcium and strontium absorption is depressed.

Food decreases strontium absorption and fasting enhances it. Raising low calcium intakes in the diet reduces strontium retention. Giving calcium and phosphorus (as in calcium phosphate) in the diet reduces strontium retention and the effect is greater than with calcium alone. Usually intestinal strontium absorption by adults ranges from 5 to 25 per cent with age changes varying from over 90 per cent in the very young to less than 10 per cent in the elderly.

Strontium is poorly retained by human beings. Excretion is via the bile and kidneys. An oral intake of 1.99mg strontium is excreted in the faeces (1.58mg) and in the urine (0.39mg) so very little is retained. In children of different ages, the strontium intakes ranged from 0.67 to 3.57mg per day from the diet and most of it was excreted in the faeces. The little quantity of strontium that is retained accumulates in the bones and teeth.

Some epidemiological evidence shows that strontium may have a protective effect against dental caries. The evidence is based on an association between caries incidence and the strontium concentration in drinking water. The higher the level of the mineral in the water, the higher the level in the dental enamel and the lower the incidence of caries. However, studies where high strontium levels were fed to experimental rats suggested that these resulted in increased caries. A human study found that strontium content was higher in decayed than in healthy teeth of Australian children. In those respects strontium appears to be similar to fluoride; a small amount is beneficial but higher intakes are damaging to the teeth. Strontium appears to have no anti-plaque activity. One study suggests it may be helpful in the treatment of osteoporosis. It may also protect the energy-producing apparatus of body cells.

A wide margin of safety exists between dietary levels of strontium likely to be ingested from ordinary foods and water supplies and those that induce toxic effects. The most serious of these is lack of mineralization of the bone by calcium. However, as calcium intakes in the diet rise, the toxic influence of strontium is reduced.

---

strontium-90, radioactive form of strontium produced by the effect of nuclear explosions. It can be dispersed over wide areas and so finds its way into plants and thence into animals and man. Like calcium it accumulates in the bones where it can continue to radiate radioactivity. With a half-life of 28 years such effects can eventually become dangerous. Strontium-90 represents the only toxic form of strontium. The non-radioactive mineral appears to be perfectly safe.

---

sugar, refined white variety is completely devoid of all vitamins.
Demerara sugar contains the following B vitamins in mg per 100g: thiamine, trace; riboflavin 0.01; nicotinic acid 2.0; pyridoxine 0.1; pantothenic acid 0.20mg. Contains also choline (2.8mg per 100g); inositol (24.0mg per 100g).
Muscovado and light muscovado sugars contain the following B vitamins in mg per 100g: thiamine 0.02; riboflavin 0.03; nicotinic acid 6.5; pyridoxine 0.06; pantothenic acid 0.8. Contains also choline (10.4mg per 100g); inositol (78mg per 100g).

Mineral
Demerara type provides significant quantities of all minerals; white variety is practically devoid of minerals. Demerara and white varieties respectively, provide (in mg per 100g): sodium 6, trace; potassium 89, 2; calcium 53,

2; magnesium 15, trace; phosphorus 20, trace; iron 0.9, trace; copper 0.06, 0.02; sulphur 14, trace; chloride 35, trace.

---

sulpha drugs,   anti-infection drugs that function by inhibiting uptake of PABA by harmful bacteria. PABA should *not* be taken as supplement whilst taking sulpha drugs. Prevent synthesis of vitamin K by destroying intestinal bacteria.

---

sulphur,   chemical symbol S. Atomic weight 32.1. Occurs in nature in the free state and in combination as sulphates and sulphides. Constitutes 0.05 per cent of the earth's crust.

As it is a constituent of all proteins it is an essential element for man, animals, plants and micro-organisms. Sulphur content of an adult body is about 100g. The greater part occurs in the three amino acids, cysteine, cystine and methionine. Some is present in the amino acid taurine. The rest appears as sulphate within body cells, either free or attached to body constituents like the anti-blood clotting substance heparin and the structural component chondroitin sulphate.

Sulphur is also present in the two vitamins thiamine and biotin; in vitamin D of milk where it occurs as a water-soluble sulphate; in fatty acid sulphates; in the enzymes that contain glutathione and coenzyme A. Sulphur-containing compounds are often prefixed by the term 'thio', derived from the Greek word for sulphur, theion. Thiosulphates and thiocyanates are present in body fluids in very small amounts where they are produced in the detoxification of cyanide present in foods, polluted atmospheres and tobacco smoke.

Body content of sulphur resides mainly in keratin, the horny layer of the skin; in fingernails; in toenails; in skin; in the joints. The characteristic smell of burning hair is due to its high sulphur content. The curliness of hair depends upon the sulphur — sulphur bonds of cystine. To straighten hair, these bonds must be opened up. During permanent waving the bonds are opened with one agent then closed again to the desired shape or pattern with another agent. Sheep's wool, which is very curly, can contain 5 per cent of its weight as sulphur.

Food sources of sulphur are (in mg per 100g): mustard powder 1280;

dried egg 630; scallops 570; lobster 510; shellfish 250-450; crab 470; nuts 150-380; garlic 370; prawns 370; poultry 200-340; meats 200-330; kidney 170-290; liver 220-270; white fish 200-300; skimmed milk 320; fatty fish 150-260; cheese 230-250; dried peaches 240; roe 240; horseradish 210; offal 140-200; mung beans 190; whole egg 180; Indian tea 180; haricot beans 170; red kidney beans 170; mustard and cress 170; peas 130-180; dried apricots 160; oatmeal 160; wholemeal flour 150; watercress 130; lentils 120; coffee 110; barley 110; wholemeal bread 81. For other foods see individual entries.

Protein supplies most of the sulphur in the diet but some comes in the form of sulphates. A good diet will provide 800mg sulphur daily. Little is known about its intermediate metabolism but excretion parallels that of nitrogen. There is no evidence of any deficiency states in animals or man.

Medicinal uses of sulphur include: a mild laxative when taken orally; a mild antiseptic in ointment form to treat acne; a parasiticide in lotion form, used to treat scabies; with lead acetate to darken grey hair; a depilatory agent to remove body hair.

Medicinal forms include: precipitated sulphur or milk of sulphur, dose 1-4g; sublimed sulphur or flowers of sulphur, dose 1-4g; sulphurated potash, a mixture of potassium polysulphide, potassium sulphite and potassium thiosulphate containing 42 per cent sulphur, used as a lotion on the skin.

---

sulphasalazine, used to treat Crohn's disease and ulcerative colitis. Prevents absorption of folic acid.

---

sulphitocobalamin, B_{12} vitamin.

---

sulphonamides, *see* sulpha drugs.

---

sunburn, vitamin E cream applied directly and take 600IU (200IU three times daily) orally to help healing and prevent scarring. Vitamin C

(1000-1500mg daily) will help healing and prevent infection. In addition 15mg zinc daily will benefit.

---

sunscreen agent,   most effective is PABA which is incorporated at 5 per cent in creams and lotions. Also may be best protectant against skin cancer induced by ultra-violet light.

---

sunshine vitamin,   *see* D vitamin.

---

surgery,   on intestinal tract may cause paralytic ileus (paralysis of the intestine) characterized by wind pains and abdominal distension. Doses of calcium pantothenate (50-100mg per day), preferably by injection, are used in prevention and treatment. Supplementary intakes of all vitamins but especially vitamin C (1000mg daily) and the mineral zinc (20mg daily) before and after surgery may help accelerate healing process. Post-surgical harmorrhage controlled by vitamin K given under medical supervision.

---

symptoms of mineral deficiencies in plants,   when minerals required by a plant are not in sufficient concentration in a soil or they are prevented from being absorbed by certain factors, specific symptoms appear. Plants in deficient soil may grow but are far from healthy. Typical symptoms are shown in Table 18.

Table 18: Symptoms of mineral deficiencies in plants

Deficient minerals	Symptoms
Nitrogen	Lack of growth and leaves yellowing. Entire plant affected.
Phosphorus	Dark green stunted plants. Delayed maturity. Entire plant affected.
Potassium	Mottled yellowing. Spots of dead areas. Weak stalks. Roots more susceptible to disease.
Sulphur	Yellowing of young leaves. Veins remain green.

Magnesium	Mottled or yellow leaves. Leaf tips turned upwards. Older leaves most affected.
Calcium	Inhibition of root development with death of shoot and root tips. Young leaves and roots most affected.
Iron	Yellowing of veins in young leaves. Stems short and slender. Buds remain alive.
Chlorine	Wilted leaves, yellowing, spots of dead areas. Stunted, thickened roots.
Manganese	Yellow, dead areas between veins. Smallest veins remain green.
Boron	Death of stem. Leaves twisted, pale at base. Swollen, discoloured root tips.
Zinc	Reduction in leaf size. Yellowing. Older leaves most affected.
Copper	Young leaves dark green, twisted, wilted, misshapen.
Molybdenum	Yellowing or twisting and death of young leaves.

T

---

talc,   purified, native hydrated magnesium silicate containing a small amount of aluminium silicate. Also known as French chalk. A food additive used as a release agent; as a lubricant in tablet making. Acceptable daily intake is not specified. Permitted as a miscellaneous additive. Excessive inhalation of talc can cause lung disease (pneumoconiosis).

---

tea, Indian,   dried leaf has useful content of some vitamins but these are drastically reduced when it is infused. Traces only of carotene and vitamin C in dried leaf but not detectable in the drink. B vitamins present are (in mg per 100g), for the dried leaf and infusion respectively: thiamine 0.14, trace; riboflavin, 1.2, 0.01; nicotinic acid 7.5, 0.1; pantothenic acid 1.3, trace.

Mineral
Dried leaf is rich in minerals but infused tea contains only traces of most minerals with high content of manganese (about 1mg per cup). Levels for dried leaf and infusion respectively (in mg per 100g) are: sodium 45, trace; potassium 2160, trace; calcium 430, trace; magnesium 250, 1; phosphorus 630, 1; iron 15.2, trace; copper 1.6, trace; zinc 3.0, trace; sulphur 180 for dried leaf; chloride 52, trace.

---

teeth,   pyridoxine may help prevent tooth decay, particularly in children, when taken at a daily dose of 10mg. Vitamins A and D essential during childhood for normal development of healthy teeth. Vitamin C, at intakes of 100mg with each meal, has been used as orthodontic supplement in children. *See also* bruxism.

---

tellurium, also known as *aurum paradoxum* and *metallum problematum*. Has the chemical symbol Te with an atomic weight of 127.60.

For over a century, ingestion of tellurium has been known to be associated with a garlic-like odour of the breath. This indicates that the mineral is absorbed by the intestine, metabolized by tissues and excreted through routes other than the faeces. In sheep and swine, at least 24 per cent of an oral dose is absorbed. After intravenous injection, urinary excretion is three times that of faecal excretion but the reverse occurs after oral administration. Hence homoeostatic mechanisms for tellurium exist in animals and humans. The usual concentration in normal human urine is $0.63\mu g$ per ml.

The toxicity of orally administered tellurium itself is relatively low. High intakes ($375-1500\mu g$ per g diet) fed to rats for 21 days gave rise to garlic odour on breath, in the urine and faeces but nothing abnormal was noted. However, if given as tellurium oxide ($375-750\mu g$ tellurium) over the same period, rats developed redness of the feet along with oedema and a temporary paralysis of the hind legs with loss of hair. All soluble tellurites and tellurates were found to be toxic at levels of 25 to $50\mu g$ per g food. Nausea, vomiting and depression of the central nervous system were typical symptoms. Other studies indicated that the level of $500\mu g$ tellurium per g food increased the incidence of vitamin E–selenium deficiency-type signs of necrosis of heart and skeletal muscle. Lower levels of tellurium apparently did not have this effect and even increased the lifespan of rats. These results suggest a possible role for tellurium at low intakes but at higher levels (as with other trace minerals) toxic effects take over.

---

temperature, *see* seasonal supplementation.

---

tetany, a condition resulting from a severe low blood calcium or a reduction in the serum ionized calcium when total blood calcium is normal. It is characterized by sensory symptoms of tingling (pins and needles) of the lips, tongue, fingers and feet; muscular spasms of the hands and feet; spasm and twitching of the face muscles. May be indicative of low body calcium or respiratory or metabolic alkalosis (excess alkali in the body). Treatment is supplementary calcium — orally in mild cases; by intravenous infusion in severe cases.

---

tetracycline,   antibiotic. Prevents formation of vitamin K by intestinal bacteria.

---

thallium,   chemical symbol Tl and atomic weight 204.37.

Thallium is a toxic mineral which has been used as a poison for rats and other rodents. In man, symptoms of acute toxicity are nausea, vomiting, diarrhoea, tingling, pain in the extremities, weakness, coma and convulsions leading to death. Chronic poisoning leads to weakness and pain in the extremities (polyneuritis) and loss of hair. Toxicity occurs because thallium salts are rapidly and completely absorbed after oral administration. The mineral accumulates in the body with age leading to autonomic dysfunction with fast heart rate and high blood pressure. Toxicity is sometimes seen in cattle who have eaten plants containing high levels of the mineral.

Thallium can serve as a cofactor in the activation of certain enzymes, including pyruvate kinase so it is possible that at very low levels it may have a function in the body.

---

thiamin(e), B_1 vitamin.

---

thrombophlebitis,   *see* phlebitis.

---

thrombosis,   *see* blood clot.

---

thymus,   gland concerned with development of immune system and resistance to infection. Fully developed at 2 years of age then slowly regressive after a period of stagnation. Full activity requires adequate vitamin A, choline; folic acid, vitamin B$_{12}$ and amino acid. Methionine essential in pregnant mother for full, efficient development of thymus in baby.

---

thyroid,   an endocrine gland found in the neck in front of and partially surrounding the thyroid cartilage and the upper end of the trachea. *See also* hyperthyroidism.

Term also applies to the thyroid gland of slaughtered animals when it is freed from connective tissue and fat then dried and powdered. Contains not less than 1.70mg and not more than 2.30mg iodine in combination per gram dried gland. One gram dried thyroid equals 5g fresh gland. In man it is used as a source of thyroid hormone in hypothyroidism. In animals it has been used in obesity; kidney failure; chronic skin conditions; and to increase spermatogenesis, libido and milk production.

---

thyrotoxicosis,   *see* hyperthyroidism.

---

thyroxine,   known also as L-thyroxine; T4. First isolated from thyroid gland by E. C. Kendall of the USA in 1919. It is a natural thyroid hormone containing 4 atoms of iodine per molecule thyroxine. Can also be obtained by chemical synthesis. Used in the treatment of hypothyroidism, particularly for long-term therapy. D-thyroxine has been used to decrease high fat levels in the blood serum. L-thyroxine has been used to treat some cases of obesity. *See* hypothyroidism; iodine; triiodothyronine.

---

tin,   chemical symbol Sn, from the Latin *stannum*. Atomic weight 118.7. Occurs in nature as cassiterite, stannite and tealite; abundance in earth's crust is 6mg per kg.

It has been considered to be an essential trace mineral for some animals since the 1960s when rats reared on a tin-free diet were found to have retarded growth. Addition of 1mg tin sulphate to each kg of their diet restored normal growth.

Functions of tin in animals believed to reside in:
1. its stimulating the transcription of RNA and DNA which determine genetic characteristics;
2. protein synthesis through RNA;
3. growth, probably a result of (1) and (2). No functions of tin have been discovered in man.

Food sources of tin are unknown because of difficulty in measurement but canned foods contain higher levels than fresh or frozen foods due to contamination from the container. Even this is reduced because insides of tins are now lacquered. Human diets can provide between 3.5 and 17mg per day, but only when some of the food is of the canned variety. The toxic level is believed to be about 6.0mg per kg body weight so fresh-food diets have a high safety margin. Legal limit of tin in canned foods in 25mg per 100g food. As the toxic amount for a 70kg adult is 420mg tin, excessive intakes of canned food can approach this level. A concentration of 300mg tin in 100g food causes toxic effects in experimental animals.

Excessive intakes in animals cause anaemia, which can be reversed by feeding extra iron and copper; depressed growth.

Absorption of tin and its salts from the gastrointestinal tract is very poor and most is excreted in the faeces.

Acute toxic effects in man include colic; distension of the abdomen (tympanites or meteorism); constipation.

Chronic toxic effects in man include nausea; colic; headache; weakness; fever; muscle pain; joint pain; tinnitus (head noises).

Inhalation over prolonged periods can cause pneumoconiosis (lung disease). Maximum permissible concentration in atmosphere is 2mg per cubic metre (inorganic tin) or 100μg cubic metre (organic tin).

Medical uses of tin and tin oxide in tablet form include the treatment of boils, carbuncles and acne; tapeworm infestation.

Metabolic Toxic Effects — high levels of tin can influence the metabolism of other minerals. For example, calcium levels in liver and femur bone are reduced; acid and alkaline phosphatase concentrations are reduced; selenium and zinc absorption is lowered, indicated by excess excretion in the faeces; no effects were derived on copper, iron, manganese faecal or urinary losses. One study has indicated that in human beings 25 to 100mg of tin had no effect on zinc intake from a 12.5mg dose of zinc. Excess tin has an adverse effect on blood formation. It interferes with the production of haemoglobin and enhances its breakdown. There is no direct effect on the blood-forming minerals iron and copper.

---

tinea versicolor, also known as pityriasis versicolor, a skin infection characterized by multiple patches of lesions varying in colour from white to brown. It is common in young adults. Tan, brown or white, slightly scaling areas are seen on the chest, neck, abdomen and occasionally on the face. These areas do not tan but appear as white `sun spots`. Treatment is application of undiluted selenium sulphide shampoo or a 2.5 per cent lotion to affected areas (avoiding the scrotum) for 3 or 4 days at bedtime, washing it off in the morning.

---

tissue salts, inorganic mineral salts, specific deficiency of which is believed to be associated with particular diseases. Also known as biochemic tissue salts. Tissue salt therapy is based upon homoeopathic principles first put forward by a German doctor, Wilhelm H. Scheussler of Oldenburg and tested by him from the years 1872 to his death in 1898. Dr Scheussler believed that the disease process was always associated with a deficiency of one or more tissue salts that are normally present, in correct balance, in body tissue cells. By supplying the deficient mineral salts a healthy balance is restored. The twelve tissue salts of Dr Schuessler are: calc. fluor. (calcium fluoride); calc. phos. (calcium phosphate); calc. sulph. (calcium sulphate); ferr. phos. (ferric phosphate or iron phosphate); kali mur. (potassium chloride); kali phos. (potassium phosphate); kali sulph. (potassium sulphate); mag. phos. (magnesium phosphate); nat. mur. (sodium chloride); nat. phos. (sodium phosphate); nat. sulph. (sodium sulphate); silica (silicon dioxide).

True deficiency of a particular mineral is not overcome by sole treatment with a tissue salt, since the quantity in its preparation is minute, based upon homoeopathic principles of dilution At this dilution the biochemic tissue salt is more likely to influence the way in which the deficient mineral is distributed throughout the body and hence rectify imbalances in that way. Biochemic tissue salts can also influence minerals when they are present in excess in body cells and tissues. Biochemic remedies may therefore be regarded as having a regulatory function on body minerals by influencing the distribution of anions and cations within body cells and in the extracellular fluids bathing those cells.

The preparation of biochemic tissue salts is based upon homoeopathic principles of serial dilution and trituration. One part of the appropriate salt is mixed with nine parts of lactose (milk sugar) and the resultant mixture is vigorously ground and mixed to ensure a completely homogeneous blend. This is termed *trituration* and comprises the first decimal potency called 1X. One part of this potency is mixed with a further nine parts of lactose and the resulting mixture is exhaustively blended to produce the homogeneous second decimal potency 2X. One part of this potency is further diluted with nine parts of lactose in the same manner as before and the resulting mix is termed the third decimal potency 3X. The process, which is known as *serial dilution* (the X simply means that each stage of the dilution is ten-fold) is carried on until the sixth decimal potency. At this stage the tissue salt has been diluted one million times and is known as potency 6X, the most commonly utilized homoeopathic potency. Further dilution to 12X is sometimes carried out but it is seldom necessary to continue beyond this. This constant serial dilution combined with exhaustive blending (trituration) is known as potentization, a term also applied to homoeopathic preparations. The potentized powder is finally highly compressed into small tablets that readily dissolve on or under the tongue.

For best effect the following precautions should be taken:

1. No food or drink should be consumed within 15 minutes of taking a biochemic remedy.
2. Teeth should not be cleaned within the same time restraint.
3. All tissue salts should be kept in containers that will not let in daylight or odours from other substances.
4. Avoid handling the tablets apart from those to be immediately consumed.
5. Transfer to other containers from those in which they are supplied should not be carried out. This is to avoid contamination of the minute amounts of salt left in the biochemic remedy.

The following observations are also important to anyone contemplating biochemic tissue salt remedies:

1. The remedies may be used to treat acute disease (usually infections) and chronic disease (inflammatory and degenerative conditions).
2. Sometimes the condition appears to worsen after taking tissue salts.

If it happens during treatment of an acute illness, like an infection, administration of the remedy should cease to allow the body to enter a healing phase. Improvement should then follow. If not, the services of a practitioner, preferably a homoeopathic one, should be sought. Similar considerations apply to treatment of a chronic condition except that worsening may occur several weeks after therapy is initiated. In the same way, therapy should cease to allow the healing phase to come into operation. If necessary when the condition persists, continued therapy at the recommended dose should be re-started.

3. All biochemic tissue salt therapy is safe but those unduly sensitive to lactose should be aware of its presence in these remedies.

4. No other complementary therapy is affected by tissue salts but the effectiveness of the latter may be reduced and professional advice should be sought.

Properties and applications of the twelve tissue salts are:

Calc. fluor. — calcium fluoride, indicated where tissues have lost their tone, e.g., varicose veins; leg ulcers; eczema; piles; poor blood circulation; constipation; backache; chronic synovitis (arthritis). May be used to treat diseases of the teeth; the bones; the skin; the nails where a surface lesion exists.

Calc. phos. — calcium phosphate, promotes healthy cells in organs and tissues; assists digestion, absorption and assimilation of foodstuffs; improves poor blood circulation; relieves chilblains; relieves generalized pruritus (itching) in the elderly; helps shrink enlarged tonsils and nose polyps. In conjunction with ferr. phos. treats simple anaemia; in alternation with kali phos. produces more rapid results in relieving pruritus.

Calc. sulph. — calcium sulphate, cleanses the blood and the tissues of the body by removing toxic and waste products. Is used in mild skin conditions; mucous membrane infections; catarrhal complaints where it supplements the action of kali mur. On its own, calc. sulph. helps relieve head pains and neuralgias in the elderly.

Ferr. phos. — ferric phosphate (or iron phosphate), maintains healthy, strong blood vessel walls; ensures the blood is rich in oxygen to maintain health;

complements other treatments for anaemia; relieves congestion, inflammation, high temperature, rapid pulse. Should be given as a standard in the early stage of all acute disorders at frequent intervals. Is an excellent all-round remedy for illnesses associated with ageing and with children. Can be regarded as a first-aid treatment for any sort of muscular or joint injury.

Kali mur. — potassium chloride, indicated for any soft glandular swelling or those associated with chronic rheumatic conditions. Should be used in conjunction with calc. sulph. which complements its action by purifying the blood. Specific for infantile eczema. When used alternatively with ferr. phos. is particularly beneficial in all children's ailments. Kali mur. is specific for any sort of thick, white, gelatinous discharges; for a sluggish, underactive liver; for reduced bile production. When alternated with ferr. phos. it is indicated for inflammatory conditions of the respiratory system like coughs, colds, sore throats, tonsillitis, bronchitis. Problems associated with the digestive system may respond to kali mur.

Kali phos. — potassium phosphate, is indicated for mild nerve complaints that cause headaches; dyspepsia; sleeplessness; depression; lethargy; reduced vitality; edginess. Regarded as a general tonic. May also help in nerve-related conditions like shingles (infection of nerve endings with herpes zoster); nervous asthma; nervous insomnia. In these conditions its beneficial action is accentuated by mag. phos. taken in conjunction with it.

Kali sulph. — potassium sulphate, acts primarily on the skin and mucous membranes of all the internal organs. It treats the feelings of extremes of cold and of heat; pain in the limbs; vague, generalized pains. Any abnormal condition of the skin and mucous membranes, particularly where there is discharge or scaling, will respond to kali sulph. Specific for catarrh, a condition of the respiratory mucous membranes. Also treats psoriasis of the skin and fungal infections of athlete's foot. In conjunction with silica it restores brittle nails to health; with silica and nat. mur. it helps maintain healthy hair.

Mag. phos. — magnesium phosphate, the anti-spasmodic tissue salt. Like kali phos. it maintains a healthy nervous system; in conjunction with this tissue salt it relieves cramping, shooting, darting and spasmodic pains. On its own, mag. phos. is indicated for the painful conditions of neuralgia, neuritis, sciatica and headache. Muscular twinges, cramps, hiccoughs, fits of coughing and any sudden, sharp pains will respond to mag. phos. It acts more rapidly when the biochemic salt tablets are taken with a sip of hot water.

Nat. mur. — sodium chloride, restores to normal any part of the system that is too wet or too dry, where water balance is upset. Typical conditions include headache; constipation; hard faeces; soreness of the anus; watery discharge of colds; dry nose and throat; sluggish digestion; thirst, excessive flow of tears and saliva as in neuralgia and toothache; watering eyes; hay fever; respiratory allergies; dryness of the skin; tiredness on waking; craving for salt and salty foods. Nat. mur. stimulates the flow and production of hydrochloric acid in the digestive system. It controls water distribution throughout the body. Has been used to make salt-free or low-salt diets more acceptable to the individual. Relieves insect bites and stings when applied directly to the affected area.

Nat. phos. — sodium phosphate, is an acid neutralizer. Excess acid can give rise to rheumatic conditions; digestive upsets; intestinal disorders; inefficient assimulation of nutrients. Nat. phos. relieves all of these states. It also helps regulate the bile content and flow and so is indicated in the treatment of jaundice, colic, sick headaches and gastric disturbances. It helps promote the absorption of water and so with nat. mur. and nat. sulph. serves to control body-water balance. Nat. phos. helps emulsify fatty acids in the digestive system so it is indicated where fat digestion and absorption is difficult. Specific for relieving gouty and allied conditions due to the deposition of uric acid in the joints. Remedies any condition giving rise to yellow exudates and discharges.

Nat. sulph. — sodium sulphate, controls the density of the extracellular fluids (which bathe the cells) by eliminating excess water. Essential for the healthy functioning of the liver by ensuring an adequate supply of bile to assist in fat digestion. Toxins from body cells are excreted through the cell membrane to the extracellular fluid from where they are eliminated through the kidneys. Nat. sulph. is concerned in this disposal so it is essential to prevent accumulation of toxins in the cells and water. For this reason it is indicated in rheumatic conditions; in biliousness; in treating influenza; in sluggish kidneys; in conditions causing a coated tongue; when there is excess bitterness in the mouth.

Silica — silicon dioxide, acts upon the organic tissues of the body including the bones, joints, glands and skin. It is indicated for any condition where there is pus formation like abscesses, styes and boils. An inflamed throat as in tonsillitis needs biochemic silica. It is also of benefit in nail and hair conditions. Silica restores a healthy skin and normalizes the perspiration. When rheumatic conditions are related to excess uric acid, as in gout, silica functions by dissolving the crystals and excreting them. The mild mental aberrations observed in old people (senile dementia) may respond to silica.

Often a combination of tissue salts is more effective at relieving a variety of related symptoms. Examples are mag. phos., nat. mur., and silica for migraine; ferr. phos., kali mur., and nat. mur. for coughs, colds and influenza; calc. fluor., calc. phos., kali phos. and nat. mur. for backache and lumbago; calc. fluor., ferr. phos. and nat. mur. for varicose veins and blood circulation problems; kali mur., kali sulph., calc. sulph. and silica for minor skin ailments; ferr. phos., kali phos. and mag. phos. for sciatica, neuralgia and neuritis; calc. phos., kali phos. and ferr. phos. for general debility and nervous exhaustion.

Titanium,   chemical symbol Ti with atomic weight 47.9. Like aluminium, titanium is abundant in the earth's crust and soil. It is poorly absorbed by both plants and animals. Most plants contain only 1µg per g. Foods are therefore poor sources, and nuts, fruits and vegetables usually provide less than 0.5mg per g. Exceptions are breadfruit (6.0); taro (80); yam (15.0); cassara (6.0); rice (2.0); avocado (1.0); dry beans (2.0) and corn (2.0). (All figures are µg per g). UK diets provide about 800µg titanium per day. There is no evidence that absorbed titanium performs any vital function in animals or that it is a dietary essential for any living organism.

Human organs and tissue contain very variable amounts of titanium. Most soft tissues contain 0.1 to 0.2µg per g with lungs being the highest at greater than 4µg per g, probably due to inhalation of titanium-containing dust.

Kidney, liver and spleen contain 1.44, 3.09 and 1.84µg per g respectively. Hair can contain between 3.5 and 20µg per g although in some cases it could not be detected. Whole blood contains only 0.03µg per g.

Titanium is essentially non-toxic in the amounts and forms that are usually ingested. When mice were fed titanium in large amounts (5µg per ml drinking water) for life, their growth, longevity and tumour incidence were not affected. Toxicity has never been found in any species. Titanium oxide is often used as a white pigment in tabletting.

---

tobacco amblyopia, *see* eyes.

---

tocopherol, E vitamin.

---

torula yeast, torulopsis utilis. Strain of yeast less bitter than baker's and brewer's varieties containing the following vitamins (in mg per 100g dried product): carotene (trace); thiamine (15.0); riboflavin (5.0); pyridoxine (3.5); nicotinic acid (50.0); pantothenic acid (10.0); biotin (0.1); folic acid (3.0). Rich source of RNA and DNA; together account for 12 per cent of dried yeast.

---

toxaemia of pregnancy, may be related in some cases to lack of pyridoxine and more importantly folic acid.

---

toxic reactions, undesirable effects of vitamin therapy are rare in the West but they have been observed, usually as a result of excessive intake of vitamins when self-administered as supplements.

For the water-soluble vitamins it is difficult to produce high tissue levels because the kidneys readily excrete the excess when blood concentrations are above a certain threshold. There is no evidence that the body is able to convert excessive quantities of the B complex into their metabolically active forms above those normally present.

Fat-soluble vitamins, however, tend to be stored both in the liver and in the fatty tissues of the body. When these vitamins spill over into the tissues, toxic reactions occur and certain symptoms become apparent, summarized as follows:

Vitamin A — first indications of acute vitamin A toxicity were reported when seamen and Arctic explorers ate polar-bear liver which is a particularly rich source of the vitamin. Symptoms included drowsiness, increased cerebrospinal fluid (which bathes the spinal column and brain) pressure, vomiting and extensive peeling of the skin. Vitamin A quantities measured in millions of units were eaten.

At least twenty cases of children under three years of age with vitamin A poisoning have been described in USA medical literature. The cause was usually misguided enthusiasm on the part of the mothers who gave their offspring from 30mg (90000IU) to 150mg (450000IU) of vitamin A daily for several months. The symptoms of these chronic intakes included loss of appetite, irritability, a dry, itching skin, coarse, sparse hair and swellings over the long bones. Usually an enlarged liver was present.

Much of our knowledge of vitamin A toxicity comes from India and the Philippines where doses of 200000IU are given to deficient patients in outlying villages once every six months. From 3-4 per cent of them suffer loss of appetite, nausea, vomiting and headache within 24 hours. These side-effects last only a few days, then as the body distributes the vitamin, deficiency symptoms disappear and the beneficial effects of the vitamins are felt.

Severe overdosage gives rise to generalized itching, redness of the skin, dry scaling of the skin and mucous membranes, cracking of the corners of the mouth and lips, inflamed tongue and gums, ulceration of the mouth and loss of hair. In addition there are fatigue, haemorrhages, retention of water, tenderness of the long bones and a tender enlarged liver. If intake is continued there is mental irritability, sleep disturbance, loss in weight and rises in the blood enzyme alkaline phosphatase which leads to calcium deposition in the blood-vessels.

Toxicity is unlikely if the daily intake is kept below 5000IU per kg body weight (i.e., 350000IU for a 70kg or 11 stone individual) for not more than 200 days. Intervals of 4 to 6 weeks between courses of treatment are recommended. These levels of intakes apply only when the vitamin is being used therapeutically and under medical supervision. There is now an increased tendency to give large daily doses of vitamin A and its analogues for skin diseases and for cancer. The symptoms mentioned above apply mainly to vitamin A alcohol (retinol) because it is stored in the liver. Retinoic acid is not stored and is used where high blood levels are needed quickly.

Synthetic retinoic acid analogues (retinoids) can induce toxicity symptoms but at intakes higher than those of vitamin A. The widely used 13-cis-retinoic acid used to treat acne gives side-effects confined to the skin, the mucous membranes of the mouth, the nose and the eyes. Toxic symptoms rapidly abate when treatment with the analogues is stopped. Reducing the intake of vitamin A and its analogues is the only treatment for overdosage.

Vitamin D — there is a narrow gap between the nutrient requirement and the toxic dose. As little as five times the recommended intake (50μg daily) taken over prolonged periods can lead to high blood calcium levels in infants and calcium deposition in the kidneys of adults.

Toxicity is more likely in children, either because of excessive doses administered by over-zealous mothers or because of increased sensitivity of some infants to fortified milk containing the vitamin. The usual signs in children are loss of appetite with nausea and vomiting. Excessive passing of urine with consequent thirst are soon evident. Constipation often alternates with diarrhoea. Frequently there are pains in the head and in the bones. The child becomes thin, irritable and depressed, eventually becoming stupored. Calcium deposits are laid down in the arteries, kidneys, heart, lungs and other soft tissues and organs. Death can result.

In adults a regular intake of more than 100000IU (2.5mg) of vitamin D for long periods is required to produce the typical symptoms of weakness, nausea, vomiting, constipation, excessive passing of urine, thirst, and dehydration. Less obvious but more serious results are deposition of calcium in the soft tissues and organs and eventually kidney failure leading to death.

High doses of vitamin D are used in treating metabolic bone disease, hypoparathyroidism, malabsorption and certain arthritic conditions. Potent preparations must be taken for long periods so close medical monitoring is essential.

The only treatment for vitamin D overdosage is to stop taking the vitamin.

Vitamin E — the only side-effect noted with this vitamin is muscle weakness in a few people taking at least 600IU daily. Many more have taken from 400 to 1600IU daily with no ill-effects. In a period spanning forty years, doctors at the Shute Institute in Canada have treated over 40000 patients with doses of vitamin E up to 5000IU daily with no discernible side-effects. Occasionally there is a transient rise in blood-pressure in susceptible people given over 800IU daily but no effect has been noted in those being treated for high blood-pressure. Both muscle weakness and the raised blood-pressure quickly disappear when the vitamin intake is stopped or reduced to 400IU daily. Occasionally contact dermatitis has occurred when people applied the pure oil to the skin or even an ointment or cream containing more than 100IU per gram. Reduction of the potency removes the allergic reaction.

Thiamine — very occasionally injections of thiamine can cause hypersensitivity reactions in susceptible people. Effects include itching and swelling at the side of injection; swelling of the tongue, lips and eyes; generalized itching and sweating; sneezing, wheezing, difficulty in breathing and cyanosis (where the skin becomes blue); nausea; low blood-pressure and, very rarely, death has resulted. No side-effects have been reported from orally-administered thiamine.

Nicotinic acid — large doses of between 3 and 10 grams daily have been prescribed to reduce blood cholesterol levels and the toxic reactions include flushing of the skin of the face, neck and chest accompanied by itching in these areas. More than one-third of patients so treated continue to suffer this flushing while undergoing this therapy. In some there are rashes, dry skin and increased pigmentation of the skin. Occasionally jaundice appears, accompanied by nausea, diarrhoea, abdominal pain and headache in as many as 20 to 40 per cent of patients treated. Gastric and duodenal ulcers can worsen.

Nicotinamide in similar doses does not cause flushing but liver damage has been recorded. Nicotinic acid must therefore be used with caution and under close monitoring in those suffering from gastric and duodenal ulcers, gout, diabetes and liver disease and in pregnant women.

Pyridoxine — until recently was believed to be non-toxic, although for some time it has been known to neutralize the effect of the drug levodopa used in treating Parkinson's disease. There are cases of toxicity reported in subjects who took more than 200mg pyridoxine daily but the most comprehensive study was as follows.

Daily intakes of at least 2000mg pyridoxine taken over 2 to 40 months have given rise to peripheral neuropathy in seven subjects. Typical symptoms started with numbness in the feet and unstable gait. This led to increasing inability to walk steadily, particularly in the dark, and difficulty in handling small objects. Numbness and clumsiness of the hands followed within months, sufficient to impair typing ability; there were also changes in the feeling in lips and tongue. Normal blood plasma levels of pyridoxine are in the range of 0.36 to 1.8μg per 100ml but those patients had levels of 3.0μg and above. After one month's abstinence from pyridoxine supplementation, the level fell to 1.7μg per 100ml plasma. In all cases, withdrawal of pyridoxine led to improvement in symptoms and tests indicated a marked recovery of the nervous system, but the process took several months. None of these patients experienced symptoms when their intake was below 2000mg pyridoxine daily. There is no evidence of harm from the more usual daily dose of 25 to 100mg taken for PMT.

Folic acid — antagonism has been reported between folic acid and the drug phenytoin used in treating epilepsy. Hence balance between drug and vitamin is critical and best left to the medical practitioner.

High folic acid intakes can deplete vitamin B_{12} stores in the body. If given to those suffering from pernicious anaemia resulting from malabsorption of vitamin B_{12}, high-dose folic acid can mask the blood anaemia symptoms but allow the spinal column nerve degeneration to continue. Hence the importance of diagnosing megaloblastic anaemia as due to either folic acid or vitamin B_{12} deficiency.

Oral therapy has given rise to loss of appetite, abdominal distension and flatulence. Occasionally injection of folic acid can cause transient rise in temperature and symptoms of fever.

Vitamin B_{12} — toxicity reactions from oral dosage have never been reported. Very rare allergic reactions have occurred following intramuscular injection of the vitamin.

Riboflavin — no reported toxicity reactions.

Pantothenic acid — no reported toxicity reactions even after long-term treatment with up to 2 grams daily in cases of rheumatoid arthritis, either orally or by injection.

Carotene — generally accepted as safe, even at intakes sufficient to impart a yellow colour to the skin.

Biotin — no adverse reactions reported even in infants given 5mg daily, orally or by injection, for skin lesions.

Vitamin C — generally regarded as one of the safest vitamins, even when taken in massive doses. There are some who should avoid large (i.e., greater than 1g daily) intakes of the vitamin because they suffer from inherited metabolic diseases giving rise to excess oxalic acid, cystine or uric acid in the blood and urine. They have a greater tendency to form kidney stones. Such disease is rare and most people can tolerate vitamin C intakes up to 3g daily and even more. Those who suffer from kidney stones and those who are taking oral anticoagulant drugs should take high-dose vitamin C with caution although intakes of up to 500mg daily can be tolerated by these people for long periods.

Physical signs of overdose are gastro-intestinal and include nausea, abdominal cramps and diarrhoea. The vitamin can also act as a diuretic causing increased urination but this can be beneficial in removing excess body water. If a high intake causes diarrhoea, reducing the amount taken by 500mg or 1g daily will often reduce the side-effect. Previous claims that high vitamin C intakes can destroy vitamin B_{12} have now been discounted.

---

trace elements,   also known as trace minerals. They are elements that occur in the body at very low concentrations, usually less than 0.01 per cent of the body's weight. At least 15 trace elements are presently recognized as essential for warm-blooded animals and birds. They are, in order of demonstrated need, iron, iodine, copper, manganese, zinc, cobalt, molybdenum, selenium, chromium, tin, vanadium, fluorine, silicon, nickel and arsenic. Man's needs for twelve of them has been demonstrated but it is likely that the other three — arsenic, nickel and tin — are also essential. Difficulty in creating deficiencies of these three in modern diets has been conducive to lack of knowledge of their specific roles in man. All trace elements can also be toxic in man but in most cases the range of intakes between needs and toxicity is wide. Some trace elements are positively harmful in man and these include cadmium, lead and mercury.

Table 19: Recommended daily intakes of selected trace elements

	Age (yrs)	Cu (mg)	Mn (mg)	F (mg)	Cr (μg)	Se (μg)	Mo (μg)
Infants	0-0.5	0.5-0.7	0.5-0.7	0.1-0.5	10-40	10-40	30-60
	0.5-1	0.7-1.0	0.7-1.0	0.2-1.0	20-60	20-60	40-80
Children and	1-3	1.0-1.5	1.0-1.5	0.5-1.5	20-80	20-80	50-100
adolescents	4-6	1.5-2.0	1.5-2.0	1.0-2.5	30-120	30-120	60-150
	7-10	2.0-2.5	2.0-3.0	1.5-2.5	50-200	50-200	100-300
	11+	2.0-3.0	2.5-5.0	1.5-2.5	50-200	50-200	150-500
Adults		2.0-3.0	2.5-5.0	1.5-4.0	50-200	50-200	150-500

(Iodine and iron recommended dietary intakes are quoted in the appropriate entries.)

The functions of trace elements in the body are as integral components of many enzymes and some hormones. Unlike the macro-elements, they play no part in the structure make-up of the body (with the possible exception of fluoride in bones and teeth), nor do they contribute to the electrolyte balance. An excess or a deficiency of trace elements can be wholly or partially responsible for a number of disorders. The toxic trace elements in particular may accumulate in the body and produce ill-effects in an insidious manner.

Estimated safe and adequate daily intakes of selected trace elements have been recommended by the Food and Nutrition Board, National Research Council — National Academy of Sciences, 1980 as shown in Table 19.

---

travel sickness, *see* nausea.

---

tretinoin, vitamin A acid; retinoic acid. Toxic effects include transitory stinging, redness, allergic dermatitis when applied to skin.

---

triamterene, diuretic. Impairs folic acid utilization.

---

trifluoperazine, antidepressant, bronchospasm relaxant, gastrointestinal sedative, sedative, anti-nausea agent. Prevents absorption of
vitamin B_{12}.

---

trigeminal neuralgia, severe, brief, lancing pain at either side of face.
Known also as facial neuralgia. Has been relieved with large doses of
thiamine (50-600mg daily).

---

triiodothyronine, known also as liothyronine; T3. First isolated from
thyroid gland by J. Gross and R. Pitt-Rivers of the UK in 1952. A natural
thyroid hormone containing 3 atoms of iodine per molecule
triiodothyronine. Can also be obtained by chemical synthesis. Used in the
initial therapy of hypothyroidism because it has a faster action and turnover
rate than thyroxine.

Elevated blood levels have been found in victims of sudden infant death
syndrome. *See* hypothyroidism; iodine; thyroxine.

---

tryptophan(e), essential amino acid normally supplied by the diet. Has
been used to treat depression in high doses along with nicotinamide,
pyridoxine and vitamin C. Precursor of nicotinic acid; 60mg tryptophane
necessary for each mg of vitamin. Tryptophane in diet will not be sufficient
to supply all nicotinic acid needs but conversion depends upon adequate
quantities of thiamine, riboflavin, pyridoxine and biotin. Precursor of
serotonin, an essential factor for nerve and brain function. Vitamin B_6
required for synthesis of serotonin, lack of which produces depression.

---

tungsten, chemical symbol W from the alternative name Wolfram.

Atomic weight is 183.85. Occurs naturally as wolframite and scheelite.

It is an essential mineral for the micro-organism Clostridium thermo-aceticum where it is a cofactor for the enzyme formate dehydrogenase. It has no known function in animals but there is interaction between tungsten and molybdenum. When rats and mice were given drinking water supplemented with 5µg per ml tungsten for life, there was a slight enhancement in growth of rats. The same treatment shortened the longevity of mice. All other criteria were normal. No effect was seen with goats fed tungsten at levels of 0.06 or 1.0µg per g food; growth, haematocrit, haemoglobin, insemination, conception, abortion rate and sex, number and mortality of kids were the same in those goats receiving low levels of tungsten as in those on the higher intake. However, the tungsten-low mothers tended to show higher mortality and an elevated reticulocyte count. Tungsten can increase the lifespan of rats deficient in vitamin E and selenium.

The UK diet supplies less than 1µg tungsten per day so any dietary requirement for the mineral would be small. Tungsten is well absorbed since after ingestion, much of it is found in the urine. The main part of the body that retains tungsten is the bone but the significance of this is not known.

U

---

ubiquinone, vitamin-like substance found in all body cells but particularly rich in heart muscle. Functions as oxygen transfer coenzyme. Synthesis dependent on vitamin E. Rich source is yeast. Known also as coenzyme Q.

---

ulcers, loss of substance on the surface of the skin or mucous membranes.

Decubitus — *see* bedsores.

Indolent — one that will not heal. May respond to oral vitamin E (400-600IU daily) plus direct application of vitamin E cream.

Leg — sometimes associated with diabetes. Treat as for indolent with vitamin E *or* folic acid, 5mg tablets three times daily and in serious cases with additional injections of 20mg twice weekly.

Gastric — has responded to 150000IU vitamin A daily for four weeks.

Mouth — prevented by adequate intakes of riboflavin (10mg daily) plus vitamin A (7500IU daily). May be treated by same regime.

Varicose — *see indolent ulcer.*

V

---

vanadium, chemical symbol V. Atomic weight 50.9. Widely distributed in ores; abundance in earth's crust 100mg per kg.

An essential trace element for rats and chicks, it may also be necessary for human beings. Deficiency in animals causes reduction in red blood cell production leading to anaemia; upset in iron metabolism; lack of growth of bones, teeth and cartilage; increased blood fat levels; increased blood cholesterol levels. It therefore functions in growth; fat metabolism; blood production; and possibly in prevention of dental caries. Feeding vanadium to deficient animals reduces blood fat and cholesterol levels.

Vanadium in the form of vanadate ions inhibit the cells' sodium pump (see entry). Vandayl ions can mimic the effect of insulin on glucose oxidation by cells in *in vitro* experiments. Similar *in vivo* experiments on rats indicate that vanadium can reduce the blood sugar of normal rats, making them hypoglycaemic. The trace mineral can also reduce the high blood sugar levels of diabetic rats to normal. Hence a simple vanadium salt, sodium metavanadate, given orally, appears to have the same effect as injected insulin in diabetic rats. These beneficial effects are only seen with very low dose vanadium — at high doses the mineral causes kidney failure. As vanadium is able to enter the brain, it also reduces the animals' desire for food, presumably by an action on the appetite centre in that organ.

Excess vanadium in man may be related to manic depression. Manic-depressives, when fed a low vanadium diet or given extra vitamin C (to remove excess vanadium) showed great improvements as their body levels of vanadium fell. Daily intakes of vanadium in the diet are probably between 100 and 300µg. Most of this passes directly through the system, unabsorbed, but some is retained in the bones and liver.

Food sources are (in µg per 100g): parsley 2950; lobster 1610; radishes 790;

dill 460; lettuce 280; gelatin 250; fish bones 240; strawberries 70; whortleberries (bilberries) 54; calf liver 11-51; sardines 46; cucumber 38; apples 33; cauliflower 9; tomatoes 4; potatoes 1. All other foods contain less than $1\mu g$ per 100g.

Processed foods may contain more than the fresh variety because of contamination from the vanadium in the stainless steel of processing plants.

Toxic effects have not been reported except the possibility that the trace mineral may be related to manic depression.

---

varicose veins, swollen, knotted and dilated condition of vein. *Bioflavonoids* (1000mg daily) plus vitamin C (500mg daily) can help reduce condition. *Vitamin* E (400-600IU) daily can reduce swelling, pain and prevent phlebitis. *Lecithin* (5-15g) daily complements actions of vitamin E.

---

vasopressin, also known as anti-diuretic hormone or ADH. A peptide hormone, produced in the pituitary gland, that increases the reabsorption of water by the kidney so preventing excessive losses from the body. Used medically to treat diabetes insipidus.

---

veganism, extreme form of vegetarianism where no product of animal, fish, fowl or insect is eaten. Practised by vegans who may be prone to vitamin B_{12} deficiency but this can be obtained from supplements which contain the vitamin produced by fermentation. Spirulina, an alga, can supply sufficient B_{12} acceptable to vegans. Possible vitamin D deficiency overcome by exposure of skin to sunshine or supplements containing the vitamin derived from yeast.

---

vegetable oils, important sources of vitamin E and the polyunsaturated fatty acid, linoleic acid.

Soft margarine made from these oils also provides useful quantities of these nutrients plus vitamins A and D.

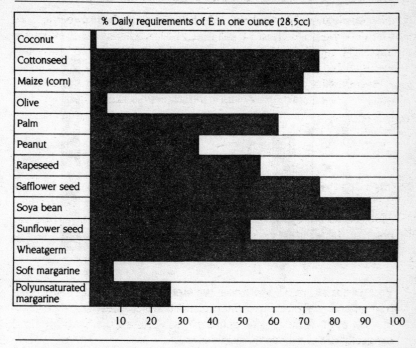

% Daily requirements of E in one ounce (28.5cc)
Coconut
Cottonseed
Maize (corn)
Olive
Palm
Peanut
Rapeseed
Safflower seed
Soya bean
Sunflower seed
Wheatgerm
Soft margarine
Polyunsaturated margarine

vegetables, completely devoid of vitamin A, but some are good source of its precursor carotene. They contain no vitamin D but usually some vitamin E. Most supply all the B vitamins except for vitamin B_{12}, but concentrations vary. Some vegetables supply good quantities of vitamin C. Carotene and vitamin E are unaffected by cooking methods. Invariably some loss of B vitamins when vegetables are cooked.

Greenleaf variety include asparagus, broccoli, Brussels sprouts, cabbage, celeriac, chicory (endive), celery, endive (chicory), leeks, cauliflower, lettuce, parsley, plantain, seakale, spinach, spring greens, turnip tops, watercress.

Root variety include artichokes, beetroot, carrots, parsnips, potatoes, pumpkin, radishes, swedes, turnips, yam to which can be added surface vegetables such as aubergine (eggplant), cucumber and marrow.

The contributions of vegetables to vitamins and minerals in the diet are shown in the accompanying charts. Also shown are the amounts of vitamins and minerals left in the vegetables after cooking.

See also pulses.

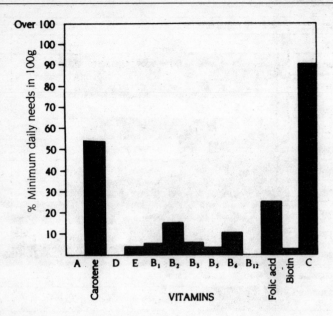

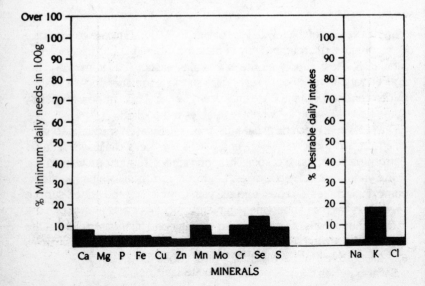

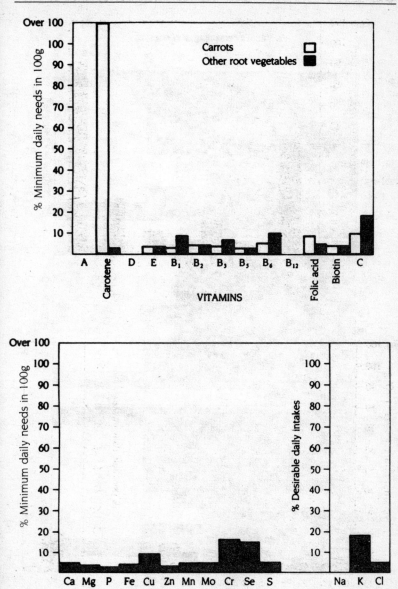

VITAMINS

MINERALS

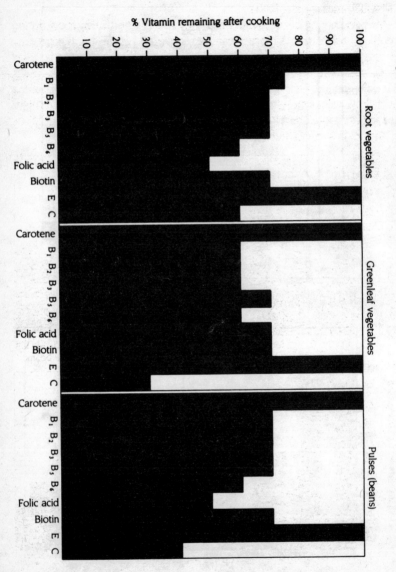

Vegetables — Vitamins remaining after boiling

Minerals remaining after boiling

Minerals cannot be destroyed but they are leached from food during cooking processes. All losses can be recovered by utilizing the cooking water.

More minerals are lost from food boiled in soft water than in hard. Losses are increased by using large volumes of water and by pressure-cooking which increases the temperature. Soaking vegetables in water overnight may also cause losses of some minerals from vegetables.

The charts indicate minerals left in the food after boiling.

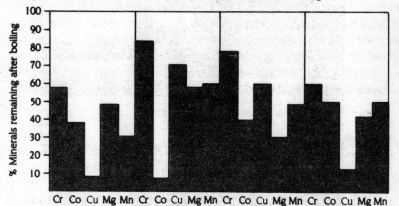

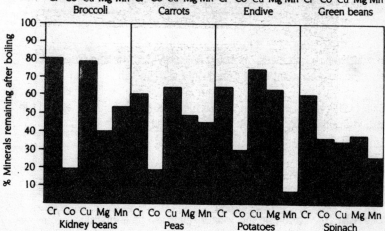

vegetarianism,   practised by those who eat no meat, fish or fowl. May benefit from vitamin B_{12} supplementation but probably obtain enough from dairy products in diet. Same source for vitamin D. Tend to receive high intakes of folic acid and vitamin C because of dietary habits.

---

veruccae,   *see* warts.

---

virus,   the smallest of parasites. Consists of central core of nucleic acid and an outer cover of protein. Wholly dependent on bacterial, plant or animal cells for reproduction. Nucleic acid represents basic infective material. Best natural defences against viruses are adequate vitamin A and vitamin C. Viral infections best supplemented with vitamin A (7500IU) and vitamin C (up to 6g daily).

---

vitamin,   derived from 'vita' (meaning life) and 'amine' (substance incorrectly assigned to all vitamins). Term first used by Polish chemist Casimir Funk in 1911. Micronutrient essential for health that cannot be synthesized in sufficient amounts by the animal or human body. Divided into fat soluble — A, D, E and K — and water-soluble — B-complex and C.
   Vitamins must satisfy three criteria:

1. adequate amounts supplied only in the diet;
2. deficiency produces discrete clinical symptoms and disease;
3. disease and symptoms cured only with specific vitamin.

Exceptions may be vitamin D (produced in skin by sunshine) and biotin and vitamin K produced by intestinal bacterial synthesis.

---

vitamin B_3,   nicotinic acid.

---

vitamin B_4,   adenine (no longer regarded as a vitamin).

---

vitamin B$_5$, pantothenic acid.

vitamin B$_7$, growth factor for micro-organisms but not for man.

vitamin B$_8$, growth factor for micro-organisms but not for man.

vitamin B$_9$, growth factor for micro-organisms but not for man.

vitamin B$_{10}$, unindentified growth and feathering factor for chicks.

vitamin B$_{11}$, unidentified growth and feathering factor for chicks.

vitamin B$_{13}$, orotic acid.

vitamin B$_{14}$, derivative of vitamin B$_{12}$.

vitamin Bc, folic acid.

vitamin BT, carnitine (no longer regarded as a vitamin).

vitamin Bx, para-aminobenzoic acid.

vitamin F, once applied to polyunsaturated fatty acids, especially linoleic acid, but now no longer used and officially not recognized.

vitamin G, B_2 vitamin.

---

vitamin H, biotin.

---

vitamin H$_3$, procaine (no longer regarded as a vitamin).

---

vitamin L$_1$, ortho-aminobenzoic acid; **L$_2$,** adenine derivative. Factors presumably necessary for lactation. Very doubtful significance in human beings.

---

vitamin M, folic acid.

---

vitamin P, old name for carotenoids but no longer accepted as a vitamin.

---

vitamin PP, nicotinic acid.

---

vitamin T, also known as tegotin, termitin, factor T, vitamin T Goetsch, Goetsch's vitamin. Complex of growth-promoting substances, originally obtained from termites. Also present in yeasts and fungi. Probably a mixture of known vitamins and growth-promoting factors but never characterized fully.

---

vitamin U, the anti-ulcer substance reported in cabbage leaves and other green vegetables. It is no longer accepted as a vitamin. Believed to be L-methionine methylsulphonium salt. Has been used to treat gastric ulcers.

---

vitamin/mineral relationships, functions where each is needed for complete utilization of the other; where both are required for a specific process. Examples are:

1. vitamin D, essential for absorption and assimilation of calcium and phosphate;
2. vitamin C, essential for absorption of iron and its incorporation into haemoglobin;
3. vitamin C, possibly needed for the absorption of calcium phosphate;
4. riboflavin (vitamin B_2), essential for iron utilization in making haemoglobin;
5. vitamin E, complements the action of selenium. Selenium is a constituent of the enzyme glutathione peroxidase but vitamin E appears to be essential for its function also.
6. zinc liberates vitamin A from the liver stores;
7. zinc is essential for absorption of folic acid;
8. calcium is necessary for absorption of vitamin B_{12};
9. zinc and vitamin B_6 are essential and function together in the production of essential brain transmitters;
10. magnesium and vitamin B_6 combine to prevent kidney-stone formation;
11. manganese is needed by intestinal bacteria for synthesis of vitamin K.

---

vitiligo, depigmentation of areas of skin which have lost ability to produce natural pigment melanin. Condition worsens on exposure to sunlight probably because non-affected areas become darker with tanning. Harmless condition apart from cosmetic blemish.

Has been treated with PABA, 50mg by injection twice daily plus 100mg twice a day orally. Condition improved after 6 to 8 months. May be complemented with additional pantothenic acid, vitamin B_6, zinc and manganese to stimulate melanin production.

W

warfarin, anti-coagulant drug. Acts by inhibiting action of vitamin K.

warts, common, benign skin eruptions caused by a virus. Known also as veruccae. Have been treated with directly applied solutions of water-solubilized vitamin A palmitate. Alternatively may respond to vitamin E oil applied directly plus oral supplement of 400IU daily.

wheat flour, May be wholemeal (or wholewheat) flour in which the whole of the wheatgrain is ground with nothing added or taken away. May also be white flour from which the bran and wheatgerm have been removed before grinding. White flour is inferior in its contents of minerals and vitamins but is fortified with calcium, iron, thiamine (B_1) and nicotinic acid (B_3).

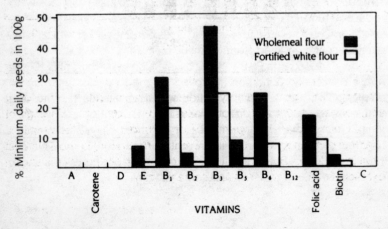

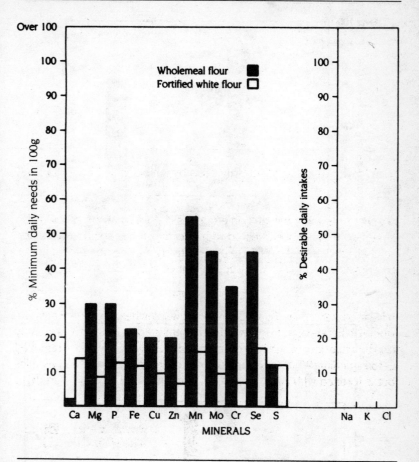

wheatgerm, germ or embryo of the wheat grain situated at the lower end; consists of root and shoot. Makes up 3 per cent of total weight of grain. Claimed that wheatgerm (60g or 2 ounces daily) plus vitamin C (2000mg daily) more effective in preventing respiratory complaints than vitamin C alone. Usually stabilized by mild heat but product is still an excellent source of minerals and some vitamins.

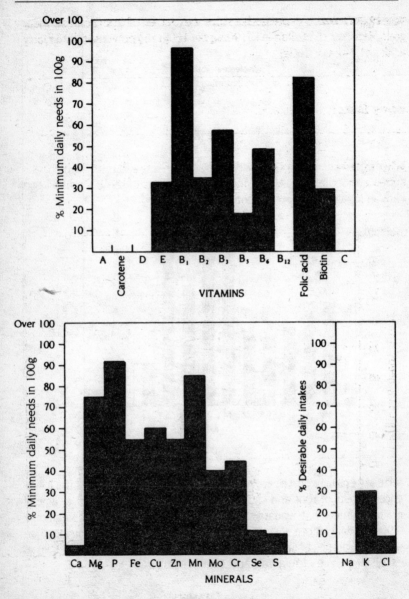

wheatgerm oil, expressed or solvent-extracted oil from germ of wheat grain. Rich source of vitamin E (190mg per 100g) and polyunsaturated fatty acids (41.54g per 100g).

---

whey factor, orotic acid.

---

wholegrains, comprise barley, oats, wheat and corn which are ingredients of muesli. All are meaningful sources of the B vitamins and vitamin E along with the essential minerals.

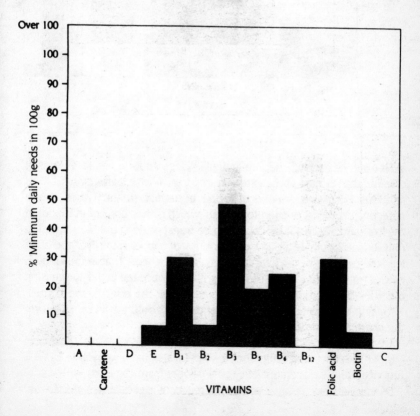

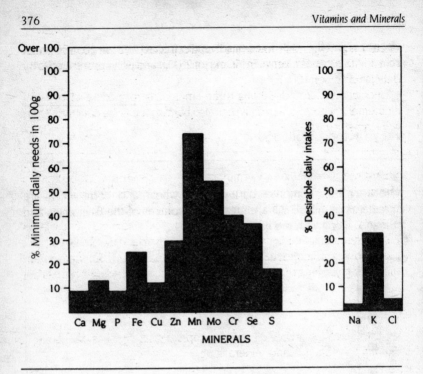

Wilson's disease, hepatolenticular degeneration. A rare familial disease that occurs most often in children whose parents are blood relations. Excessive amounts of copper accumulate in the tissues, due to defective synthesis of caeruloplasmin (which carries copper in blood) in the liver and hence allows copper to be transported in the blood plasma only loosely bound to albumen. Deposition of copper in the liver and brain leads to cirrhosis of the liver and brain disturbances. That in the kidneys causes renal dysfunction. The mineral is also deposited in the eye causing a golden-brown or grey-green pigment ring at the edge of the cornea. Radiating brownish spokes of copper deposits on the lens capsule form the characteristic sunflower cataract.

Treatment is by avoidance of foods high in copper; chelation of the excess copper with chelating drugs such as D-penicillamine or ethylene diamine tetraacetate; displacement of excess copper from the body with zinc.

D-penicillamine can cause acute toxic reactions in about one-third of those treated, e.g., fever, rash, low white blood cell count and low blood platelet count. Vitamin B_6 is given at the intake of 25-50mg daily to prevent possible deficiency.

Zinc sulphate, 200 or 300mg three times daily (providing 45 or 68mg elemental zinc three times daily) has also been found to be effective. There were no side-effects.

women, have different vitamin and mineral needs to men because of menstrual cycle. May have requirements for pyridoxine ten days or so before menstruation far above those supplied by the diet. Usually minimum of 25mg daily. Extra needs for vitamin C, folic acid, vitamin B_{12} and vitamin E to ensure maximum incorporation of iron into haemoglobin to replace blood losses of menstrual flow. Extra requirements of all vitamins and minerals whilst pregnant and during period of breast feeding. Those taking contraceptive pill have increased requirements for certain vitamins.

wound healing, accelerated by supplementary intakes of vitamin C, vitamin E, vitamin A and mineral zinc.

Mineral
Needs many micro-nutrients including iron, zinc, vitamins A and C with adequate protein in the diet. The key healing nutrient is zinc which functions in:

1. rapid cell division, dependent on DNA synthesis, which supplies new cells to close the wound;
2. the synthesis of collagen which toughens up the newly laid-down cells by meshing these with existing old tissue cells; this process also needs vitamin C;
3. liberation of vitamin A from the liver; this vitamin is also needed for the rapid rate of production of new tissue cells;
4. stabilizing cell membranes, keeping them strong and resilient under stress.

To ensure maximum healing rate, supplementation should provide at least 15mg zinc element daily and possibly double this. Excessive quantities of zinc will not cause faster healing so there is no point in taking more than the recommended supplement.

X

xerophthalmia, drying and degenerative disease of the transparent part of the eye associated with vitamin A deficiency.

Y

yeast, excellent source of all minerals but particularly rich in the trace minerals including chromium and selenium. Torula variety is similar but devoid of chromium and selenium. Useful source of B vitamins apart from B_{12}. *See* individual variety.

yeast extract, very rich source of most of the B vitamins but completely devoid of carotene, vitamin E and vitamin C. B vitamins present are (in mg per 100g): thiamine 3.1; riboflavin 11; nicotinic acid 67; pyridoxine 1.3. Folic acid level is 1010μg per 100g; vitamin B_{12} content is 0.5μg per 100g but this is probably added.

yogurt, useful source of some B vitamins plus fat-soluble variety. Higher potencies than milk because of bacterial synthesis, providing (in mg per 100g): vitamin A 0.008; carotene 0.005; thiamine 0.05; riboflavin 0.26; nicotinic acid 1.16; pyridoxine 0.04; folic acid 0.002; vitamin E 0.03; vitamin B_{12} trace; vitamin D trace.

Mineral
Excellent source of calcium, potassium, phosphorus and chloride. Small but useful amounts of the trace minerals and only moderate amounts of sodium. Mineral levels vary, according to variety, in the following ranges (in mg per 100g): sodium 64-76; potassium 220-240; calcium 160-180; magnesium 17-20; phosphorus 140; iron 0.09-0.24; copper 0.04-0.10; zinc 0.60-0.69; chloride 150-180.

Z

zinc, chemical symbol Zn, atomic weight 65.4. Essential trace mineral for plants, animals and human beings.

Body Content

Adult contains between 2 and 3g zinc. Highest concentration in prostate, semen and sperm but muscle, liver and kidney also have high concentrations. Muscles and bones contain 63 per cent of body zinc; skin contains further 20 per cent. Some also in hair — when zinc is lacking hair growth slows or stops.

Excretion

Mainly via the faeces but some lost in urine. Low intakes cause less losses; high intakes, excess is simply excreted.

Excessive loss in:
Alcoholism
Kidney disease
Liver disease

Drugs cause extra losses e.g., diuretics of thiazide type or lower losses e.g., diuretics of frusemide type.

Relationship to Other Minerals

Zinc accompanies calcium in the mineralization of bone and when calcium is lost from bone.

High copper content of blood can depress zinc absorption from the intestine; high zinc intakes can reduce copper absorption. Increase in copper: zinc dietary ratio from normal 4 to 14 or 20 causes increased blood cholesterol leading to atherosclerosis.

Cadmium, a toxic non-essential mineral, antagonizes zinc intake from food. Zinc can help detoxify high cadmium body levels.

Best Food Sources
in mg per 100g

Oysters	70.0
Liver	7.8
Dried brewer's yeast	7.8
Shellfish	5.3
Meats	4.3
Hard cheese	4.0
Canned fish	3.0
Wholemeal bread	2.0
Eggs	1.5
Pulses (beans)	1.0
Wholegrain cereals	1.0
Rice	0.4
Greenleaf vegetables	0.3
Potatoes	0.3

Absorption From Food

On average, 20 per cent of zinc in food is absorbed. Zinc from animal and fish sources is better absorbed than that from vegetables and fruits. This is due to high cysteine content of animal-derived foods.

Factors Reducing Dietary Zinc

Two most important are:
  Food refining
  Food processing

e.g. production of white flour from wholemeal causes 77 per cent loss of zinc; refining unpolished brown rice to white rice causes 83 per cent loss; processing cereals from wholegrains causes 80 per cent loss.

Factors Limiting Absorption

Phytic acid in cereals and
  vegetables
High dietary fibre intakes
Polyphosphates, used as food
  additives
Ethylene diamine tetra-acetate
  (EDTA), used in food
  processing
TVP (textured vegetable
  protein) products eaten in
  excess
Supplementation with zinc
  required in all above

Zinc Supplements (zinc in mg per 100mg)

Zinc amino acid chelate (10); zinc gluconate (13); zinc orotate (17); zinc sulphate (22.7).

Functions

Growth
Insulin activity
Release vitamin A from liver
In metabolism of pituitary,
  adrenals, ovaries and testes
Development of skeleton,
  nervous system and brain
  in growing foetus
Maintaining healthy liver
  function

Deficiency Symptoms

Eczema of face and hands
Hair loss
Mental apathy
Defects in reproductive organs,
  particularly testes
Decreased growth rate
Impaired mental development
Post-natal depression
Congenital abnormalities in
  new-born
Loss of sense of taste
Loss of sense of smell
White spots on nails
Pica-eating of dirt and
  strange substances by
  children
Susceptibility to infections

Recommended Daily Intakes

Should be between 15 and
20mg zinc but see separate
entry.

Deficiency

In man, gives rise to condition
characterized by lack of
physical, mental and sexual
developments. Can be
reversed in pre-puberty girls
and boys with increased zinc
intakes.

Causes also growth failure,
impaired sense of taste, poor
appetite, all of which are
reversed with zinc treatment.

Deficiency

Has caused impotence in men
on long-term kidney dialysis.

Causes acrodermatitis
enteropathica, a rare skin
disease of infancy.

Therapeutic Uses

Treating acne, eczema,
  psoriasis, rosacea
Prevention and treatment of
  prostate problems
Treating mild mental
  complaints
Decreasing blood fat levels
Supplementing schizophrenics
Supplementing hyperactive
  children
Treating the common cold
  with zinc gluconate in
  suckable preparations
Treating anorexia nervosa

Effects of Excess Oral Zinc

Toxic effects of supplementary oral zinc at intakes up to 150mg daily have not been reported. Very high doses may cause mild gastric irritation and vomiting.

---

zirconium, chemical symbol Zr with an atomic weight of 91.22. Occurs in the mineral zircon and has an abundance in the earth's crust of 0.023 per cent. Zircon is present in all human tissues and organs which contain between 0.01 and 0.06μg per g fresh tissue. It is often concentrated in the fat (18.7μg per g).

Meat, dairy products, vegetables, cereal grains and nuts generally provide 1 to 3μg zirconium per g fresh weight. Lower levels are present in fruits and seafoods. UK diets provide 20 to 80μg per day.

There are few studies on the metabolism in the human body. Its presence in blood and tissue indicates that it is absorbed from the diet. There is none detected in urine so secretion is mainly via the intestine. When given by injection, most of the zirconium accumulates in the bone.

Zirconium salts have a low order of toxicity for rats and mice whether injected or given orally. When the mineral was fed in the drinking water (5μg per ml) for life, there were no adverse effects on growth of the mice but there was a small reduction in survival time. There was no accumulation in the tissue when given by this route. A similar experiment carried out on rats caused increased copper levels in the liver and kidneys but no other abnormalities were seen.
